Uterine Cancer

Uterine Cancer

Edited by

David M. Luesley
Birmingham Women's Hospital
Birmingham, U.K.

Frank G. Lawton
Guy's, King's and St Thomas' Hospitals
London, U.K.

Andrew Berchuck
Duke University Medical Center
Durham, North Carolina, U.S.A.

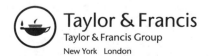

Taylor & Francis
Taylor & Francis Group
New York   London

Published in 2006 by
Taylor & Francis Group
270 Madison Avenue
New York, NY 10016

International Standard Book Number-10: 0-8247-5951-6 (Hardcover)
International Standard Book Number-13: 978-0-8247-5951-3 (Hardcover)

Library of Congress Cataloging-in-Publication Data

Catalog record is available from the Library of Congress

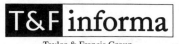

Taylor & Francis Group
is the Academic Division of T&F Informa plc.

Visit the Taylor & Francis Web site at
http://www.taylorandfrancis.com

Preface

In the developed world, endometrial cancer is the most common gynecological malignancy. Overall survival rates of approximately 75% suggest that this cancer has a favorable prognosis, but with one-quarter of patients dead within five years of diagnosis, this is no time for therapeutic complacency. Our knowledge about extrauterine spread of disease apparently confined to the uterus has led to changes in staging criteria, and a therapeutic as well as a diagnostic role for lymphadenectomy has been suggested. The role of radiotherapy has been defined further and it is accepted by many that "postoperative radiotherapy for (nearly) all" is not necessary. However, we do not know the best treatment for serous papillary or clear cell tumors and the place of cytotoxic, and for that matter hormonal therapy, has not been established. Molecular biology findings suggest that endometrial cancer evolves through a number of pathways—inactivation of tumor suppressor genes, activation of oncogenes, etc. Further studies should lead to improvements in prevention, detection, and treatment. This may be particularly true in cases of endometrial cancer associated with hereditary nonpolyposis colorectal cancer. Most cases of endometrial cancer are estrogen associated and tamoxifen is a known endometrial mutagen. Tamoxifen use is likely to increase as more women are screened for breast cancer and women at high risk of the disease are treated prophylactically. In addition to chapters reviewing our present knowledge of all aspects of endometrial cancer, some authorities have been asked to predict future directions in management.

David M. Luesley
Frank G. Lawton
Andrew Berchuck

Contents

Preface . . . . *iii*
Contributors . . . . *xi*

1. **Epidemiology** *1*
   David M. Purdie
   Incidence and Mortality 1
   Cancer Subtypes 2
   Risk Factors for Endometrial Cancer 2
   References 6

2. **Screening in Endometrial Cancer** *13*
   Thomas Hogberg
   What Does Cancer Screening Actually Mean? 13
   Cancer Screening Traps 14
   Screening for Endometrial Cancer? 15
   Screening Tests for Endometrial Cancer 16
   What Could Be Gained by Screening for Endometrial
       Cancer? 18
   The Natural Course of Endometrial Cancer—Premalignant
       Conditions? 19
   Risk Groups 22
   Preliminary Screening Trials 22
   Conclusions 26
   References 26

3. Pathology of Endometrial Hyperplasia and Neoplasia *31*
Terry Rollason and Raji Ganesan
Introduction 31
Endometrioid Carcinoma 34
Mucinous Carcinoma 38
Serous Carcinomas 39
Clear Cell Carcinoma 41
Mixed Carcinomas 42
Undifferentiated Carcinoma 43
Other Rare Types of Endometrial Carcinoma 43
Tumors Metastatic to the Endometrium 43
References 49

4. Pathology of Uterine Sarcoma *53*
Nafisa Wilkinson
Introduction 53
Staging of Uterine Sarcomas 54
Endometrial Stromal Sarcoma 54
Immunohistochemistry of Uterine Sarcomas 58
Hormonal Aspects of Stromal Sarcomas 59
Myxoid Leiomyosarcoma 61
Epithelioid Leiomyosarcoma 62
Carcinosarcoma: A Metaplastic Carcinoma or
   Sarcoma? 62
Pure Sarcomas 63
Tamoxifen and its Role in Uterine Sarcoma 63
References 63

5. The Molecular Genetics of Endometrial Cancer *69*
G. Larry Maxwell, John I. Risinger, J. Carl Barrett, and
Andrew Berchuck
Introduction 69
Somatic Genetic Alterations 70
Hereditary Endometrial Cancer 76
Epigenetics in Endometrial Carcinoma 76
Microarray 80
Summary of the Molecular Biology of Endometrial
   Cancer 81
References 83

6. **Clinical Presentation and Investigation: The "One-Stop" Clinic, Endometrial Sampling, Hysteroscopy, Vaginal Ultrasound** *91*
   Christopher Lee and Davor Jurkovic
   Introduction 91
   Investigations 92
   The Rapid Access Clinic 97
   Conclusion 100
   References 100

7. **Imaging Endometrial Cancer** *107*
   Moji Balogun and Julie Olliff
   Magnetic Resonance Imaging 112
   References 126

8. **Surgery for Uterine Cancer** *131*
   Neville F. Hacker and Donald E. Marsden
   Endometrial Cancer 131
   Prognostic Factors That May Help Determine the Appropriate
      Surgery for Endometrial Cancer 133
   Diagnosis 136
   Preoperative Work Up 137
   The Surgical Procedure 137
   Uterine Sarcomas 142
   Summary 144
   References 144

9. **Risk Factors and the Role of Radiotherapy in the Treatment of Endometrial Cancer** *149*
   Ida Ackerman and Helen Steed
   History of Radiation 149
   Staging and Prognostic Factors 150
   Stage I Disease 153
   Stage II Disease 160
   Stage III and IV Disease 161
   Palliative Radiotherapy 165
   Uterine Papillary Serous Carcinoma 165
   Uterine Sarcomas 166
   Irradiation Technique and Dose 166
   Radiotherapy Toxicity 167

Conclusions   168
References   168

10. **Chemotherapy for Uterine Cancer** *177*
Kathryn F. Chrystal, Kerry A. Cheong, and Peter G. Harper
Introduction   177
Endometrioid Adenocarcinoma   178
Conclusion   182
Serous Carcinoma   182
Uterine Sarcomas   184
Conclusions   188
References   188

11. **Minimal Access Surgery in Endometrial Cancer** *199*
Robbert Soeters and Lynette Denny
Introduction   199
The Role of Vaginal Hysterectomy in the Management of
    Endometrial Cancer   200
Laparoscopic-Assisted Vaginal Hysterectomy
    (LAVH)   200
Laparoscopic Lymphadenectomy   201
Application of LAVH and Lymphadenectomy for Endometrial
    Cancer   201
Complications of Laparoscopy   202
Clinical Outcome of Laparoscopic Versus Open Abdominal
    Surgical Approach to Management of Endometrial
    Cancer   203
Cost Benefit of Laparoscopic Surgery   203
Contraindications to Laparoscopic Surgery for Treatment of
    Endometrial Cancer   204
Setting up for Laparoscopic Surgery   204
Laparoscopic Surgery   205
References   208

12. **Follow-Up and Detection of Relapsed Disease in Uterine**
    Cancer *211*
Fabio Landoni, Angelo Maggioni, and Guilherme Cidade Crippa
Background   211
Patterns of Recurrence   213
Recurrence Risk Groups   216

Prognosis After Recurrence 218
Detection and Surveillance 220
Conclusions 228
References 231

13. **The Role of Surgery in Advanced and
    Relapsed Disease** *233*
    J. Michael Straughn and Ronald D. Alvarez
    Importance of Surgical Staging 233
    Role of Radical Hysterectomy 234
    Role of Primary Cytoreduction in Patients with Advanced
        Disease 235
    Role of Secondary Cytoreduction in Patients with Relapsed
        Disease 238
    Role of Pelvic Exenteration in Patients with Relapsed
        Disease 239
    Conclusion 239
    References 240

14. **Endometrial Carcinoma and Hormone Replacement
    Therapy** *243*
    Michael S. Marsh
    Endometrial Cancer and Unopposed Estrogen Use 243
    Vaginal Estrogen Treatment 244
    The Addition of Progestogens 245
    Tibolone and Endometrial Cancer Risk 248
    Selective Estrogen Receptor Modulators (SERMs) 249
    ERT Use in Women with Previous Endometrial
        Carcinoma 249
    Summary Points 251
    References 251

15. **Future Developments in Radiation Therapy for Endometrial
    Carcinoma** *255*
    Carien L. Creutzberg and Jan G. Aalders
    Reducing Indications for Pelvic Radiotherapy 256
    The Role of Lymphadenectomy and Its Combination with
        Radiotherapy 257
    The Increasing Use of Vaginal Brachytherapy Alone 258

The Use of Both Adjuvant Radiotherapy and Chemotherapy in
   High-Risk Disease 259
The Use of New RT Techniques to Reduce
   Morbidity 261
Conclusions 262
References 262

16. **Future Directions: Chemotherapy and Novel Agents
    for Uterine Cancer** **267**
    Stacy D. D'Andre and Karl C. Podratz
    Introduction 267
    Adjuvant Chemotherapy 268
    Combined Modality Therapy: Radiosensitizing
       Chemotherapy 268
    Chemotherapy for Advanced Disease 268
    Paclitaxel 270
    Topotecan 271
    Doxil® 271
    Docetaxel 271
    Oxaliplatin 272
    Novel Agents 272
    Conclusions 274
    References 274

17. **Combined Therapy in Uterine Cancer:
    Future Directions** **281**
    Howard D. Homesley
    Whole Abdominal Radiation Versus Chemotherapy 281
    High-Risk Stage I Endometrial Carcinoma 282
    Hormonal Therapy 283
    The GOG Chemotherapy Trials in Endometrial
       Cancer 285
    Alternative Chemotherapy Combinations 285
    Current GOG Combined Radiation and Chemotherapy
       Trial 287
    Combined Hormonal, Chemotherapy, and Radiation
       Therapy 287
    References 288

Index 291

Contributors

Jan G. Aalders Department of Gynecological Oncology, University Medical Center Groningen, Groningen, The Netherlands

Ida Ackerman Department of Radiation Oncology, Toronto Sunnybrook Regional Cancer Centre, University of Toronto, Ontario, Canada

Ronald D. Alvarez Division of Gynecologic Oncology, University of Alabama, Birmingham, Alabama, U.S.A.

Moji Balogun Department of Radiology, Birmingham Women's Hospital, Birmingham, U.K.

J. Carl Barrett Laboratory of Biosystems and Cancer, National Cancer Institute, Bethesda, Maryland, U.S.A.

Andrew Berchuck Division of Gynecologic Oncology, Duke University Medical Center, Durham, North Carolina, U.S.A.

Kerry A. Cheong Department of Medical Oncology, Guy's Hospital, London, U.K.

Kathryn F. Chrystal Department of Medical Oncology, Guy's Hospital, London, U.K.

Guilherme Cidade Crippa European Institute of Oncology, Milan, Italy

Carien L. Creutzberg Department of Clinical Oncology, Leiden University Medical Center, Leiden, The Netherlands

Stacy D. D'Andre Department of Hematology–Oncology, University of California, Davis, California, U.S.A.

Lynette Denny Department of Obstetrics and Gynaecology, Groote Schuur Hospital, Cape Town, South Africa

Raji Ganesan Department of Histopathology, Birmingham Women's Healthcare NHS Trust, Birmingham, U.K.

Neville F. Hacker Gynaecological Cancer Centre, Royal Hospital for Women, Randwick, and, School of Obstetrics and Gynaecology, University of New South Wales, New South Wales, Australia

Peter G. Harper Department of Medical Oncology, Guy's Hospital, London, U.K.

Thomas Hogberg Department of Oncology, Division of Gynaecologic Oncology, University Hospital, Linkoping, Sweden

Howard D. Homesley Brody School of Medicine, East Carolina University, Greenville, North Carolina, U.S.A.

Davor Jurkovic Early Pregnancy and Gynaecology Assessment Unit, Kings College Hospital, London, U.K.

Fabio Landoni European Institute of Oncology, Milan, Italy

Christopher Lee Early Pregnancy and Gynaecology Assessment Unit, Kings College Hospital, London, U.K.

Angelo Maggioni European Institute of Oncology, Milan, Italy

Donald E. Marsden Gynaecological Cancer Centre, Royal Hospital for Women, Randwick, and School of Obstetrics and Gynaecology, University of New South Wales, New South Wales, Australia

Michael S. Marsh Guy's, Kings, and St. Thomas' Medical School, London, U.K.

G. Larry Maxwell Division of Gynecologic Oncology, Walter Reed Army Medical Center, Washington, D.C., U.S.A.

Julie Olliff Department of Radiology, University Hospital NHS Trust, Birmingham, U.K.

Karl C. Podratz   Division of Gynecologic Surgery, Mayo Clinic, Rochester, Minnesota, U.S.A.

David M. Purdie   Population and Clinical Sciences Division, Queensland Institute of Medical Research, Royal Brisbane Hospital, Queensland, Australia

John I. Risinger   Laboratory of Biosystems and Cancer, National Cancer Institute, Bethesda, Maryland, U.S.A.

Terry Rollason   Department of Histopathology, Birmingham Women's Healthcare NHS Trust, Birmingham, U.K.

Robbert Soeters   Department of Obstetrics and Gynaecology, Groote Schuur Hospital, Cape Town, South Africa

Helen Steed   Department of Gynecology, Cross Cancer Institute, Edmonton, Alberta, Canada

J. Michael Straughn   Division of Gynecologic Oncology, Birmingham, Alabama, U.S.A.

Nafisa Wilkinson   Department of Histopathology, St. James University Hospital, Leeds, U.K.

1

Epidemiology

David M. Purdie

Population and Clinical Sciences Division, Queensland Institute of Medical Research, Royal Brisbane Hospital, Queensland, Australia

INCIDENCE AND MORTALITY

Endometrial cancer (cancer of the uterine corpus) is the most common gynecologic cancer. It ranks fourth in terms of incident cancers in women and eighth in terms of age-adjusted mortality (1). Endometrial cancer accounted for around 6% of all incident cancers and 2% of cancer deaths in women in the United States in 1999. In Western populations, endometrial cancer is most commonly found between the ages of 50 and 65 years, and is rare before the age of 40. The peak incidence occurs in the postmenopausal age group (2).

Endometrial cancer mortality rates have declined by around 60% since the 1950s. The incidence, however, showed a marked increase in the early 1970s, followed by a reduction in the early 1980s back to previous levels (2,3). Since the mid-1980s, the incidence has remained steady. The increasing age of developed populations, however, will lead to greater numbers of new cases and deaths from endometrial cancer each year.

The incidence of endometrial cancer varies greatly between countries. High rates are seen in Europe, the United Kingdom, the United States (Caucasian population), Canada, New Zealand, and Australia. Consistently lower rates are seen in Africa, Central and South America, and Asia (2). There is also regional variation within racial groups, with black and Asian women living in the United States having much higher rates than their racial counterparts in other countries (2). This racial and geographic variation suggests that there are important genetic and environmental factors that influence the development of endometrial cancer. While there are some data available concerning the role of different environmental risk factors, very little is known regarding the relation between germ line genetic factors and risk of endometrial cancer, except that an increased risk of endometrial cancer among relatives suggests that a strong inherited component exists.

CANCER SUBTYPES

From a histological and molecular pathology perspective, at least two major types of endometrial tumors can be distinguished. Type I tumors are mostly endometrioid carcinomas and are generally associated with endometrial hyperplasia (4,5). Type II tumors are more often serous papillary, clear cell, or adenosquamous carcinomas; generally develop from atrophic endometrial tissues in older women (6); and are associated with a much more aggressive phenotype (5). The molecular profile of the two tumor types also appears to be distinct. Type I carcinomas are associated with mutations in the PTEN tumor suppressor gene (up to 83% of tumors), mutations in the ras proto-oncogene (10–46%), and mismatch repair defects (9–45%). In contrast, the majority of type II tumors have mutations in the *p53* tumor suppressor gene (90%), but none of the molecular features of type I carcinomas. The proportion of type II tumors is reported to range from 20% to 50% (4), and although there is evidence to suggest that there may be heterogeneity within this group, this has not been systematically investigated at the molecular level (5). Few epidemiological studies have distinguished between the two tumor types, and these studies have included relatively small numbers of type II tumors. There is evidence that endocrine and nutritional lifestyle factors affect the risk of type I but not type II tumors, with age being the only recognizable risk factor for type II cancer (4,5).

RISK FACTORS FOR ENDOMETRIAL CANCER

Menstrual Factors

Early age at menarche and late age at menopause are consistently seen to be positively associated with risk of endometrial cancer (7,8). Studies that have examined the effect of "menstruation span" (years between menarche and menopause, excluding pregnancy-related time) found that cases had a longer mean menstruation span than controls (9). An association with long or irregular menstrual cycles has also been reported (10).

Reproductive Factors

Nulliparity is associated with a two- to three-fold increased risk of endometrial cancer, and risk appears to be decreased with increasing number of children (9,11). Unlike breast cancer, endometrial cancer is not consistently associated with age at first birth (8,12). Older age at last birth, however, has been found to significantly reduce the risk of endometrial cancer (12).

It is not certain whether spontaneous and induced abortions influence a woman's risk of endometrial cancer. Some studies find no association (13) and others find a significant negative association (11). An increased risk of endometrial cancer associated with induced abortions has also been reported (9).

Nulliparity is also a manifestation of infertility, which in turn has been separately identified as a risk factor for endometrial cancer (8). Conditions associated with infertility, such as Stein–Leventhal syndrome (polycystic ovary syndrome) (14) and granulosa-thecal cell ovarian tumors (15), have independently been linked to the occurrence of endometrial cancer.

Hormone Replacement Therapy

One of the most consistent factors to be associated with endometrial cancer is use of estrogen replacement therapy. Nearly all case–control and cohort studies that have examined the issue have found use of estrogen replacement therapy to be predictive of endometrial cancer. A meta-analysis that combined both case–control and cohort studies found a summary relative risk of endometrial cancer of 2.3 [95% confidence interval (CI) 2.1–2.5] for women who used estrogen at any time compared to women who never used estrogen (16). Risk of endometrial cancer also increases with increasing duration of use of estrogen therapy (17). Summary relative risk estimates suggest increases in risk of about 40% associated with a year or less of estrogen therapy and up to a 10-fold increase for 10 or more years of use (16). Risk also increases with increasing dose of conjugated estrogen (17), although moderate increased risks have been seen in women taking low-dose estrogen preparations (i.e., 0.3 mg/day) (18).

Despite some studies noting that the size of the risk decreases after cessation of estrogen therapy (19), an increased risk persists for many years (20). Summary estimates suggest that risk of endometrial cancer remains raised about two-fold for five or more years after discontinuation of use (16).

Administration of cyclic progesterone (for at least 10 days of each treatment cycle) appears to mitigate the continuous mitotic stimulation of the endometrium by unopposed estrogen therapy and its incomplete shedding (17). Progesterone antagonizes the effects of estrogen by decreasing estrogen receptors and increasing the activity of enzymes that metabolize oestradiol to less potent metabolites (21). The Women's Health Initiative randomized controlled trial of combined estrogen plus progestin therapy found no apparent increased risk of endometrial cancer based on 47 cases (hazard ratio = 0.83, 95% CI 0.29–2.32) (22).

Oral Contraceptives

The combined oral contraceptive pill (estrogen plus progestin) has consistently been reported to reduce the risk of endometrial cancer (11,23). Long-term use of combined oral contraceptives appears to further reduce risk (23), and the protective effect lasts for 20 or more years after discontinuation (23). Results of some studies, but not all (24), suggest that the protective effect of the combined oral contraceptive pill does not depend on the dose of progestin: risk is similar whether the progestin content is high or low (25).

Body Mass

Large body mass in general, and obesity in particular, has been linked to increased risk of endometrial cancer in many studies (26–29). Relative risks associated with obesity range from 2 to 10. It has also been suggested that central- or upper-body weight is more important than peripheral body weight with significant increasing risk being seen with increasing measures of central adiposity, after adjustment for body mass index (BMI) (30,31). The association between large body mass and endometrial cancer is possibly stronger or more consistent in postmenopausal women (26), or does not apply to premenopausal women (11).

A substantial portion of the international variation in the incidence of endometrial cancer is thought to be explained by differences in rates of obesity between populations. Comparisons of rates of endometrial cancer with rates of obesity among women in developed and developing countries suggest that obesity may account for up to 40% of the worldwide variation in occurrence of endometrial cancer (32).

An association with obesity is biologically plausible. Postmenopausal obese women are known to have higher endogenous estrogen levels than lean women (33) due to the aromatization of androstenedione in adipose tissue (34). Obesity is also associated with reduced levels of sex-hormone-binding globulin (35), which would further increase the amount of bioavailable estrogen.

Diabetes and Hypertension

Diabetes mellitus is another condition long known to be associated with endometrial cancer (8,19,29,36,37), as has hypertension (19,36,38,39). One possible explanation is that these conditions are simply markers of obesity (40). Some studies have found that both associations became less consistent after adjustment for body mass (41), others that only the association with diabetes persisted (8), though others have found both to persist after adjustment not only for body mass, but for other confounding factors as well, including parity, estrogen replacement therapy, and smoking (36,37,42). It has also been suggested that the increased risk associated with diabetes and hypertension may be restricted to obese or overweight women (29).

Whether the association with endometrial cancer differs between insulin-dependent (Type 1) or non-insulin-dependent (Type 2) diabetes mellitus has not been established. One study found significant differences in the effect of the two types, with an OR of 1.5 (95% CI 1.0–2.1) for Type 2 diabetes as opposed to 13.3 (3.1–56.4) for Type 1 (29). Others have suggested the risk is greater for diabetes in older women (usually Type 2) (37). Hyperinsulinemia and higher levels of insulin-like growth factor I (IGF-I) are proposed to play a role in the diabetes–endometrial cancer association (37,43). Studies have shown that serum estradiol concentrations are positively correlated with IGF-I (44).

Smoking

Women who have ever smoked have been found to have a reduced risk of endometrial cancer (45,46), although some studies have suggested that this association is restricted to postmenopausal women (46,47). Relative risks associated with ever smoking are in the range of 0.2–0.9. Evidence is not consistent regarding the association in current compared with ex-smokers (48). The protective effect of smoking has been found to increase with increasing smoking duration and intensity (46).

The reduced risk of endometrial cancer in smokers is thought to provide further evidence of an anti-estrogenic effect of smoking. Other evidence is the earlier age at menopause among smokers as well as increased osteoporosis and hip fractures, all thought to be the result of lowered estrogen levels (49). Others have suggested that rather than affecting risk of endometrial cancer by reducing estrogen, smoking may act by increasing levels of circulating androgen (50).

Cigarette smoking has also been considered as a possible effect modifier of the associations between factors such as estrogen use and obesity and endometrial cancer. Some studies have found the protective effect of smoking to be greater among postmenopausal estrogen users than among non-users (51), although others have found no significant interaction between smoking and estrogen replacement therapy (48). Some authors have suggested that smoking reduces the effect of obesity on endometrial cancer (45). Clearly, interactions of this kind can occur by chance and require confirmation from large studies with enough power to detect such complex associations.

Diet, Alcohol, and Exercise

Diets high in fat and low in complex carbohydrates and fiber have been shown to increase a woman's risk of endometrial cancer (28,52,53). Although diets of these kinds are often associated with greater body mass, the association with diet persists after adjustment for body mass as well as other risk factors (28,53). Diets with high intakes of fruits and vegetables or carotene have also consistently been seen to reduce the risk of endometrial cancer (28,52,54). The biological mechanism underlying the associations with diet can once again be tied to endogenous estrogen levels. Several studies have found lower levels of urinary estriol and plasma concentrations of estrogen in vegetarian compared with non-vegetarian women (55,56), the conclusion being that low-fat diets are associated with a reduction in bioavailable estrogens. Studies have also shown that serum estrogen levels were reduced in women on low-fat diets (57), although others have not observed an association between estrogen levels and diet (58,59).

High levels of alcohol consumption have also been linked to increased estrogen levels (58), prompting several studies to specifically investigate the effect of alcohol consumption on risk of endometrial cancer. The majority have found either no association or a protective effect (13,52,60–62), though positive associations have also been reported (63).

On the reverse side of energy intake is energy expenditure in the form of physical activity. The close relationship between diet, physical activity, and body mass has made it difficult to assess the independent risks of the three on endometrial cancer. Increased levels of physical activity reduce serum estrogen levels (64), and some studies have found that a sedentary lifestyle increases risk of endometrial cancer after adjustment for BMI and caloric intake (62,65). Whether physical activity plays a role via its association with obesity, or whether it has an independent effect on risk of endometrial cancer, is not clear.

Genetic Risk Factors

A limited number of population-based studies have demonstrated an increased risk of endometrial cancer, up to three-fold, for women reporting a family history among first-degree relatives (66–69). This risk is greater for younger women (aged < 50 years) (11,67) as would be expected for individuals harboring a genetic predisposition to disease. Young women with a family history of colorectal cancer also appear to be at increased risk of endometrial cancer (67), most likely attributable to genes that cause hereditary nonpolyposis colorectal cancer (HNPCC) (70). Endometrial cancer is a feature of this syndrome, and women with a mutation in one of the HNPCC genes usually develop endometrial cancer before 50 years of age (71). It has been estimated that up to 7% of incident endometrial cancers among women aged 20–54 may be due to relatively high risk genetic mutations which account for these two distinct forms of heritable cancer (67). However, a thorough examination of the genetic basis of the disease within such families has not been carried out.

REFERENCES

1. Landis SH, Murray T, Bolden S, Wingo PA. Cancer Statistics 1999; Cancer Statistics 1999; 49:8–31.

2. Parkin DM, Whelan SL, Ferlay J, Raymond L, Yound J. Cancer Incidence in Five Continents Volume VII. IARC Scientific Publications. Vol. 143. Lyon: IARC, 1997.

3. Muir CS, Waterhouse J, Mack T, Powell J, Whelan S. Cancer Incidence in Five Continents Volume V. IARC Scientific Publications. Vol. 88. Lyon: IARC, 1987.

4. Emons G, Fleckenstein G, Hinney B, Huschmand A, Heyl W. Hormonal interactions in endometrial cancer. Endocr Relat Cancer 2000; 7:227–242.

5. Sherman ME. Theories of endometrial carcinogenesis: a multidisciplinary approach. Mod Pathol 2000; 13:295–308.

6. Bokhman JV. Two pathogenetic types of endometrial carcinoma. Gynecol Oncol 1983; 15:10–17.

7. Ewertz M, Schou G, Boice JD Jr. The joint effect of risk factors on endometrial cancer. Eur J Cancer Clin Oncol 1988; 24:189–194.

8. Brinton LA, Berman ML, Mortel R, Twiggs LB, Barrett RJ, Wilbanks GD, Lannom L, Hoover RN. Reproductive, menstrual, and medical risk factors for endometrial cancer: results from a case-control study. Am J Obstet Gynecol 1992; 167:1317–1325.

9. McPherson CP, Sellers TA, Potter JD, Bostick RM, Folsom AR. Reproductive factors and risk of endometrial cancer. The Iowa Women's Health Study. Am J Epidemiol 1996; 143:1195–1202.

10. Henderson BE, Casagrande JT, Pike MC, Mack T, Rosario I, Duke A. The epidemiology of endometrial cancer in young women. Br J Cancer 1983; 47: 749–756.

11. Parslov M, Lidegaard O, Klintorp S, Pedersen B, Jonsson L, Eriksen PS, Ottesen B. Risk factors among young women with endometrial cancer: a Danish case-control study. Am J Obstet Gynecol 2000; 182:23–29.

12. Lambe M, Wuu J, Weiderpass E, Hsieh CC. Childbearing at older age and endometrial cancer risk (Sweden). Cancer Causes Control 1999; 10:43–49.

13. Kalandidi A, Tzonou A, Lipworth L, Gamatsi I, Filippa D, Trichopoulos D. A case-control study of endometrial cancer in relation to reproductive, somatometric, and life-style variables. Oncology 1996; 53:354–359.

14. Jafari K, Javaheri G, Ruiz G. Endometrial adenocarcinoma and the Stein–Leventhal syndrome. Obstet gynecol 1978; 51:97–100.

15. Mansell H, Hertig AT. Granulosa-theca cell tumors and endometrial cancer: a study of their relaionship and a survey of 80 cases. Obstet gynecol 1955; 6: 385–395.

16. Grady D, Gebretsadik T, Kerlikowske K, Ernster V, Petitti D. Hormone replacement therapy and endometrial cancer risk: a meta-analysis. Obstet gynecol 1995; 85:304–313.

17. Weiderpass E, Adami HO, Baron JA, Magnusson C, Bergstrom R, Lindgren A, Correia N, Persson I. Risk of endometrial cancer following estrogen replacement with and without progestins. J Natl Cancer Inst 1999; 91: 1131–1137.

18. Cushing KL, Weiss NS, Voigt LF, McKnight B, Beresford SA. Risk of endometrial cancer in relation to use of low-dose, unopposed estrogens. Obstet gynecol 1998; 91:35–39.

19. Hulka BS, Fowler WC Jr, Kaufman DG, Grimson RC, Greenberg BG, Hogue CJ, Berger GS, Pulliam CC. Estrogen and endometrial cancer: cases and two control groups from North Carolina. Am J Obstet Gynecol 1980; 137:92–101.
20. Shapiro S, Kelly JP, Rosenberg L, Kaufman DW, Helmrich SP, Rosenshein NB, Lewis JL Jr, Knapp RC, Stolley PD, Schottenfeld D. Risk of localized and widespread endometrial cancer in relation to recent and discontinued use of conjugated estrogens. N Engl J Med 1985; 313:969–972.
21. Tseng L, Gurpide E. Effects of progestins on estradiol receptor levels in human endometrium. J Clin Endocrinol Metab 1975; 41:402–404.
22. Rossouw JE, Anderson GL, Prentice RL, LaCroix AZ, Kooperberg C, Stefanick ML, Jackson RD, Beresford SA, Howard BV, Johnson KC, Kotchen JM, Ockene J. Risks and benefits of estrogen plus progestin in healthy postmenopausal women: principal results From the Women's Health Initiative randomized controlled trial. JAMA 2002; 288:321–333.
23. Weiderpass E, Adami HO, Baron JA, Magnusson C, Lindgren A, Persson I. Use of oral contraceptives and endometrial cancer risk (Sweden). Cancer Causes Control 1999; 10:277–284.
24. Hulka BS, Chambless LE, Kaufman DG, Fowler WC Jr, Greenberg BG. Protection against endometrial carcinoma by combination-product oral contraceptives. JAMA 1982; 247:475–477.
25. Voigt LF, Deng Q, Weiss NS. Recency, duration, and progestin content of oral contraceptives in relation to the incidence of endometrial cancer (Washington, USA). Cancer Causes Control 1994; 5:227–233.
26. Tornberg SA, Carstensen JM. Relationship between Quetelet's index and cancer of breast and female genital tract in 47,000 women followed for 25 years. Br J Cancer 1994; 69:358–361.
27. Olson SH, Trevisan M, Marshall JR, Graham S, Zielezny M, Vena JE, Hellmann R, Freudenheim JL. Body mass index, weight gain, and risk of endometrial cancer. Nutr Cancer 1995; 23:141–149.
28. Goodman MT, Hankin JH, Wilkens LR, Lyu LC, McDuffie K, Liu LQ, Kolonel LN. Diet, body size, physical activity, and the risk of endometrial cancer. Cancer Res 1997; 57:5077–5085.
29. Weiderpass E, Persson I, Adami HO, Magnusson C, Lindgren A, Baron JA. Body size in different periods of life, diabetes mellitus, hypertension, and risk of postmenopausal endometrial cancer (Sweden). Cancer Causes Control 2000; 11:185–192.
30. Schapira DV, Kumar NB, Lyman GH, Cavanagh D, Roberts WS, LaPolla J. Upper-body fat distribution and endometrial cancer risk. JAMA 1991; 266: 1808–1811.
31. Swanson CA, Potischman N, Wilbanks GD, Twiggs LB, Mortel R, Berman ML, Barrett RJ, Baumgartner RN, Brinton LA. Relation of endometrial cancer risk to past and contemporary body size and body fat distribution. Cancer Epidemiol Biomarkers Prev 1993; 2:321–327.
32. Akhmedkhanov A, Zeleniuch-Jacquotte A, Toniolo P. Role of exogenous and endogenous hormones in endometrial cancer: review of the evidence and research perspectives. Ann N Y Acad Sci 2001; 943:296–315.

33. Austin H, Austin JM Jr, Partridge EE, Hatch KD, Shingleton HM. Endometrial cancer, obesity, and body fat distribution. Cancer Res 1991; 51:568–572.
34. Enriori CL, Reforzo Membrives J. Peripheral aromatization as a risk factor for breast and endometrial cancer in postmenopausal women: a review. Gynecol Oncol 1984; 17:1–21.
35. Davidson BJ, Gambone JC, Lagasse LD, Castaldo TW, Hammond GL, Siiteri PK, Judd HL. Free estradiol in postmenopausal women with and without endometrial cancer. J Clin Endocrinol Metab 1981; 52:404–408.
36. Elwood JM, Cole P, Rothman KJ, Kaplan SD. Epidemiology of endometrial cancer. J Natl Cancer Inst 1977; 59:1055–1060.
37. Parazzini F, La Vecchia C, Negri E, Riboldi GL, Surace M, Benzi G, Maina A, Chiaffarino F. Diabetes and endometrial cancer: an Italian case-control study. Int J Cancer 1999; 81:539–542.
38. Weiss NS, Farewall VT, Szekely DR, English DR, Kiviat N. Oestrogens and endometrial cancer: effect of other risk factors on the association. Maturitas 1980; 2:185–190.
39. Soler M, Chatenoud L, Negri E, Parazzini F, Franceschi S, la Vecchia C. Hypertension and hormone-related neoplasms in women. Hypertension 1999; 34:320–325.
40. Jung RT. Obesity as a disease. Br Med Bull 1997; 53:307–321.
41. Kelsey JL, LiVolsi VA, Holford TR, Fischer DB, Mostow ED, Schwartz PE, O'Connor T, White C. A case-control study of cancer of the endometrium. Am J Epidemiol 1982; 116:333–342.
42. La Vecchia C, Negri E, Franceschi S, D'Avanzo B, Boyle P. A case-control study of diabetes mellitus and cancer risk. Br J Cancer 1994; 70:950–953.
43. Troisi R, Potischman N, Hoover RN, Siiteri P, Brinton LA. Insulin and endometrial cancer. Am J Epidemiol 1997; 146:476–482.
44. Poehlman ET, Toth MJ, Ades PA, Rosen CJ. Menopause-associated changes in plasma lipids, insulin-like growth factor I and blood pressure: a longitudinal study. Eur J Clin Invest 1997; 27:322–326.
45. Elliott EA, Matanoski GM, Rosenshein NB, Grumbine FC, Diamond EL. Body fat patterning in women with endometrial cancer. Gynecol Oncol 1990; 39:253–258.
46. Parazzini F, La Vecchia C, Negri E, Moroni S, Chatenoud L. Smoking and risk of endometrial cancer: results from an Italian case-control study. Gynecol Oncol 1995; 56:195–199.
47. Stockwell HG, Lyman GH. Cigarette smoking and the risk of female reproductive cancer. Am J Obstet Gynecol 1987; 157:35–40.
48. Levi F, La Vecchia C, Gulie C, Franceschi S, Negri E. Oestrogen replacement treatment and the risk of endometrial cancer: an assessment of the role of covariates. Eur J Cancer 1993; 29a:1445–1449.
49. Terry PD, Rohan TE, Franceschi S, Weiderpass E. Cigarette smoking and the risk of endometrial cancer. Lancet Oncol 2002; 3:470–480.
50. Baron JA, Comi RJ, Cryns V, Brinck Johnsen T, Mercer NG. The effect of cigarette smoking on adrenal cortical hormones. J Pharmacol Exp Ther 1995; 272:151–155.

51. Franks AL, Kendrick JS, Tyler CW Jr. Postmenopausal smoking, estrogen replacement therapy, and the risk of endometrial cancer. Am J Obstet Gynecol 1987; 156:20–23.
52. Levi F, Franceschi S, Negri E, La Vecchia C. Dietary factors and the risk of endometrial cancer. Cancer 1993; 71:3575 3581.
53. Shu XO, Zheng W, Potischman N, Brinton LA, Hatch MC, Gao YT, Fraumeni JF Jr. A population-based case-control study of dietary factors and endometrial cancer in Shanghai, People's Republic of China. Am J Epidemiol 1993; 137:155–165.
54. Barbone F, Austin H, Partridge EE. Diet and endometrial cancer: a case-control study. Am J Epidemiol 1993; 137:393–403.
55. Goldin BR, Adlercreutz H, Gorbach SL, Warram JH, Dwyer JT, Swenson L, Woods MN. Estrogen excretion patterns and plasma levels in vegetarian and omnivorous women. N Engl J Med 1982; 307:1542–1547.
56. Barbosa JC, Shultz TD, Filley SJ, Nieman DC. The relationship among adiposity, diet, and hormone concentrations in vegetarian and nonvegetarian postmenopausal women. Am J Clin Nutr 1990; 51:798–803.
57. Bennett FC, Ingram DM. Diet and female sex hormone concentrations: an intervention study for the type of fat consumed. Am J Clin Nutr 1990; 52:808–812.
58. Katsouyanni K, Boyle P, Trichopoulos D. Diet and urine estrogens among postmenopausal women. Oncology 1991; 48:490–494.
59. London S, Willett W, Longcope C, McKinlay S. Alcohol and other dietary factors in relation to serum hormone concentrations in women at climacteric. Am J Clin Nutr 1991; 53:166–171.
60. Austin H, Drews C, Partridge EE. A case-control study of endometrial cancer in relation to cigarette smoking, serum estrogen levels, and alcohol use. Am J Obstet Gynecol 1993; 169:1086–1091.
61. Swanson CA, Wilbanks GD, Twiggs LB, Mortel R, Berman ML, Barrett RJ, Brinton LA. Moderate alcohol consumption and the risk of endometrial cancer. Epidemiology 1993; 4:530–536.
62. Terry P, Baron JA, Weiderpass E, Yuen J, Lichtenstein P, Nyren O. Lifestyle and endometrial cancer risk: a cohort study from the Swedish Twin Registry. Int J Cancer 1999; 82:38–42.
63. Parazzini F, La Vecchia C, D'Avanzo B, Moroni S, Chatenoud L, Ricci E. Alcohol and endometrial cancer risk: findings from an Italian case-control study. Nutr Cancer 1995; 23:55–62.
64. Cauley JA, Gutai JP, Kuller LH, LeDonne D, Powell JG. The epidemiology of serum sex hormones in postmenopausal women. Am J Epidemiol 1989; 129:1120–1131.
65. Levi F, La Vecchia C, Negri E, Franceschi S. Selected physical activities and the risk of endometrial cancer. Br J Cancer 1993; 67:846–851.
66. Parazzini F, La Vecchia C, Moroni S, Chatenoud L, Ricci E. Family history and the risk of endometrial cancer. Int J Cancer 1994; 59:460–462.
67. Gruber SB, Thompson WD. A population-based study of endometrial cancer and familial risk in younger women. Cancer and Steroid Hormone Study Group. Cancer Epidemiol Biomarkers Prev 1996; 5:411–417.

68. Sandles LG, Shulman LP, Elias S, Photopulos GJ, Smiley LM, Posten WM, Simpson JL. Endometrial adenocarcinoma: genetic analysis suggesting heritable site- specific uterine cancer. Gynecol Oncol 1992; 47:167–171.
69. Schildkraut JM, Risch N, Thompson WD. Evaluating genetic association among ovarian, breast, and endometrial cancer: evidence for a breast/ovarian cancer relationship. Am J Hum Genet 1989; 45:521–529.
70. Watson P, Vasen HF, Mecklin JP, Jarvinen H, Lynch HT. The risk of endometrial cancer in hereditary nonpolyposis colorectal cancer. Am J Med 1994; 96:516–520.
71. Berends MJ, Kleibeuker JH, de Vries EG, Mourits MJ, Hollema H, Pras E, van der Zee AG. The importance of family history in young patients with endometrial cancer. Eur J Obstet gynecol Reprod Biol 1999; 82:139–141.

2

Screening in Endometrial Cancer

Thomas Hogberg

*Department of Oncology, Division of Gynaecologic Oncology, University Hospital,
Linkoping, Sweden*

WHAT DOES CANCER SCREENING ACTUALLY MEAN?

Usually in medicine a patient initiates a consultation to get advice and treatment because he/she has experienced some symptoms. In a cancer screening program, however, people are invited because they belong to a certain risk group (e.g., age). With few exceptions, they are all, by definition, asymptomatic. In an ideal situation, the cancer screening test will tell if a subject has the disease or not. There is, however, no perfect test. There is an inherent inverse relationship between the ability of a test to detect disease (sensitivity) and the ability of a test to detect the absence of disease (specificity). At times, all screening tests will miss some cases with disease (i.e., false negative results), and at times, all screening tests will suggest the presence of disease where none exists (i.e., false positive results) (1). More often, though, the test merely tells something about the *risk* of having or contracting a disease. For those testing positive, further tests have to be done to confirm or exclude disease. Most of those testing positive will be worried without reason and will be subject to unnecessary investigations with associated possible adverse effects. In the end, the diagnosis will be confirmed in some cases and definite treatment of the cancer disease can be instituted. The majority of those individuals are the winners in the screening game. But a minority of those would never have been troubled by their cancer, and thus are loosers. They may have a slowly developing cancer and could well die of other causes before having

13

symptoms from their screen-detected cancer even if it remains untreated. Some of those testing negative will still have an increased risk, or have the disease, but will be falsely reassured. In some cases, the cancer would, in spite of screening, be detected in an advanced stage when curative treatment is no longer possible. "It is the small proportion who would die of their disease in the absence of screening, but who if their cancer is screen detected, go on to die of another condition later who really benefit from screening" (2).

There is a fundamental difference between an offer from society to investigate a person free of symptoms and the situation when a person with symptoms seeks the help of a practitioner. If a patient asks a medical practitioner for help, the doctor does the best he/she can. The individual practitioner is not responsible for defects in medical knowledge. If, however, society initiates screening procedures, the situation is very different. The majority of those screened do not get any benefit from the investigation and the investigation can convert a participant to a patient with all its consequences. This means that the demands on the methods used in screening are far greater than in a medical consultation. Conclusive evidence that screening can alter the natural history of disease in a significant proportion of those screened is an absolute requirement.

A screening program against any disease should be founded on evidence-based knowledge. This means that ideally a cancer screening program should be evaluated by at least one randomized study with mortality as an end point (2). Unless the effects of screening on mortality are expected to be very dramatic, these studies have to be performed in large populations. For the evaluation of ovarian cancer screening, 37,000 women were randomized in the United States and 200,000 are planned to be randomized in the United Kingdom. The time between initiation and evaluation of these studies is much longer than we are used to in randomized clinical studies testing drug effects. For the United States ovarian cancer study, it will be about 23 years and the results are expected around 2015 (3). A formal randomized study can prove the efficacy of a screening procedure. The cost benefit for the host society and for participants should also be evaluated. Finally, the effectiveness, or the real-life results, of a proposed screening program has to be documented. This last evaluation includes compliance, organization, economy, and outcomes (2).

CANCER SCREENING TRAPS

In Non-Randomized Trials

Lead Time Bias

There will always be an interval between the screen detection of a condition and the time when the condition would have been diagnosed because of symptoms. This will automatically increase the time between screen detection and the end point (e.g., death) for screen-detected cases, whether or not the time for the end point has actually been postponed by screening.

Length Bias

Screen-detected cases, especially in periodic screening programs, tend to have longer preclinical intervals. The preclinical interval is the period between the time point a screening test could detect a condition and the time point when a patient would seek help because of symptoms. A screening program could result in a selection of cases with longer preclinical intervals and presumably slower-developing tumors that are less aggressive and with better prognoses.

Overdiagnosis Bias

A screening program can detect cases that would never develop into an invasive tumor giving symptoms. This bias and the two mentioned above might lead to an overestimation of the effects of a screening program on survival.

Selection Bias

The selection of the population targeted for screening can in turn result in the detection of selected subpopulations of tumors with better or worse prognoses. This bias can work both ways when evaluating the effect of a screening program on survival.

In Randomized Trials

Internal Validity—Contamination

Some of the patients in the control group may be subject to "wild screening."

Internal Validity—Dilution

Some of the patients in the experimental arm who are offered screening may not accept the screening procedure.

External Validity—Representativity

Controlled, randomized trials may not model reality.

SCREENING FOR ENDOMETRIAL CANCER?

Wilson and Jungner (4) summarized the basic principles of screening as follows:

- The condition sought should be an important health problem: Endometrial cancer is the most common gynecologic cancer and in many countries the fraction of the elderly population is growing.

This suggests that the number of cases of endometrial cancer will increase even if the age-specific incidence may be stable or even decrease (5).

- There should be an accepted treatment for patients with recognized disease: Surgery with hysterectomy and bilateral salpingo-oophorectomy, with pelvic and para-aortic lymph node exploration in selected cases, is the accepted primary treatment.
- Facilities for diagnosis and treatment should be available: The diagnosis and treatment of endometrial cancer requires basic health care resources that exist in most countries.
- There should be a recognizable latent or early symptomatic stage: It is doubtful that there is a precursor stage, although atypical hyperplasia in many cases is associated with endometrial cancer, usually of a less malignant type. The more malignant types arise in an atrophic endometrium and may be heralded by metaplastic changes.
- There should be a suitable test or examination: Endometrial biopsies or vaginal ultrasound examinations have been used in endometrial cancer screening tests. Both, however, are more resource-demanding tests than are usually accepted in screening programs.
- The test should be acceptable to the population: Endometrial biopsies have proved to be a fairly acceptable method in studies on endometrial screening.
- The natural history of the disease, including latent to declared disease, should be adequately understood: Little is actually known about this. The performed screening trials suggest that the preclinical phase could be several years.
- There should be an agreed policy on who to treat as patients: It is accepted that individuals with atypical hyperplasia and early endometrial cancer should be treated.
- The cost of case-finding (including diagnosis and treatment of patients diagnosed) should be economically balanced in relation to possible expenditure on medical care as a whole: This is the most doubtful point. Analysis of the Japanese experience of screening (see below) will hopefully provide an answer, although this screening program has been implemented without forgoing randomized trials.
- Case-finding should be a continuing process and not a "once and for all" project: Currently there is a lack of knowledge of suitable screening intervals for endometrial cancer.

SCREENING TESTS FOR ENDOMETRIAL CANCER

A prerequisite for screening is that there is a reliable test that is acceptable to the potential subjects of screening. In the case of endometrial cancer, there is no test as simple as the Pap smear for cervical cancer. Pap smears can be used to diagnose atypical cells of possible endometrial origin, but the sensitivity for the definitive diagnosis of an endometrial cancer is low (6,7). There are several methods for endometrial sampling, both for cytology and histology. These samples can be acquired in an outpatient setting without anesthesia or analgesia. In 95% of the cases, the subjects rate the pain and mild discomfort as acceptable (8). However, it is a technically more demanding procedure than a Pap smear, as an instrument has to be introduced into the endometrial cavity. The investigation must be done by a doctor and is therefore resource-demanding. As the patients are usually elderly with associated genital atrophy, it is not possible to introduce the instrument in the endometrial cavity in 10–15% of the cases (6–8). Examples of endometrial cancer have been found among such cases (7). In around 10% of the cases no interpretable material is obtained in spite of the fact that the instrument has been successfully introduced (7). Most investigators have evaluated tests where the investigator regards the procedure as successful but no material has been obtained as signifying an atrophic endometrium. An ultrasound investigation may be helpful to select cases that should be further investigated by dilation and curettage (D & C).

In an extensive literature review, Voupala (6) found a diagnostic accuracy of 88.5% for cytology of endometrial aspirations in 12,480 patients, 81.6% for endometrial lavage in 2805 patients, and 87.4% for the endometrial brush technique in 1354 patients. The jet wash technique with direct smear rendered 87% accuracy in 2258 patients, 75% for the Millipore filter technique ($n = 1234$), and 88% for the cell block technique. For histological methods, Voupala found 87% accuracy for endometrial biopsies with different metal or plastic cannulas or curettes in 1679 patients and 98% for Vabra vacuum curettage in 1135 patients (92% for hyperplasia). Methods with effective vacuum suction seem to obtain a larger portion of the endometrium than other methods. The mean percent of endometrial surface sampled with the Pipelle device was 4.2% (range 0–12%) and with the Vabra aspirator 42% (range 0–79%) (9). Clearly, focal lesions can be missed even with a conventional blindly performed dilatation and curettage; a false-negative rate of 2–6% has been reported (10–13). Hysteroscopically directed biopsies should improve the detection of focal lesions, but even with this method a false-negative rate of 3% has been reported (14).

Although the false-positive rate of a test is as important when screening diseases with low prevalence, little reference is made to this in the available literature.

Measuring endometrial thickness with ultrasound has a high negative predictive value ($\geq 99\%$) (15–17). In women who have the examination because of irregular bleeding and who are deemed negative, no case of endometrial cancer has been registered during a follow-up period of at least 10 years after the examination. However, the positive predictive value of a thick endometrium is low (2–3%), disqualifying measurement of endometrial thickness with ultrasound as a candidate for a primary screening method (15–17).

One can only speculate about suitable future tests. Interesting results have been published regarding analysis of proteomic patterns in serum to identify ovarian cancer (18). In endometrial cancer, it may also be possible to analyze lavage fluid from the endometrial cavity. More insight into the molecular changes involved in endometrial cancer are required in order to design new tests.

WHAT COULD BE GAINED BY SCREENING FOR ENDOMETRIAL CANCER?

The aim of screening for cancer is to improve survival by an early diagnosis, which makes it possible to treat the disease in an early stage or even before invasive cancer has occurred. Presumptions for this are that there exist usable tests to identify the disease in an early or precursor stage, that the disease actually has an identifiable precursor state and/or a sufficiently long preclinical phase, and that an effective treatment exists.

It is accepted that there are two types of endometrial cancers. Type I is estrogen-dependent and the histological type is well or moderately differentiated endometrioid adenocarcinoma. Atypical endometrial hyperplasia frequently coexists with, or heralds, type I disease. Mutations of K-*ras*, PTEN, β-cathenin, and microsatellite instability are more common with type I tumors (19). The prognosis is usually good for patients with type I disease (20,21). Type II disease, on the other hand, is estrogen-independent and develops in an atrophic endometrium and is not preceded by hyperplasia but rather intraepithelial metaplasia. Mutations of *p*53 and Her-2-*neu* are more common in type II lesions and seem to develop early in the disease course. The histological types are poorly differentiated endometrioid, serous, or clear cell carcinoma (19). The prognosis for type II disease is worse than for type I disease (20,22,23).

In clinical practice without screening programs, the diagnosis of an endometrial cancer is made when the disease is in stages I–IIA in 76% of the cases and the five-year survival rate for this group is 88% (24). About 80% of patients in stages I–IIA have type I tumors. The prognosis for those patients is very good and their survival rate seems to be very close to that for the general female population with the same age distribution (20,21,25). Patients with type II tumors in stages I–IIA constitute about 20% and have around 70% five-year survival rate (20). Twenty-four percent of the patients are diagnosed with stages IIB–IV disease and their five-year survival rate is 54% (24). Patients surviving five years without recurrence are unlikely to subsequently die of endometrial cancer.

The patients that would potentially benefit from screening are the 24% who today are diagnosed with stages IIB–IV disease and possibly the 15%

with type II disease in stages I–IIA. Together these women comprise around 40% of the total number of patients diagnosed with endometrial cancer. The incidence of endometrial cancer in Sweden in 2001 was 28/100,000 woman-years (26). Endometrial cancer is practically never diagnosed before the age of 45. The Swedish incidence for women older than 44 years was 52/100,000 woman-years in 2001. The incidence of cases for which an early detection could affect the outcome would then be 40% or 21/100,000 woman-years for women aged over 44. The five-year survival rate for those cases would be around 58%. Hypothesize that we do a prevalence screen of 1,000,000 women aged over 44 with a perfect method. Suppose that this method detects all cases that would have been diagnosed in the first and second year following the screen. We would then expect to diagnose a total of 1040 cases with 420 of those being of type II, stages I–IIA or stages IIB–IV (0.04% of the screened population). Suppose the five-year survival rate for these screen-detected cases would be as good as for type I, stages I–IIA tumors (88%). About 370 instead of 244 women would then survive five years. The majority of these women will also survive until they die of other causes. The median age for the diagnosis of endometrial cancer in Sweden was almost 70 years in 2001 and the median survival rate for all women in the population was 85 years. This would translate to 1890 years of life saved. If we accept a cost of US $50,000/year of life saved, which incidentally is the estimated cost for ovarian cancer screening (28), it would require a budget of US $94,500,000 for screening 1,000,000 women, which translates to around US $95 per person. This would be a tight budget. These figures presuppose an ideal test that would identify every patient with a stage I-IIA type II or high-stage endometrial cancer and very successful therapy for those cases. A real screening procedure would realistically save fewer years of life and the budget would be even tighter. On the other hand, the number of cases detected by screening may be underestimated (Table 1). This hypothetical example is intended to show that if a disease is fairly unusual and has a relatively good survival rate without screening, the potential gains of screening are small and the costs will be high. From the perspective of health care providers, other measures with better cost-benefit ratios might seem more attractive than screening for endometrial cancer.

THE NATURAL COURSE OF ENDOMETRIAL CANCER—PREMALIGNANT CONDITIONS?

Estrogen-dependent type I lesions are associated with atypical endometrial hyperplasia. Patients with atypical endometrial hyperplasia have a high risk of developing endometrial cancer within a few years (28). Hyperplastic lesions have traditionally been regarded as precursors of type I endometrial cancer. However, screening trials do not support the hypothesis that endometrial hyperplasia is a precursor, since usually the number of cases

Table 1 Screening Studies

Author year (ref)	Setting	Number of subjects	Diagnostic method	Number of cases with endometrial cancer	Detection rate of endometrial cancer
Horwitz 1981 (29)	Autopsy study. Previously unsuspected EC in asymptomatic women aged ≥45	8998	Autopsy	24	267/100,000
Koss 1984 (36)	Asymptomatic women ≥45 years. 1st screen	2586	Mi-Mark helix or aspiration biopsy (Isaacs cannula)	16[*]	619/100,000
Koss 1984 (36)	2nd screen after 1 year, 3rd screen after 2 years	1567 (2nd screen) 187 (3rd screen)	Mi-Mark helix or aspiration biopsy (Isaacs cannula)	1[**]	27/100,000
Osmers 1990 (16)	Asymptomatic PM women	283	Vaginal US + curettage if ≥4 mm endometrial thickness	10	3534/100,000
Archer 1991[a]	Asymptomatic peri- or PM women before enrollment in HRT-study	801	Endometrial biopsy	1	125/100,000
Gronroos 1993 (36)	Asymptomatic women aged from 45–69 with diabetes and/or hypertension	597	Aspiration biopsy (Vabra)	0[***]	0
Vuento 1995 (8)	2nd screen 8 years after the first of women with diabetes from Gronroos (1993)	78	Aspiration biopsy (Pistolet aspiration)	0	0

Study	Description	N	Method	Cases	Rate
Vuento 1995 (8)	Control group from Gronroos (1993), diabetic and not previously screened	148	Aspiration biopsy (Pistolet aspiration)	1	556/100,000
Korhonen 1997[b]	Asymptomatic peri- or PM women before enrollment in HRT-study	2964	Aspiration biopsy (Vabra)	2	67/100,000
Fleischer 2001 (15)	Asymptomatic PM women eligible for osteoporosis prevention study	1792	Vaginal US + aspiration biopsy	2	112/100,000
Nakagawa-Okamura 2002 (37)	Mass screening of women at high risk****	217,827	Endocyte endometrial smears	238	109/100,000
Patai 2002[c]	High-risk women ≥35 years	72	Vaginal US, aspiration biopsy (Tis-U-Trap)	2	2778/100,000
Total (1st screen)*****		227,070		272	120/100,000

Articles otherwise not referenced in text.

[a] Archer DF, McIntyre-Seltman K, Wilborn WW, Dowling EA, Cone F, Creasy GW, Kafrissen ME. Endometrial morphology in asymptomatic postmenopausal women. Am J Obstet Gynecol 1991; 165(2):317–322.

[b] Korhonen MO, Symons JP, Hyde BM, Rowan JP. Histologic classification and pathologic findings for endometrial biopsy specimens obtained from 2964 perimenopausal and postmenopausal women undergoing screening for continuous hormones as replacement therapy (CHART 2 study). Am J Obstet Gynecol 1997; 176(2):377–380.

[c] Patai K, Szentmariay IF, Jakab Zs, Szilagyi G. Early detection of endometrial cancer by combined use of vaginal ultrasound and endometrial vacuum sampling. Int J Gynecol Cancer 2002; 12(3):261–264.

*2 cases of endometrial cancer missed.
**2 cases of endometrial cancer missed.
***2 cases of adenocarcinoma in situ.
****High risk defined as at least one of age ≥50, PM, nulligravid with irregular menstruation.
*****excluding 1. Horwitz 1981 (autopsy study), 3. Koss 1984 (2nd and 3rd screen), 7. Vuento (1995 2nd screen).

Abbreviations: HRT: hormone replacement therapy, PM: postmenopausal.

diagnosed with hyperplasia is only 1-1.5 times those with endometrial cancer (7,8). If hyperplasia is a precursor lesion, one would expect more cases of hyperplasia detected in the screening trials. Two screening trials (7,8) indicate that the preclinical phase of endometrial cancer may be rather long. Few cases of endometrial cancer were discovered in the secondary screening rounds of these trials, one, two, or eight years after the first. The detection and treatment of cases in the first screening rounds probably explain the low rate of endometrial cancer in the secondary screening rounds.

Autopsy studies show that for many cancer types, it is not unusual to find malignant tumors that were not diagnosed during life. A large study on endometrial cancer demonstrated that for 9098 females aged 45 or more with an intact uterus, 24 patients had occult endometrial cancer. No history of symptoms related to endometrial cancer could be found in their records. After a comparison with the tumor registry of the region (Connecticut State Tumor Registry, U.S.A.), the authors conclude that their results indicated that there were at least three asymptomatic cases of endometrial cancer for every diagnosed case (29). Suen et al. (30) reported an autopsy study on 3535 patients over 65 years of age. Of those, 1693 were women. They found 52 cases of endometrial cancer of which seven (13.5%) were not suspected during life and did not contribute to the patient's demise.

RISK GROUPS

Selection of groups considered to be at increased risk is one approach that may make screening more cost-effective. Obesity, diabetes, late menopause, nulliparity, and unopposed estrogen hormone replacement therapy are recognized risk factors for endometrial cancer (31,32). Tamoxifen treatment is a well-known risk factor for endometrial cancer (33). A fraction of cases with endometrial cancer have a genetic background. Hereditary nonpolypous colorectal cancer (HNPCC) is a condition with a very high lifetime risk (approaching 40%) for endometrial cancer. In some countries, those patients are already offered screening, although there is no evidence-based support for this (34).

PRELIMINARY SCREENING TRIALS

There are many screening trials that merely test a method for the diagnosis of an endometrial cancer and apply that to a population. This is important to test the efficacy of the method of diagnosis, and may also provide data with regard to the prevalence of the disease in the population. Table 1 shows some examples of screening trials.

The next test of the efficacy of a screening procedure is a second screen of the population to see if the prevalence has decreased or to at least serve as a prolonged follow-up after the first screen. Few studies of screening in endometrial cancer have addressed this issue. One Finnish study (8) has performed a repeat screen and an American study (7) two repeat screens, both suggesting that a single screen could be effective. There is also a Swedish study (35) where the initial screen was done with ultrasound and dilation and curettage in a population of postmenopausal women who were investigated because of bleeding. In 178 women who had an endometrial mucosal thickness of <4 mm, no case of endometrial cancer was diagnosed in relation to the screening round or during a follow-up period of at least 10 years. The risk of endometrial cancer in the total cohort of 339 women referred for postmenopausal bleeding was 66 times higher than the risk for the female population with the same age distribution from the same region of Sweden according to tumor registry data. Koss et al. (7) reported on a cohort of 2586 asymptomatic women over 45 years of age, who were screened once, of whom 1567 were screened twice and 187 were screened three times. The patients were recruited either by general practitioners or were volunteers. The inclusion criteria were:

- age 45 or older,
- an intact uterus,
- absence of symptoms referable to the genital tract, such as vaginal bleeding, and
- willingness to sign an informed consent form.

Endometrial samples were obtained either with Mi-Mark Helix or the Isaacs cannula. The choice of sampling device was randomly assigned. A vaginal pool smear was also taken. Subjects with atypical, suspicious, or positive results on histology or cytology underwent either endometrial biopsy or formal curettage. A clinically satisfactory sample was achieved in 93% of the subjects; Mi-Mark performed less well with an 86% success rate. The overall rate of satisfactory interpretation was 86% where an attempt at sampling was included as the denominator. Sixteen endometrial carcinomas were found in the first screening round and two further cases with recurrent vaginal bleeding were found to have endometrial cancer during the first year after the screening. This corresponds to a rate of 70/10,000 women. The rate of hyperplasia and polyps with hyperplasia was only slightly higher, 81/10,000 women. In the second and third screening rounds, one and two years after the first, one further case of endometrial cancer was discovered and two cases were missed. This translates to an incidence of 17/10,000 woman-years. The incidence according to the cancer registries of Connecticut and New York during the same time was 9/10,000 woman-years for women aged 45 and above. A positive diagnosis was rendered in nine cases with carcinoma. The endometrial material was suspicious in another seven patients and repeatedly atypical in one. In two additional patients, the positive diagnosis remained unproven and they were considered as false positives. Nine additional patients had a suspicious diagnosis. In four of them, endometrial hyperplasia was observed; in five, no lesions could be found. The occurrence of atypical hyperplasia was not stated. Thus, between five and nine samples were false-positives. There were 125 women with atypical endometrial findings. In one woman with cytologically atypical endometrial smears, endometrial carcinoma was diagnosed. In 17 patients, hyperplasia or polyps were found in biopsy or curettage samples. The number of false-positives was in total between 114 and 135, which translates to a positive predictive value for endometrial carcinoma and atypical hyperplasia between 11% and 13%. Koss et al. (7) speculated that the probable duration of the preclinical interval for endometrial cancer could be four years. They arrived at this conclusion by dividing their prevalence rate by their incidence rate. In an earlier study, they had arrived at a figure of 6.6 years. Koss et al. (7) do not specify figures for sensitivity or specificity. For endometrial cancer, the sensitivity would be 17/21 or 0.81. The figures for specificity and negative predictive values are harder to calculate with any degree of certainty from the data provided.

The first part of the Finnish study was reported by Gronroos et al. (36). They invited 1578 asymptomatic women with diabetes and/or hypertension aged 45–65 years identified through a Social Insurance Registry, where they could identify individuals with reimbursed medication for diabetes and hypertension. Seven hundred and twelve subjects were studied: 235 with diabetes, 284 with both diabetes and hypertension, and 193 with only hypertension. The samples were taken with a Vabra vacuum suction curettage. The catheter could be inserted in the endometrial cavity in 597 women (84%). Four of the women with diabetes had adenocarcinoma in situ and two had atypical hyperplasia; another 13 had nonatypic hyperplasia. Vuento et al. reported the second part of the study (8) in which 462 patients with diabetes were chosen from the Social Insurance Registry. Of these, 237 were invited for first screening and 225 remained as a control group. From the description in the paper, it is very hard to deduct how the groups in this report related to the groups in the first report. For example, the existence of a control group was not mentioned in the first study. Despite this lack of detail, it appeared that 85 women who were screened in the first study (36) during 1980 and 1981 and 175 women from the control group accepted an invitation for a screen during 1988 and 1989; 34 were excluded because they had had hysterectomies in the interim (seven in group one because of pathologies detected at the first screen and 27 in the control group). After the exclusions, there were 78 females in the rescreen group and 148 in the control group. This time the endometrial biopsies were taken with a Pistolet aspiration sampling device. A histologic sample was obtained in 193 cases. The endometrial cavity could be sampled in 85% of the cases. In the 72 samples that could be obtained from the rescreen group, no pathologic lesions of the endometrium could be found, while one case of endometrial carcinoma (0.8%), two cases of nonatypical complex hyperplasia (1.6%), four cases of endometrial polyps (3.3%), and one case of inflammatory change (0.8%) were diagnosed among the 121 samples from the control group. Vuento et al. (8) also made a record linkage to the Finnish Cancer Registry for the time between the first screen and 1994. One case of endometrial cancer was found in the rescreen group in a patient who had declined the first screening round. Two cases of endometrial cancer were found in the control group. One case was symptom-diagnosed in the interval between 1981 and the second screen round; the other case was screen-detected in the 1988–1989 screening.

In Japan, there has been an organized mass screening for endometrial cancer in selected women who have participated in the cervical cancer screening program since 1987 (37). Gynecologists select the participants from the cervical cancer screening program who they believe are at high risk for endometrial cancer and invite them to participate in a screening program for endometrial cancer. Women at high risk are those who have had abnormal vaginal bleeding within the previous six months and meet at least one of the following criteria:

- Age ≥ 50 years,
- Postmenopausal, and
- Nulligravid with irregular menstruation.

The screening is done with Endocyte endometrial smears that are classified as positive, suspicious, or negative. If the result is suspicious or positive, a dilatation and fractional curettage is performed. According to official Japanese statistics cited in the article, 217,827 women participated in endometrial cancer screening in 1995, of whom 4219 (1.9%) were referred for D&C, and 238 (0.1%) were diagnosed as having endometrial cancer. This corresponds to a positive predictive value of 5.1% for the primary screening test. There is no information to determine whether this was a single screen or if it was repeated. Nakagawa-Okamura et al. (37) compared 167 patients with screen-detected endometrial cancer with a control group consisting of 1069 patients with symptom-diagnosed endometrial cancer who were not participating in the screening program at the same hospitals. The five-year disease-specific survival rate was 95% for the screen-detected group and 86% for controls ($p = 0.041$). In a Cox univariate analysis, the hazard ratio was 0.47 (95% confidence interval 0.23–2.08) without controlling for stage, age at diagnosis, and geographic region. In the subsequent multivariate analyses, the hazard ratio was the same after correction for age at diagnosis and geographic region, but was almost one (0.96; CI 0.45–2.08) after correction for stage. The authors concluded that the survival benefit for the screen-detected group was due largely to the fact that the screening program detected cancer cases at earlier stages. The authors confess that the comparison is not free from lead-time bias, length bias, or other uncontrolled factors that could affect the result. The health economics of the screening program have yet to be analyzed, although it will, in the absence of randomized data, be difficult to decide the effect of the program in terms of life years saved.

CONCLUSIONS

Considering the available knowledge about the disease and the available tests, it seems unlikely that screening will be implemented in the near future. This has also been the view expressed in statements from official organizations such as the International Union Against Cancer (UICC) (38) and American Cancer Society (39). There are a few uncontrolled studies lending some support to the efficacy of screening programs (7,8,37). No randomized trials have been published. No health economic data have been presented in relation to the published reports. In spite of the lack of evidence-based support, general screening is organized for high-risk women in Japan (37). In some countries women with a hereditary risk (HNPCC) are offered screening. Screening of women on tamoxifen therapy with ultrasound or endometrial biopsies is not recommended (40). Even if new candidate tests emerge, the process of evaluating them and then evaluating screening will take decades. It seems unlikely that mass screening aimed at endometrial cancer can be recommended during the first decades of the 21st century.

REFERENCES

1. Galen RS, Gambino SR. Beyond Normality, the Predictive Value and Efficiency of Medical Diagnoses. New York, London, Sydney, Toronto: John Wiley & Sons, 1975.
2. Day NE. The theoretical bais for cancer screening. In: Miller AB, ed. Advances in Cancer Screening. Boston/Dordrecht/London: Kluwer Academic Publishers, 1996:9–24.
3. PCLO-trial. http://www3.cancer.gov/prevention/plco/news/winter-2001/notes.html.
4. Wilson JMG, Jungner G. Principles and practice of screening for disease. In: Wilson JMG, Jungner G, eds. Principles and Practice of Screening. Geneva: World Health Organization, 1968.
5. Moller B, Fekjaer H, Hakulinen T, Tryggvadottir L, Storm HH, Talback M, Haldorsen T. Prediction of cancer incidence in the Nordic countries up to the year 2020. Eur J Cancer Prev 2003; 11(Suppl 1):S1–S96.
6. Voupala S. Diagnostic accuracy and clinical applicability of cytological and histological methods for investigating endometrial carcinoma. Acta Obstet Gynecol Scand 2003; 56(Suppl.70):1–72.
7. Koss LG, Schreiber K, Oberlander SG, Moussouris HF, Lesser M. Detection of endometrial carcinoma and hyperplasia in asymptomatic women. Obstet Gynecol 1984; 64(1):1–11.
8. Vuento MH, Maatela JI, Tyrkko JE, Laippala PJ, Gronroos M, Salmi TA. A longitudinal study of screening for endometrial cancer by endometrial biopsy in diabetic females. Int J Gynecol Cancer 1995; 5(5):390–395.
9. Rodriguez GC, Yaqub N, King ME. A comparison of the Pipelle device and the Vabra aspirator as measured by endometrial denudation in hysterectomy

specimens: the Pipelle device samples significantly less of the endometrial surface than the Vabra aspirator. Am J Obstet Gynecol 1993; 168(1 Pt 1):55–59.

10. Stovall TG, Solomon SK, Ling FW. Endometrial sampling prior to hysterectomy. Obstet Gynecol 1989; 73(3 Pt 1):405–409.

11. Stock RJ, Kanbour A. Prehysterectomy curettage. Obstet Gynecol 1975; 45(5):537–541.

12. Guido RS, Kanbour-Shakir A, Rulin MC, Christopherson WA. Pipelle endometrial sampling. Sensitivity in the detection of endometrial cancer. J Reprod Med 1995; 40(8):553–555.

13. MacKenzie IZ, Bibby JG. Critical assessment of dilatation and curettage in 1029 women. Lancet 1978; 2(8089):566–568.

14. Gimpelson RJ, Rappold HO. A comparative study between panoramic hysteroscopy with directed biopsies and dilatation and curettage. A review of 276 cases. Am J Obstet Gynecol 1988; 158(3 Pt 1):489–492.

15. Fleischer AC, Wheeler JE, Lindsay I, Hendrix SL, Grabill S, Kravitz B, MacDonald B. An assessment of the value of ultrasonographic screening for endometrial disease in postmenopausal women without symptoms. Am J Obstet Gynecol 2001; 184(2):70–75.

16. Osmers R, Volksen M, Schauer A. Vaginosonography for early detection of endometrial carcinoma? Lancet 1990; 335(8705):1569–1571.

17. Langer RD, Pierce JJ, O'Hanlan KA, Johnson SR, Espeland MA, Trabal JF, Barnabei VM, Merino MJ, Scully RE. Transvaginal ultrasonography compared with endometrial biopsy for the detection of endometrial disease. Postmenopausal Estrogen/Progestin Interventions Trial. N Engl J Med 1997; 337(25): 1792–1798.

18. Petricoin EF, Ardekani AM, Hitt BA, Levine PJ, Fusaro VA, Steinberg SM, Mills GB, Simone C, Fishman DA, Kohn EC, Liotta LA. Use of proteomic patterns in serum to identify ovarian cancer. Lancet 2002; 359(9306):572–577.

19. Inoue M. Current molecular aspects of the carcinogenesis of the uterine endometrium. Int J Gynecol Cancer 2001; 11(5):339–348.

20. Hogberg T, Fredstorp-Lidebring M, Alm P, Baldetorp B, Larsson G, Ottosen C, Svanberg L, Lindahl B. A prospective population-based management program including primary surgery and postoperative risk assessment by means of DNA ploidy and histopathology. Adjuvant radiotherapy is not necessary for the majority of patients with FIGO stage I–II endometrial cancer. Int J Gynecol Cancer 2004; 14(3):437–450.

21. Poulsen HK, Jacobsen M, Bertelsen K, Andersen JE, Ahrons S, Bock J, Bostofte E, Engelholm SA, Holund B, Jakobsen A, Kiaer H, Nyland M, Pedersen PH, Stroyer I. Adjuvant radiation therapy is not necessary in the management of endometrial carcinoma stage I, low-risk cases. Int J Gynecol Cancer 1996; 6(1):38–43.

22. Abeler VM, Vergote IB, Kjorstad KE, Trope CG. Clear cell carcinoma of the endometrium. Prognosis and metastatic pattern. Cancer 1996; 78(8): 1740–1747.

23. Rosenberg P, Risberg B, Askmalm L, Simonsen E. The prognosis in early endometrial carcinoma. The importance of uterine papillary serous carcinoma

(UPSC), age, FIGO grade and nuclear grade. Acta Obstet Gynecol Scand 1989; 68(2):157–163.

24. Creasman WT, Odicino F, Maisonneuve P, Beller U, Benedet JL, Heintz APM, Ngan HYS, Sideri M, Pecorelli S. Carcinoma of the corpus uteri in 24th vol of the Annual Report on the Results of Treatment in Gynecological Cancer. J Epidem Biostat 2001; 6(1):45–86.

25. Burke TW, Heller PB, Woodward JE, Davidson SA, Hoskins WJ, Park RC. Treatment failure in endometrial carcinoma. Obstet Gynecol 1990; 75(1):96–101.

26. The National Board of Health and Welfare—Centre for Epidemiology. Cancer Incidence in Sweden 2001 (http://www.sos.se/FULLTEXT/42/2003-42-6/ 2003-42-6.pdf). Stockholm 2003.

27. Kurman RJ, Kaminski PF, Norris HJ. The behavior of endometrial hyperplasia. A long-term study of "untreated" hyperplasia in 170 patients. Cancer 1985; 56(2):403–412.

28. Urban N, Drescher C, Etzioni R, Colby C. Use of a stochastic simulation model to identify an efficient protocol for ovarian cancer screening. Control Clin Trials 1997; 18(3):251–270.

29. Horwitz RI, Feinstein AR, Horwitz SM, Robboy SJ. Necropsy diagnosis of endometrial cancer and detection-bias in case/control studies. Lancet 1981; 2(8237):66–68.

30. Suen KC, Lau LL, Yermakov V. Cancer and old age. An autopsy study of 3,535 patients over 65-years-old. Cancer 1974; 33(4):1164–1168.

31. Schottenfeld D. Epidemiology of endometrial neoplasia. J Cell Biochem 1995; 23Suppl:151–159.

32. Kvale G, Heuch I, Ursin G. Reproductive factors and risk of cancer of the uterine corpus: a prospective study. Cancer Res 1988; 48(21):6217–6221.

33. Rutqvist LE, Johansson H, Signomklao T, Johansson U, Fornander T, Wilking N. Adjuvant tamoxifen therapy for early stage breast cancer and second primary malignancies. Stockholm Breast Cancer Study Group. J Natl Cancer Inst 1995; 87(9):645–651.

34. Burke W, Petersen G, Lynch P, Botkin J, Daly M, Garber J, Kahn MJ, McTiernan A, Offit K, Thomson E, Varricchio C. Recommendations for follow-up care of individuals with an inherited predisposition to cancer. I. Hereditary nonpolyposis colon cancer. Cancer Genetics Studies Consortium. JAMA 1997; 277(11):915–919.

35. Gull B, Karlsson B, Milsom I, Granberg S. Can ultrasound replace dilation and curettage? A longitudinal evaluation of postmenopausal bleeding and transvaginal sonographic measurement of the endometrium as predictors of endometrial cancer. Am J Obstet Gynecol 2003; 188(2):401–408.

36. Gronroos M, Salmi TA, Vuento MH, Jalava EA, Tyrkko JE, Maatela JI, Aromaa AR, Siegberg R, Savolainen ER, Kauraniemi TV. Mass screening for endometrial cancer directed in risk groups of patients with diabetes and patients with hypertension. Cancer 1993; 71(4):1279–1282.

37. Nakagawa-Okamura C, Sato S, Tsuji I, Kuramoto H, Tsubono Y, Aoki D, Jobo T, Oomura M, Hisamichi S, Yajima A. Effectiveness of mass screening for endometrial cancer. Acta Cytol 2002; 46(46):277–283.

38. Miller AB, Chamberlain J, Day NE, Hakama M, Prorok PC. Report on a workshop of the UICC project on evaluation of screening for cancer. Int J Cancer 1990; 46(5):761–769.
39. Smith RA, Cokkinides V, Eyre HJ. American Cancer Society guidelines for the early detection of cancer, 2003. CA Cancer J Clin 2003; 53(1):27–43.
40. Runowicz CD. Gynecologic surveillance of women on tamoxifen: first do no harm. J Clin Oncol 2000; 18(20):3457–3458.

3

Pathology of Endometrial Hyperplasia and Neoplasia

Terry Rollason and Raji Ganesan

Department of Histopathology, Birmingham Women's Healthcare NHS Trust, Birmingham, U.K.

INTRODUCTION

Endometrial carcinoma is the fifth most common cancer in women world-wide—approximately 150,000 new cases are diagnosed each year (1). The incidence of endometrial carcinoma is higher in the developed world, with highest rates occurring in North America and Europe (the incidence in whites is twice as high as in blacks). In Japan and the developing countries, the rate is four to five times lower. Endometrial carcinoma of the more common endometrioid type is associated with a hormone-dependent precursor lesion—endometrial hyper-plasia. This is a condition resulting from unopposed estrogen stimulation. It has been demonstrated that, in postmenopausal women, high estrone and albumin-bound estradiol levels are associated with increased risk in comparison with similar levels in premenopausal women (2).

A strong relationship between hormone replacement therapy and endometrial carcinoma development has been noted (3,4). When the hormone replacement is with unopposed estrogen, the risk of carcinoma development is two to three times that of the general population. However, when combined with progestins this risk is nullified (5).

Protection against endometrial carcinomas is afforded by long-term oral contraceptive usage. In one large case control study, the use of oral contraceptives for a period of one year reduced risk by 50% and this effect persisted for up to 15 years (6).

The relationship between tamoxifen usage and endometrial cancer has generated a great deal of conflicting data. Some large studies show an increased risk with usage, which is dependent on dosage and duration of use (7,8). There is a lack of uniformity in the type of cancers reported with some reports indicating that such cancers are predominantly low-grade while others report a predominance of high-grade carcinomas (9).

Obesity is a well-recognized predisposing factor for endometrial carcinoma with a relative risk of 2–10 times (1). Although the increase in risk is partly due to increased availability of circulating estrogens due to aromatization of androgens by adipose tissue, the risk associated with obesity appears partly independent of the hormonal status (10).

Diabetes is associated with an elevated risk of endometrial carcinoma independent of other variables such as obesity (1,11). Other risk factors for endometrial carcinoma include hypertension, early menarche, late menopause, and nulliparity associated with anovulation. Certain dietary factors have also been linked to increase in risk but do not appear to be independent of obesity. It should be noted that the above comments on obesity and hormonal effects relate to endometrioid carcinoma and its variants.

Classification of Endometrial Carcinomas

Clear variations are seen between different types of endometrial carcinoma, making classification mandatory. The widely used World Health Organization (WHO) classification is based on the histological cell type and pattern (Table 1). The main criticism of the WHO classification is the usage of the term papillary in the description of serous carcinomas. A papillary pattern of growth is seen in serous carcinomas but is also seen in other carcinomas with better prognosis and the term papillary can send mixed signals to clinicians. The other inconsistency is the classification of malignant mesodermal mixed tumors (MMMT) under the umbrella of mixed epithelial and nonepithelial tumors. It has been shown by molecular genetic data that both components are better considered to be of epithelial origin and the treatment given is now usually similar to that for a high-grade carcinoma. Accordingly MMMTs are better classified as epithelial cancers with "sarcomatous metaplasia."

Conventionally, a second component of less than 10% in an endometrioid carcinoma does not alter its classification. But it is increasingly recognized that the presence of serous, clear cell, small cell, or undifferentiated carcinoma may affect prognosis even when present in modest proportions (certainly above 25%) and it is regarded as good practice to mention these components in the report, whatever be their relative amounts (12).

Type of cell

Table 1 WHO Classification of Epithelial Tumors and Related Lesions of the Uterine Corpus

---

Endometrial carcinoma
Endometrioid adenocarcinoma
   Secretory variant
   Villoglandular variant
   Ciliated cell variant
   Variant with squamous differentiation
Mucinous adenocarcinoma
Serous adenocarcinoma
   Clear cell adenocarcinoma
   Mixed cell adenocarcinoma
   Squamous cell carcinoma
   Transitional cell carcinoma
   Small cell carcinoma
   Undifferentiated carcinoma
Others
Endometrial hyperplasia
Non-atypical hyperplasia
Simple
Complex (adenomatous)
Atypical hyperplasia
Simple
Complex
Endometrial polyp
Tamoxifen-related lesions

Source: From Ref. 69.

Types 1 and 2 Carcinoma

Endometrial carcinomas are broadly categorized as types 1 and 2 carcinomas. Type 1 carcinoma occurs in younger perimenopausal women and is associated with unopposed estrogenic stimulation, coexistent and/or preceding endometrial hyperplasia, and the histology is typically low-grade, low-stage endometrioid carcinoma (13,14). The prototypic type 2 carcinoma is serous carcinoma. These cancers occur in older postmenopausal women and are not associated with estrogen stimulation, arising on a background atrophic endometrium.

The molecular pathology of type 1 (endometrioid carcinoma and variants) is different from that of type 2 (nonendometrioid carcinomas) (15). In the former, microsatellite instability as well as mutations of the PTEN, k-RAS, and β-catenin genes are seen. One of these changes—loss of normal PTEN—can be detected by lack of immunostaining in neoplastic glands. Type 2 carcinomas show alteration in the *p53* gene and loss of heterozygosity

(LOH) in several chromosomes. These presumed pathways are, however, not mutually exclusive of each other.

The existence of a third type of carcinoma, postmenopausal endometrioid carcinoma arising on a background of endometrial atrophy, has been put forward in the past but has not gained acceptance.

ENDOMETRIOID CARCINOMA

This is the most common form of endometrial carcinoma and accounts for about 75% of all cases. Endometrioid carcinoma, by definition, should not contain more than 10% of other histological types. These carcinomas commonly present with abnormal vaginal bleeding in postmenopausal women. They have uncommonly been noted in women under the age of 30 years (16). The presence of abnormal endometrial cells in cervical smears reveals some cases. The sensitivity and specificity of this technique is low and is not cost-effective in population screening (17).

The gross appearances of endometrioid carcinomas do not differ from most other types of endometrial carcinomas (Fig. 1). They present as exophytic, sometimes polypoid masses that bulge into and distend the endometrial cavity. The lesion may be focal, multifocal, or global. Associated myometrial invasion when present can be identified as firm gray-white areas in the muscle deep to the exophytic tumor. It is rare, particularly in atrophic

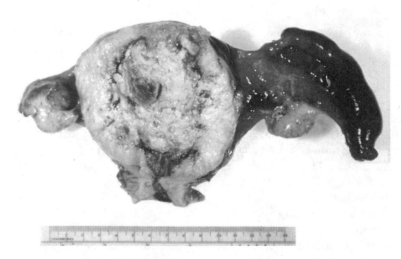

Figure 1 This is a macroscopic photograph of the uterus, tubes, and ovaries showing an enlarged globoid uterus. There is a mass filling the endometrial cavity and infiltrating through the wall of the uterus. At the fundus, the tumor extends through to the serosa.

uteri, that diffuse myometrial invasion may be grossly discernible. Although cervical involvement is noted in about a fifth of cases this may not be macroscopically detectable.

The tumors histologically resemble proliferative phase endometrium— hence their designation as endometrioid. They are characterized typically by tubular glands that are usually uniform in size but can show a wide variation. These glands are closely packed with little or no intervening stroma (Fig. 2). The stroma in myoinvasive tumors is often desmoplastic. Pseudostratified columnar cells with rounded nuclei and variably prominent nucleoli line the glands. The cytoplasm is usually pale or lightly esinophilic. Intracellular mucin is typically absent although minor foci of mucinous differentiation can be recognized in about 40% of tumors (18). Luminal mucin may, however, be prominent. Ciliated cells can be occasionally seen lining the neoplastic glands especially in well-differentiated endometrioid carcinomas (17). Focal squamous differentiation is found commonly in endometrioid carcinomas and can present as rounded luminal aggregates referred to as morules or as squamous pearls with keratinization (Fig. 3). Infiltrating nests of malignant-appearing squamous cells can be seen. Some workers put endometrioid tumors with focally malignant squamous elements as adenosquamous carcinomas and consider these more aggressive than pure endometrioid examples. Other patterns of squamous differentiation are plaque-like foci, groups of cells with vacuolization related to glycogen content, and individual cell keratinization. Sometimes whorls or

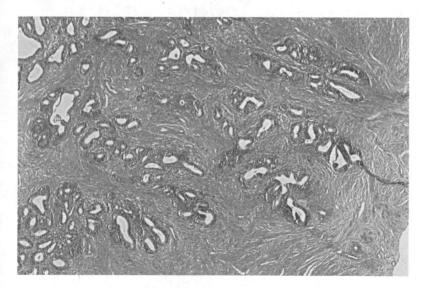

Figure 2 Well-differentiated myoinvasive endometrioid adenocarcinoma consisting of closely packed glands of varying shapes and sizes lined by pseudostratified atypical epithelium. No solid areas are seen.

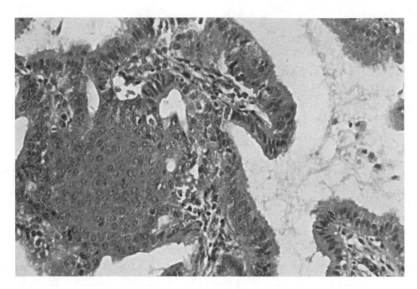

Figure 3 Well-differentiated endometrioid adenocarcinoma showing a focus of squamous differentiation.

eddies of spindled cells are present which may show features of immature squamous metaplasia or intercellular bridges.

Necrosis and foamy macrophages may be present within gland lumens. Stromal foamy histiocytes are found in about 15% of endometrioid carcinomas (19). Hyperplasia of the endometrium can be noted in the non-neoplastic endometrium.

Variants of Endometrioid Carcinoma

Secretory Carcinoma

This variant is characterized by the presence of glycogen vacuoles in a supranuclear and/or subnuclear location (in the majority of neoplastic cells) resembling early secretory endometrium. Focal areas with such appearance can be occasionally seen in otherwise typical endometrioid carcinomas but tumors classifiable as secretory carcinomas are quite rare. In these cases, the adjacent uninvolved endometrium often shows early secretory changes. The outcome is similar to other well-differentiated endometrioid carcinomas. It is important to differentiate this good prognosis variant from clear cell carcinoma which has high-grade nuclear features and a poorer prognosis.

Villoglandular Carcinoma

This variant of endometrioid carcinoma is characterized by long delicate papillae with a lining of pseudostratified cells showing no more than moderate nuclear atypia. The villous pattern is seen mainly in the superficial part of the tumor. A variable proportion of carcinoma of typical endometrioid glandular pattern is seen usually in the deeper part of the lesion. These tumors are usually not deeply invasive. Prognosis is similar to that of conventional endometrioid carcinoma. There is some evidence in the literature that this similarity may be confined to intraendometrial lesions. Myoinvasive villoglandular carcinomas possibly have a higher incidence of vascular invasion and lymph node involvement (20) than "usual" endometrioid myoinvasive tumors. Villoglandular carcinomas should be distinguished from other papillary tumors, especially from serous carcinomas. The primary papillae in the latter are broad and densely fibrotic. The cells in serous carcinoma are rounded, sometimes hobnailed and have highly atypical hyperchromatic nuclei.

Ciliated Carcinoma

In this variant, the neoplastic cells are ciliated, contradicting the common misconception that the presence of cilia in epithelial proliferations of the endometrium implies a benign lesion. A distinctive pattern of ciliated carcinoma with a cribriform appearance has been described (21). The behavior of this rare tumor is similar to endometrioid carcinomas of the usual type.

Endometrioid Carcinoma with Squamous Differentiation

The patterns of squamous differentiation in endometrioid carcinomas have already been described (see Fig. 3). These tumors were formerly divided into adenoacanthomas (where the squamous elements appear benign) and adenosquamous carcinomas (where the squamous elements are malignant), but recent evidence suggests that the outcome in these tumors is dependent on the grade of the non-squamous component of the tumor and the depth of myoinvasion rather than the appearance of the squamous component (22). Metastases from these cancers often contain both glandular and squamous components (23). It is not unusual to note squamous elements alone within vascular spaces.

Other Recently Described Variants

Endometrioid carcinomas with small non-villous papillae: This variant, described by Murray et al. (24), is important to recognize due to its potential to be confused with serous carcinomas. The variant is characterized by the presence of small papillae within the glandular spaces of otherwise typical endometrioid carcinomas. They are seen as buds of cells with ample pink cytoplasm and low-grade nuclear features. They lack vascular cores and typically show focal squamous differentiation. The pink cytoplasm noted in the papillae may be a feature of abortive squamous differentiation.

Endometrioid carcinomas with a microglandular pattern: Young and Scully have described a small series of endometrioid carcinomas with a microglandular pattern (25) occurring in postmenopausal women (Fig. 4).

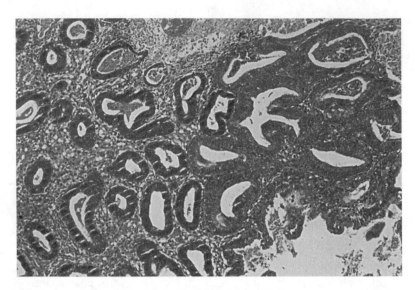

Figure 4 A focus of gland crowding with cellular atypia—constituting atypical hyperplasia—is seen (*right of photograph*) in a background of endometrial hyperplasia. The presence of necrosis and luminal debris raises the possibility that this lesion is already an established carcinoma.

The main importance in recognition of this entity is that they may be mistaken for cervical microglandular hyperplasia (MGH), which is a benign condition (26). This variant is noted to have a pattern of small coalescent glandular spaces lined by neoplastic cells. The resemblance to MGH is heightened by the presence of esinophilic luminal secretions and acute inflammatory cells. This pattern in the tumor is usually seen to merge with more conventional areas of endometrioid carcinoma.

   Sertoliform endometrioid carcinomas: Endometrioid carcinomas may show a focal or predominant pattern of short cords of cells with solid or hollow tubules resembling a Sertoli cell tumor of the ovary (27). The nuclei are generally bland. When focal, these areas merge with more conventional areas of endometrioid carcinomas. When diffuse, the possibility of uterine stromal sarcoma with sex cord elements and uterine tumor resembling ovarian sex cord tumor arises. Immunohistochemistry is helpful as Sertoliform carcinomas are positive for vimentin, cytokeratin, and epithelial membrane antigen, but not for actin, desmin, or CD10.

MUCINOUS CARCINOMA

Mucinous carcinoma, defined as a tumor showing more than 50% mucinous differentiation, is an uncommon form of endometrial carcinoma. The clinical

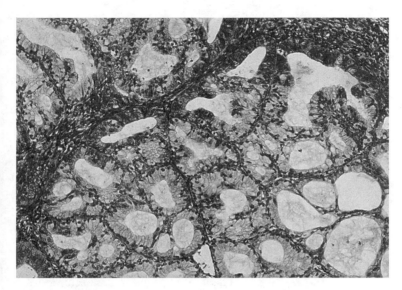

Figure 5 Mucinous carcinoma composed of closely packed glands. Most of the glands contain intracytoplasmic mucin and have an appearance reminiscent of endocervical epithelium. A few glands at the periphery have endometrioid morphology.

profile of patients with these tumors is similar to that of usual endometrioid carcinoma. On microscopy there are glands of varying sizes, often with many dilated glands, containing intraluminal mucin with acute inflammatory cells (Fig. 5). The lack of atypia may lead to misdiagnosis as a benign metaplastic process. The lining cells show nuclear stratification with usually modest nuclear atypia. Mucin is present intracellularly and can be better identified when special stains such as PAS-diastase are used. Hyperplasia and mucinous metaplasia are often seen in the non-neoplastic endometrium. The appearance of this tumor is similar to that of a primary endocervical carcinoma and it can be difficult to determine the site of origin of the cancer from curettings alone. Immunohistochemistry or mucin histochemistry is rarely helpful (28) and correlation with imaging and clinical findings is necessary. When adjusted for stage and grade, mucinous carcinomas of the endometrium behave in a fashion similar to endometrioid carcinomas of the same site.

SEROUS CARCINOMAS

These are carcinomas with a poor prognosis. Typically they arise in the atrophic uteri of postmenopausal women, i.e., in an older age group than women with endometrioid carcinomas. The tumors are not hormone-dependent.

On gross examination, unlike the uteri with endometrial carcinoma, these uteri appear small. The tumor may also be small and is usually exophytic with a fronded surface. Invasion tends not to be easily recognized macroscopically and, therefore, the depth invasion cannot always be assessed grossly. Microscopically, the tumors typically have a fine papillary pattern with hierarchical branching of papillae (Fig. 6). Detachment of cellular clusters at the tips of the papillae is seen. Psammoma bodies can be present. The cells have a hobnail appearance with the nucleus bulging into the luminal aspect beyond apparent cytoplasm. They show significant pleomorphism, clumped chromatin, prominent nucleoli, and a brisk mitotic activity. There may be nuclear pooling. This discordance of nuclear grade with architecture is distinctive of serous carcinomas.

Serous carcinoma of the endometrium is associated with frequent myometrial invasion, lymphovascular invasion, and peritoneal implantation (29,30). Even very small tumors, apparently confined to polyps, may have a poor prognosis. In a study from Norway, 5- and 10-year survival rates for serous carcinomas of the uterus were 36% and 18%, respectively (31). Even for stage I carcinomas, the five-year survival figures reported in literature have been as low as 40% (32). Similar results for survival have been reported even when the serous component is as low as 25% in a mixed tumor (29). This underscores the importance of recognition of even small foci of this histological type of carcinoma.

Atypical cells identical to those constituting the serous carcinoma can line the endometrium surface and glands adjacent to the invasive serous

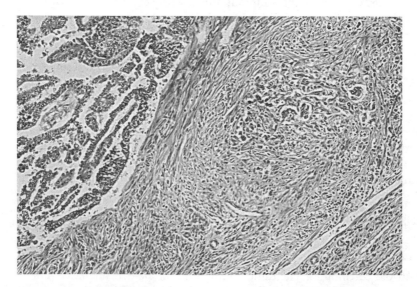

Figure 6 Serous adenocarcinoma is seen invading the myometrium. The invasive malignancy is less differentiated than the luminal component of the tumor.

carcinomas and at other foci away from the tumor. These cells can sometimes form micropapillary processes (33). This is termed endometrial intraepithelial carcinoma (EIC). Sometimes the glands lined by the highly atypical cells are confluent or have an infiltrative pattern with a desmoplastic stromal reaction but no definite myometrial or vascular invasion. These tumors are sometimes referred to as superficial serous carcinomas. The distinction between EIC and this lesion can be difficult and subjective, but they behave in a similar fashion when they are confirmed on full surgical staging as stage IA tumors and, therefore, it has been proposed that EIC and serous carcinomas measuring less than 1 cm in maximum dimension are referred to as minimal uterine serous carcinomas (34). It must be stressed that perhaps 40% of serous carcinomas are understaged. Perhaps 13% of serous carcinoma confined to the endometrium will have para-aortic nodal metastases and meticulous staging is imperative.

CLEAR CELL CARCINOMA

Most studies show that clear cell carcinomas occur in women with a similar clinical profile to that of serous carcinoma. There are no distinctive gross features. Microscopically, the tumor is characterized by clear cells, hobnail cells, or both (Fig. 7). These cells may be arranged in solid, acinar, or papillary patterns. The papillae in clear cell carcinomas generally have hyaline cores (Fig. 8). Extracellular hyaline globules are common. Nuclear atypia

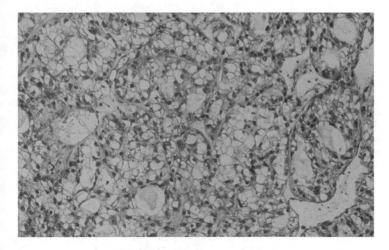

Figure 7 Clear cell adenocarcinoma composed of glands of varying sizes interspersed with solid areas. The constituent epithelium has clear cytoplasm with pleomorphic, hyperchromatic nuclei.

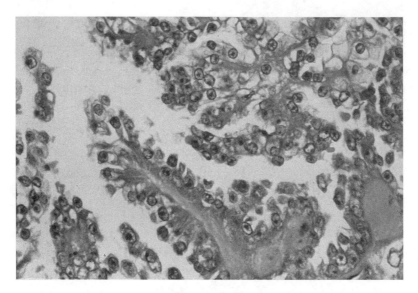

Figure 8 Clear cell carcinoma showing papillae with hyaline cores lined by pleomorphic cells. Some of the hyperchromatic nuclei are protruding leading to a "hobnailed" appearance. At the tips of the papillae the pleomorphic cells typically fall away from the stromal cores.

is generally striking. Mitotic index is high and abnormal mitotic forms are readily found.

Clear cell carcinomas have a similar poor prognosis to serous carcinomas (35). They may, however, be less likely to implant on peritoneal surfaces. Histological differential diagnosis of clear cell carcinoma includes yolk sac tumor and mesonephric carcinoma. Unlike clear cell carcinomas, yolk sac tumors are more common in young women, contain characteristic Schiller–Duval bodies, and express α-fetoprotein in blood and tissue. Mesonephric carcinomas usually arise in the cervix, occur in a younger age group, and have relatively bland cytological features. They are positive with CD10 and calretinin on immunohistochemistry.

MIXED CARCINOMAS

By convention, a mixed carcinoma is a tumor that has a minor component or components occupying more than 10% of the entire lesion. Except for carcinomas with a serous component of 25% or greater, where prognosis is known to be adversely affected (29), there are no studies in the literature to address the clinical relevance of this category. It is possible that, except for serous, clear cell, and undifferentiated components, the presence of different types of tumor does not have any clinical impact.

UNDIFFERENTIATED CARCINOMA

These are tumors that do not show glandular or squamous differentiation and are generally present as solid groups of large or small cells. The latter may be positive with neuroendocrine markers. Usually undifferentiated carcinomas are cytokeratin positive. The cells in some cases may also show positivity with neuroendocrine markers. Small cell carcinomas with neuroendocrine expression tend to behave aggressively (36). Primitive neuroectodermal tumors (PNETs) of the uterine corpus have also been reported (37). Histological, immunohisto-chemical, and in some cases ultrastructural examination revealed typical PNETs that exhibited variable degrees of neural, glial, ependymal, and medulloepithelial differentiation. In the small number of cases reported, the outcome appeared to be stage dependent.

OTHER RARE TYPES OF ENDOMETRIAL CARCINOMA

These include squamous cell carcinomas, glassy cell carcinomas, giant cell carcinomas, choriocarcinomas, transitional cell carcinomas, and signet ring carcinomas (38). In general, their prognosis is poor especially for squamous carcinomas and tumors with a choriocarcinomatous component.

TUMORS METASTATIC TO THE ENDOMETRIUM

Breast cancer, especially lobular carcinoma of the breast, is the most common metastasis from an extragenital site. Other cancers include gastric adenocarcinoma, melanoma, lung carcinoma, colonic carcinoma, and pancreatic carcinoma.

Ovarian carcinoma may precede or coexist with endometrial carcinoma and the question of synchronicity, metachronicity, or metastasis is often raised. This is a difficult question to answer. It has been suggested that when the two tumors are endometrioid in type and the endometrial tumor is noninvasive, then it is likely that these are synchronous primary tumors (39). On the other hand, if both ovaries are involved and show vascular invasion or fallopian tube involvement with an endometrial tumor with deep myometrial invasion, the ovarian lesion is metastatic (40). Association with endometriosis is also suggestive of independent primary carcinomas. Various molecular methods have been used to attempt to differentiate simultaneously noted primary carcinomas from metastases. Methods used include LOH, gene mutation studies, and clonal X-inactivation analysis (41). In the study of Fujii and others, 35% of synchronous tumors were monoclonal and 47% were polyclonal. They also concluded that molecular genetic studies correlate favorably with histopathological observations.

Pathologic Prognostic Factors for Endometrial Carcinomas

Stage

Stage of the disease is the most important prognostic factor within individual tumor types.

Almost three-quarters of all endometrial carcinomas are stage I and these tend to be endometrioid in type. Although treatment and outcome is stage dependent, the importance of grade and type must be stressed.

Grade

Grading of endometrial carcinomas is mostly applicable to endometrioid carcinomas and its variants, mucinous, and some other rare tumors. Serous and clear cell carcinomas are inherently high-grade irrespective of architecture or nuclear features as are undifferentiated carcinomas, which clearly cannot be graded. The architectural grade of the tumor is determined by the extent to which recognizable glands compose the tumor in comparison with solid areas. The three-tiered grading system is depicted in Table 2.

Tumors tend to have heterogeneity of appearance and the architectural grade is based on the overall histology of the tumor.

The most recent revision of the International Federation of Gynecology and Obstetrics (FIGO) (Table 3) guidelines recommends the grading of the tumor by both architectural and nuclear grades. Architectural grade 1 or 2 tumors should under this protocol have their grade increased by one grade if there is "notable" or "excessive" nuclear atypia. Others suggest upgrading only if the tumors have grade 3 nuclear features. These are defined as marked nuclear pleomorphism, coarse chromatin, and prominent nucleoli. Although the grading of nuclear features is subjective and prone to interobserver variation, significant discordance between nuclear and architectural grades is not usually a feature of endometrioid carcinomas and when present should raise the suspicion of a serous carcinoma. A number of alternative grading systems have been proposed with purported lower interobserver variation and significant correlation to outcome (42,43).

It has been shown that the FIGO grade on hysterectomy specimens can differ from the grade of the tumor on biopsy and this is irrespective of sampler type, time lapse between procedures, reporting pathologist, and patient age (44).

Table 2 Architectural Grading of Endometrial Carcinomas

Grade 1: 5% or less solid areas
Grade 2: 6–50% solid areas
Grade 3: more than 50% solid areas

Table 3 FIGO Staging of Cancer of the Uterine Corpus

Stage 1: tumor confined to corpus
  a. Intraendometrial
  b. <50% myometrial invasion
  c. >50% myometrial invasion
Stage IIa: tumor extending to cervix involving only glands
Stage IIb: tumor involving cervical stroma
Stage IIIa: Vaginal metastases
Stage IIIb: metastases to pelvic/para-aortic lymph nodes
Stage IVa: invasion of bladder and/or bowel mucosa
Stage IVb: distant metastases including intra-abdominal and/or inguinal lymph nodes

---

Histological Type

This has been extensively highlighted in the previous section.

Myometrial Invasion

This is an important component of FIGO staging and is reported as the proportion of the uterine wall invaded by tumor (inner or outer half). Due to variation in the thickness of the myometrial wall it is best also to indicate in reports the depth of invasion (in millimeters) and the full thickness of the muscle wall (in millimeters) at that site, i.e., indicating the tumor-free distance from the serosa. The distance from the uterine serosa has been noted in studies to be the most useful in correlation with survival (45). Tumors in vascular spaces beyond the deepest point of invasion have not used in-depth measurement by some workers, but the position remains unclear and vessel invasion is known to carry prognostic importance.

The patterns of myoinvasion include an expansile pattern with a pushing margin and single glands infiltrating the myometrium. The glands do not elicit a stromal response and this is referred to as a diffusely infiltrating pattern. There has been some conflicting data in the literature with regard to outcome in cases showing diffuse infiltration. Some studies show a poorer prognosis (46,47) in this group while others show no relation to prognosis (48).

Depth of myometrial invasion is probably the single most important predictor of outcome in early stage endometrial carcinoma (49). In a gynecologic oncology group (GOG) study, recurrence of the tumor was seen twice as often with deep invasion as with no myometrial invasion in endometrioid carcinomas. When grade was not corrected it was noted that only 1% of patients with no myometrial invasion recurred against 7.7% with inner third invasion and 15% recurrence with invasion of the outer third of the myometrium (50). Lymph node metastasis is also more common with deep muscle invasion (49).

Cervical Involvement

Tumors with cervical involvement have an increased risk of relapse in the absence of extrauterine disease. However, this has not been shown to be a definite independent risk factor and is related to higher grade, depth of myometrial invasion, and tumor volume (49).

Peritoneal Cytology

The literature is conflicting with regard to whether positive peritoneal cytology has a relation to prognosis in endometrial carcinomas. In one large study of 567 patients with stages I and II of the disease (51), only 7% of patients with negative cytology recurred while 32% of patients with malignant cells in the peritoneal washings recurred.

Lymph Node Metastases

Presence of metastatic tumor in aortic lymph nodes is important in predicting prognosis (49). The five-year tumor-free survival in node-negative patients is more than twice that of node-positive patients. The presence of metastatic carcinoma in pelvic lymph nodes is predictive of para-aortic nodal disease.

Concepts in Early Endometrial Neoplasia

Endometrial Hyperplasia

The WHO classifies hyperplasia into four types: simple hyperplasia, with and without atypia, and complex hyperplasia, with and without atypia, but a simplified system of simple, complex, and atypical hyperplasia is in use. Simple hyperplasia is generally diffuse, but complex and atypical hyperplasias are typically focal and associated with cytological atypia. Whereas outcome data for cases of hyperplasia show wide variation, in general it is accepted that rates of progression to carcinoma for simple hyperplasia are very low (a figure of 1% is often quoted) but for complex hyperplasia without cellular atypia the rates vary from 2–27% (the lower figure is probably more accurate) and 25–82% for atypical hyperplasia (after excluding those cases that already have carcinoma the lower figure is again probably the more accurate). Hysterectomy findings in women diagnosed with atypical hyperplasia in curettings have shown that in about 15–50% of the cases, an endometrial carcinoma is already present in the uterus (52,53). More alarmingly, in one study, 43% of the carcinomas detected were found to be stage Ic or higher (54).

Distinction of atypical hyperplasia from well-differentiated carcinoma: A fairly common problem is one of differentiating atypical hyperplasia from grade I endometrioid carcinoma in diagnostic samples. The criteria proposed by Hendrickson et al. (55) include a complex or cribriform glandular pattern, a bizarre glandular outline, intraglandular bridging, nuclear abnormalities, and mitotic activity. Kurman and Norris (56) have proposed a stricter set of criteria that include stromal desmoplastic change, gland confluence, and an extensive papillary pattern, which must occupy at least half of a low power field. Essentially these are criteria predictive of myoinvasive carcinoma rather than atypical hyperplasia/intraendometrial carcinoma. Despite these observations and recommendations, the problem persists and sometimes the only recourse available to the reporting pathologist may be to comment that a well-differentiated carcinoma cannot be excluded.

Endometrial Intraepithelial Neoplasia

This concept was put forward some years ago by Fox and Buckley (54). It has recently been put on a firmer footing by Mutter et al., who used cytoplasmic and nuclear pattern assessments, together with degrees of gland complexity assessments semi-quantitatively, to identify a group of lesions with a presumed increased risk of progression to carcinoma (57,58). This semi-objective method has been suggested to reduce the interobserver variation in diagnosis of atypia in hyperplasia of the endometrium. It is loosely based on the morphometric studies of Baak et al. (59). Their studies show excellent reproducibility and accuracy for simple morphometric scoring (the D-score) in endometrial hyperplasia.

Endometrial Intraepithelial Carcinoma

This is the putative precursor lesion of carcinomas not related to estrogenic stimulation. The prototypic carcinoma in this category is serous carcinoma. EIC is characterized by markedly atypical nuclei lining the surface of atrophic endometrium. The surface may have a papillary outline and the cells have hyperchromatic nuclei with vesicular chromatin and mitotic activity. On immunohistochemistry, these atypical cells are positive for *p53* (60). EIC has a propensity to be associated with established serous carcinoma. Up to 90% of cases with EIC show serous carcinoma elsewhere in the uterus. Two recent limited studies (61,62) have shown that when the EIC was associated with extrauterine disease, all patients were either dead or alive with disease at 27 months from diagnosis. Therefore, if EIC is found it should prompt a meticulous examination of the uterus and complete staging procedure.

Important Issues in Interpretation of Endometrial Biopsies

Benign disorders that mimic carcinoma   *Artifacts.*   Tissue artifacts related to the process of curetting or pipelle biopsy can result in appearances that can mimic hyperplasia or carcinoma. Isolated strips of surface epithelium, especially from atrophic endometria, can be mistaken for the surface aspect of a villoglandular carcinoma. The focal preserved dense atrophic stroma when present and bland monolayer of inactive epithelium are clues to the benign nature of the lesion. Sometimes curettage-related compaction of proliferative glands could be confused with hyperplasia. Stromal breakdown at menstruation, sometimes with syncytial metaplasia of surface epithelium, and the occasional presence of menstrual endometrium in vessels can be mistaken for carcinoma. Fragmentation-related artifacts also occur in curettings containing adenocarcinoma. Here the high-grade epithelial changes are not associated with menstrual-type stromal breakdown.

Endometrial metaplasias. The normal endometrium can show a wide variety of metaplastic changes (63). These metaplasias can also occur in neoplastic endometrium. The most frequent form of metaplasia is squamous metaplasia. It is important to be aware that cytologically and behaviorally benign squamous epithelium can show central necrosis and this should not be mistaken for tumor necrosis. The second common metaplastic change is esinophilic metaplasia, characterized by a transformation of the glandular lining epithelium into large cells with abundant cytoplasm with round nonstratified nuclei. Whenever one encounters metaplastic change in the endometrium, the architecture of the glandular component and other cytological features should be evaluated. Apparently, bland mucinous epithelium from the endometrium must always be treated with caution and well-differentiated mucinous carcinoma must be excluded as such tumors may show minimal atypia.

Pregnancy-related changes. Hobnail and clear cell change in pregnancy or progestogen-altered endometrium is a component of the Arias Stella reaction. Focal nuclear pleomorphism is also seen. These changes can be mistaken for clear cell carcinoma. In Arias Stella reaction, in addition to clinical evidence of pregnancy, the nuclear pleomorphism is random, the nuclei are "smudgy," and the underlying glandular architecture, although often complex, is not irregularly crowded.

Atypical polypoid adenomyoma. Atypical polypoid adenomyoma (APA) is a rare entity that usually affects premenopausal patients (64). These tumors are commonly exophytic and occur as polypoid lesions typically in the lower uterine corpus. On histology, crowded endometrial glands, most of which show squamous metaplasia, are seen intermingling with a smooth muscle stroma. The stromal cells may be atypical and mitotically active. Unfamiliarity with this entity can easily cause a misdiagnosis of myoinvasive adenocarcinoma. No tumor-related deaths have been noted, but about half the patients treated conservatively had recurrences (65).

The correct diagnosis rests on the recognition of the absence of overtly malignant features in the glands as well as the lack of organization of the muscle element in comparison with myometrium.

Therapy-related changes. Radiation-induced atypia can result in nuclear pleomorphism that can be mistaken for carcinoma. The appearances indicative of benignancy are the absence of architectural abnormality, random arrangement of smudgy atypical nuclei, lack of mitotic activity, and presence of radiation changes in the stroma and vessels.

Progestogens can reduce or completely mask cellular atypia in endometrial carcinomas. Squamous metaplasia can be striking and stromal pseudodecidualization is usually seen. These latter features in association with architectural abnormality must arouse suspicion.

REFERENCES

1. Parazzini F, Franceschi S, La Vecchia C, Chatenoud L, Di Cintio E. The epidemiology of female genital tract cancers. Int J Gynecol Cancer 1997; 7: 169–181.
2. Potischman N, Hoover RN, Brinton LA, Siiteri P, Dorgan JF, Swanson CA, et al. Case-control study of endogenous steroid hormones and endometrial cancer. J Natl Cancer Inst 1996; 88:1127–1135.
3. McDonald TW, Annegers JF, O'Fallon WM, Dockerty MB, Malkasian GDJ, Kurland LT. Exogenous estrogen and endometrial carcinoma: case-control and incidence study. Am J Obstet Gynecol 1977; 127:572–580.
4. Shapiro S, Kaufman DW, Slone D, Rosenberg L, Miettinen OS, Stolley PD, et al. Recent and past use of conjugated estrogens in relation to adenocarcinoma of the endometrium. N Engl J Med 1980; 303:485–489.
5. Persson I, Adami HO, Bergkvist L, Lindgren A, Petersson B, Hoover R. Risk of endometrial cancer after treatment with estrogens alone or in conjunction with progestogens: results of a prospective study. Br Med J 1989; 298:147–151.
6. Anonymous. Combination oral contraceptive use and the risk of endometrial cancer. The Cancer and Steroid Hormone Study of the Centers for Disease Control and the National Institute of Child Health and Human Development. JAMA 1987; 257:796–800.
7. Rutqvist LE, Johansson H, Signomklao T, Johansson U, Fornander T, Wilking N. Adjuvant tamoxifen therapy for early stage breast cancer and second primary malignancies. Stockholm Breast Cancer Study Group. J Natl Cancer Inst 1995; 87:645–651.
8. van Leeuwen FE, Benraadt J, Coebergh JW, et al. Risk of endometrial cancer after tamoxifen treatment of breast cancer. Lancet 1994; 343:448–452.
9. Silva EG, Jenkins R. Serous carcinoma in endometrial polyps. Mod Pathol 1990; 3:120–128.
10. Enriori CL, Reforzo-Membrives J. Peripheral aromatization as a risk factor for breast and endometrial cancer in postmenopausal women: a review. Gynecol Oncol 1984; 17:1–21.
11. Parazzini F, La Vecchia C, Bocciolone L, Franceschi S. The epidermiology of endometrial cancer. Gynecol Oncol 1991; 41:1–16.
12. Clement PB, Young RH. Endometrioid carcinoma of the uterine corpus: a review of its pathology with emphasis on recent advances and problematic aspects. Adv Anat Pathol 2002; 9(3):145–184.
13. Bokhman JV. Two pathogenetic types of endometrial carcinomas. Gynecol Oncol 1983; 15:10–17.
14. Sherman ME, Sturgeon S, Brinton LA, et al. Risk factors and hormone levels in patients with serous and endometrioid uterine carcinomas. Mod Pathol 1997; 10:963–968.
15. Matias-Guiu X, Catasus L, Bussaglia E, et al. Molecular pathology of endometrial hyperplasia and carcinoma. Hum Pathol 2001; 32(6):569–577.
16. Fujiwara H, Tortolero-Luna G, Mitchell MF, Koulos JP, Wright TCJ. Adenocarcinoma of the cervix. Expression and clinical significance of estrogen and progesterone receptors. Cancer (Phila) 1997; 79:505–512.

17. Mitchell H, Giles G, Medley G. Accuracy and survival benefit of cytological prediction of endometrial carcinoma on routine cervical smears. Int J Gynecol Pathol 1993; 12:34–40.
18. Ross JC, Eifel PJ, Cox RS. Primary mucinous adenocarcinoma of the endometrium. A clinicopathologic and histochemical study. Am J Surg Pathol 1983; 7:715–729.
19. Haibach H, Oxenhandler RW, Luger AM. Ciliated adenocarcinoma of the endometrium. Acta Obstet Gynecol Scand 1985; 64:457–462.
20. Ambros RA, Ballouk F, Malfetano JH, et al. Significance of papillary (villoglandular) differentiation in endometrioid carcinoma of the uterus. Am J Surg Pathol 1994; 18:569–575.
21. Hendrickson MR, Kempson RL. Ciliated carcinoma—a variant of endometrial adenocarcinoma: a report of 10 cases. Int J Gynecol Pathol 1983; 2:1–12.
22. Zaino RJ, Kurman RJ. Squamous differentiation in carcinoma of the endometrium: a critical appraisal of adenocanthoma and endosquamous carcinoma. Semin Diagn Pathol 1988; 5:154–171.
23. Ng AB, Reagan JW, Storaasli JP, Wentz WB. Mixed adenosquamous carcinoma of the endometrium. Am J Clin Pathol 1973; 59:765–781.
24. Murray SK, Young RH, Scully RE. Uterine endometrioid carcinoma with small nonvillous papillae: an analysis of 26 cases of a favorable-prognosis tumor to be distinguished from serous carcinoma. Int J Surg Pathol 2000; 8: 279–289.
25. Young RH, Scully RE. Uterine carcinomas simulating microglandular hyperplasia: a report of six cases. Am J Surg Pathol 1992; 16:1092–1097.
26. Leslie KO, Silverberg SG. Microglandular hyperplasia of the cervix: unusual clinical and pathologic presentations and their differential diagnosis. Prog Surg Pathol 1984; 5:95–114.
27. Eichhorn JH, Young RH, Clement PB. Sertoliform endometrial adenocarcinoma: a study of four cases. Int J Gynecol Pathol 1996; 15:9–26.
28. Ross JC, Eifel PJ, Cox RS, Kempson RL, Hendrickson MR. Primary mucinous adenocarcinoma of the endometrium. A clinicopathologic and histochemical study. Am J Surg Pathol 1983; 7:715–729.
29. Sherman ME, Bitterman P, Rosenshein NB, Delgado G, Kurman RJ. Uterine serous caricnoma. A morphologically diverse neoplasm with unifying clinicopathologic features. Am J Surg Pathol 1992; 16:600–610.
30. Wheeler DT, Bell KA, Kurman RJ, Sherman ME. Minimal uterine serous carcinoma: diagnosis and clinicopathologic correlation. Am J Surg Pathol 2000; 24:797–806.
31. Abeler VM, Kjorstad KE. Serous papillary carcinoma of the endometrium: a histopathological study of 22 cases. Gynecol Oncol 1990; 39:266–271.
32. Carcangiu ML, Chamers JT. Uterine papillary serous carcinoma: a study on 108 cases with emphasis on the prognostic significance of associated endometrioid carcinoma, absence of invasion, and concomitant ovarian carcinoma. Gynecol Oncol 1992; 47:298–305.
33. Ambros RA, Sherman ME, Zahn CM, Bitterman P, Kurman RJ. (1995) Endometrial intraepithelial carcinoma: a distinctive lesion specifically associated with tumors displaying serous differentiation. Hum Pathol 1992; 26:1260–1267.

34. Sherman ME, Bur ME, Kurman RJ. p53 in endometrial cancer and its putative precursors: evidence for diverse pathways of tumorigenesis. Hum Pathol 1995; 26:1268–1274.
35. Sakuragi N, Hareyama H, Todo Y, et al. Prognostic significance of serous and clear cell adenocarcinoma in surgically staged endometrial carcinoma. Acta Obstet Gynecol Scand 2000; 79:311–316.
36. Huntsman DG, Clement PB, Gilks CB, Scully RE. Small-cell carcinoma of the endometrium. A clinicopathological study of sixteen cases. Am J Surg Pathol 1994; 18:364–375.
37. Ng SB, Sirrampalam K, Chuah KL. Pimitive neuroectodermal tumors of the uterus: a ase report with cytological correlation and review of the literature. Pathology 2002; 34(5):455–461.
38. Ronnett BM, Zaino RJ, Ellenson LH, Kurman RJ. Endometrial Carcinoma in Blaustein's Pathology of the Female Genital Tract. 5th ed. Springer: Berlin, 2002.
39. Eifel P, Hendrickson M, Ross J, Ballon S, Martinez A, Kempson R. Simultaneous presentation of carcinoma involving the ovary and the uterine corpus. Cancer (Phila) 1982; 50:163–170.
40. Ulbright TM, Roth LM. Metastatic and independent cancers of the endometrium and ovary: a clinicopathologic study of 34 cases. Hum Pathol 1985; 16:28–34.
41. Fujii H, Matsumoto T, Yoshida M, et al. Genetics of synchronous uterine and ovarian endometrioid carcinoma: combined analyses of loss of heterozygosity, PTEN mutation, and microsatellite instability. Hum Pathol 2002; 33(4):421–428.
42. Takeshima N, Hirai Y, Hasumi K. Prognostic validity of neoplastic cells with notable nuclear atypia in endometrial cancer. Obstet Gynecol 1998; 92:119–123.
43. Lax SF, Kurman RJ, Pizer ES, et al. A binary architectural grading system for uterine endometrial endometrioid carcinoma has superior reproducibility compared with FIGO grading and identifies subsets of advance-stage tumors with favorable and unfavorable prognosis. Am J Surg Pathol 2000; 24:1201–1208.
44. Mitchard J, Hirschowitz L. Concordance of FIGO grade of endometrial adenocarcinomas in biopsy and hysterectomy specimen. Histopathology 2003; 42(4): 372–378.
45. Kaku T, Tsuruchi N, Tsukamoto N, Hirakawa T, Kamura T, Nakano H. Reassessment of myometrial invasion in endometrial carcinoma. Obstet Gynecol 1994; 84(6):979–982.
46. Mittal KR, Barwick KW. Diffusely infiltrating adenocarcinoma of the endometrium: a subtype with a poor prognosis. Am J Surg Pathol 1988; 12:754–758.
47. Lee KR, Vacek PM, Belinson JL. Traditional and nontraditional histopathologic predictors of recurrence in uterine endometrioid adenocarcinoma. Gynecol Oncol 1994; 54:10–18.
48. Longacre TA, Hendrickson MR. Diffusely infiltrative endometrial adenocarcinoma. An adenoma malignum pattern of myoinvasion. Am J Surg Pathol 1999; 23:69–78.
49. Morrow CP, Bundy BN, Kurman RJ, et al. Relationship between surgical-pathological risk factors and outcome in clinical stage I and II carcinoma of the endometrium: a Gynecologic Oncologyogy Group study. Gynecol Oncol 1991; 40:55–65.
50. Morrow CP, Bundy BN, Kurman RJ, Creasman WT, Heller P, Homesley HD. Relationship between surgical-pathological risk factors and outcome in clinical

stage I and II carcinoma of the endometrium: a Gynaecologic Oncology Group study. Gynaecol Oncol 1991; 40:55–65.

51. Turner DA, Gershenson DM, Atkinson N, Sneige N, Wharton AT. (1989) The prognostic significance of peritoneal cytology for stage I endometrial cancer. Obstet Gynecol 1991; 74:775–780.

52. Kurman RJ, Kaminski PF, Norris HJ. The behaviour of endometrial hyperplasia. A long-term study of "untreated" hyperplasia in 170 patients. Cancer 1985; 56:403–412.

53. Widra EA, Dunton CJ, McHugh M, Palazzo JP. Endometrial hyperplasia and risk of carcinoma. Int J Gynaecol Cancer 1995; 5:233–235.

54. Fox H, Buckley CH. The endometrial hyperplasias and their relationship to endometrial neoplasia. Histopathology 1982; 6(5):493–510.

55. Hendrickson MR, Ross J, Kempson RL. Toward the development of morphologic criteria for well-differentiated adenocarcinoma of the endometrium. Am J Surg Pathol 1983; 7:819–838.

56. Kurman RJ, Norris HJ. Evaluation of criteria for distinguishing atypical endometrial hyperplasia from well-differentiated carcinoma. Cancer 1982; 49:2547–2559.

57. Mutter GL. The Endoemtrial Collaborative Group. Endometrial intraepithelial neoplasia (EIN): will it bring order to chaos. Gynecol Oncol 2000; 76:287–290.

58. Mutter GL, Baak JPA, Crum CP, Richart RM, Ferenczy A, Faquin WC. Endometrial precancer diagnosis by histopathology, clonal analysis and computerised morphometry. J Pathol 2000; 190:462–469.

59. Baak JP, Orbo A, van Diest PJ, et al. Prospective multicenter evaluation of the morphometric *D*-score for prediction of the outcome of endometrial hyperplasias. Am J Surg Pathol 2001; 25(7):930–935.

60. Wheeler DT, Bell KA, Kurman RJ, Sherman ME. Minimal uterine serous carcinoma. Diagnosis and clinicopathologic correlation. Am J Surg Pathol 2000; 24:726–732.

61. Soslow RA, Pirog E, Isaacson C. Endometrial intraepithelial carcinoma with associated peritoneal carcinomatosis. Am J Surg Pathol 2000; 24:726–732.

62. Hendrickson MR, Kempson RL. Endometrial epithelial metaplasia: proliferations frequently misdiagnosed as adenocarcinoma. Report of 89 cases and proposed classification. Am J Surg Pathol 1980; 4:525–542.

63. Mazur MT. Atypical polypoid adenomyomas of the endometrium. Am J Surg Pathol 1982; 5:473–482.

64. Longacre TA, Chung MH, Rouse RV, Hendrickson MR. Atypical polypoid adenomyofibromas (atypical polypoid adenomyoma) of the uterus. A clinicopathologic study of 55 cases. Am J Surg Pathol 1996; 20:1–20.

65. Silver SA, Sherman ME. Morphologic and immunophenotypic characterization of foam cells in endometrial lesions. Int J Gynecol Pathol 1998; 17:140–145.

66. Announcements. FIGO stages—1988 revision. Gynecol Oncol 1989; 35:125–127.

67. Zaino RJ, Kurman RJ, Diana KL, et al. The unity of the revised International Federation of Gynecology and Obstetrics histologic grading of endometrial adenocarcinoma using a defined nuclear grading system. A Gynecology Oncology Group study. Cancer 1995; 75:81–86.

68. Kuman RJ, Kaminski PF, Norris HJ. The behaviour of "untreated" hyperplasia in 170 patients. Cancer 1985; 56:403–412.

69. Tavassoli Devilee. Pathology and genetics of tumors of the breast and female genital organs. WHO Classification of Tumors 2003.

4

Pathology of Uterine Sarcoma

Nafisa Wilkinson

Department of Histopathology, St. James University Hospital, Leeds, U.K.

INTRODUCTION

Uterine sarcomas are either pure sarcomas derived from mesenchymal elements (endometrial stromal cells or smooth muscle cells) or mixed tumors composed of epithelial and mesenchymal elements. In malignant mixed tumors, both components are usually malignant (carcinosarcoma). They have historically been thought of and treated as uterine sarcomas, but presently the view is that they are metaplastic carcinomas in the majority of cases. Rare sarcomas comprise heterologous sarcomas; in these the sarcomatous element is one that is usually associated with an organ other than the uterus such as rhabdomyosarcomas.

The main problem in the diagnosis of leimoyomasarcomas occurs in those rare instances where leiomyosarcoma variants morphologically mimic features that overlap with those of leiomyosarcoma. In these cases, it can be very difficult to make the diagnosis of malignancy. These diagnostic dilemmas can usually be resolved by thorough sampling of the main tumor, paying particular attention to the periphery of the tumor, where its relationship with the adjacent myometrium can be assessed. An irregular margin with features of myometrial infiltration may become obvious and the tumor may be observed in lymphovascular spaces.

The other problematic area is that of the diagnosis of an endometrial stromal lesion and its distinction from a cellular smooth muscle neoplasm. While most of these cases can be distinguished in hysterectomy specimens, they can be rather difficult or impossible to distinguish in curettage material. Interpretation can become even more difficult if the patient is taking gonado-tropin-releasing hormone (GnRH) agonist preparations and there is shrink-age of the cytoplasm in cellular smooth muscle lesions.

STAGING OF UTERINE SARCOMAS

The modified Internation Federation of Gynecology and Obstetrics (FIGO) staging for endometrial carcinoma is used as given below, but there is no specific staging system for sarcomas (1).

> *Stage I*: Sarcoma confined to the uterine corpus
> *Stage II*: Sarcoma confined to the uterine corpus and cervix
> *Stage III*: Sarcoma confined to the pelvis
> *Stage IV*: Extrapelvic sarcoma

ENDOMETRIAL STROMAL SARCOMA

This neoplasm accounts for 10–15% of malignant mesenchymal tumors of the uterus, being much rarer than smooth muscle neoplasms (2–5). The cells of endometrial stromal neoplasms mimic the architecture and cytology of the stromal cells of proliferative-phase endometrium. They are characterized by cells with little cytoplasm and round to oval nuclei. The vascular pattern is characteristic in typical cases comprising a network of small vessels resembling spiral arterioles seen in the proliferative-phase stroma of normal endometrium.

High-Grade Stromal Sarcoma and the Controversies in Classification

Endometrial stromal neoplasms were classified by Norris and Taylor in 1966 (6) into endometrial stromal nodule and endometrial stromal sarcoma. The stromal sarcomas were further divided into two categories based solely on their mitotic index. A low-grade group comprising tumors exhibiting less that 10 mitotic figures (MF)/10 high-power field (HPF) and a high-grade group comprising tumors exhibiting more than 10 MF/10 HPF.

These diagnostic criteria were used for some three decades. Using the Norris and Taylor criteria, it became evident that many of the neoplasms in the high-grade category were aggressive tumors that occurred in postmeno-pausal women and that lead to death within a few months or years of diag-nosis. These tumors tended to show destructive stromal invasion rather than the typical permeative vascular invasion characteristic of low-grade stromal sarcomas. They exhibited marked cytological atypia with no resemblance to the cells of proliferative-phase of endometrial stroma, and were associated with zones of necrosis and a brisk mitotic rate including atypical mitoses.

Evans (7) designated these tumors as poorly differentiated endometrial sarcomas and suggested that these tumors were closely related to the pleomorphic mesenchymal component of malignant mixed mullerian tumors, both morphologically and in their aggressive behavior. In these sarcomas, it is difficult to establish a stromal genesis as they lack the prerequisite morphological feature, that is, resemblance to the proliferative-phase of endometrial stroma.

In a small number of cases, high-grade stromal sarcoma is seen adjacent to low-grade stromal sarcoma suggesting that in these cases high-grade stromal sarcoma is indeed likely to be of endometrial stromal origin and has probably undergone high-grade transformation (8). In Evans' series of high-grade endometrial sarcomas, six of the seven patients died between 10 and 34 months of diagnosis and there were no cases with evidence of an intermediary form or with transition between high-grade and low-grade tumors.

The controversy regarding the classification of high-grade tumors is not resolved. Chang et al. (9) concluded from a study of 117 cases of stromal sarcoma that stratification into low-grade and high-grade based on MF was not helpful. Silverberg and Kurman (10), however, recognized three categories: low-grade endometrial stromal sarcoma, high-grade endometrial stromal sarcoma, and undifferentiated sarcoma. The important point here in the distinction of high-grade stromal sarcoma from undifferentiated sarcoma is the morphology of the cells, which must closely resemble those of the stroma of proliferative-phase endometrium. High-grade stromal sarcoma must be separated from low-grade by more cellular pleomorphism, larger nuclei, chromatin clumping, a high mitotic rate (> 10, often > 20 per 10 HPF) and a destructive pattern of invasion rather than the typical "endolymphatic pattern" used in the past to describe the permeative plugging of lymphatics and veins by tumor cells, which is a well recognized and characteristic pattern of invasion of low-grade stromal sarcoma.

The treatment and prognosis of the high-grade and undifferentiated sarcomas remains the same. Progestational agents are of no value in these high-grade neoplasms (11).

Endometrial Stromal Sarcoma— "Low Grade"

Low-grade stromal sarcomas occur largely in premenopausal women although rare cases have been documented in adolescents (12–14) and children. They are usually confined to the uterus at the time of diagnosis. A proportion of women are cured by hysterectomy alone; however, one-third to one-half will develop recurrences. Abdominal, pelvic, and even pulmonary recurrences pursue an indolent course sometimes presenting several years after hysterectomy. A recent study documents the metastatic sites in endometrial stromal sarcoma with unusual histologic features to include retroperitoneum, right atrium/inferior vena cava, colon, and ovaries (15).

The etiology is unknown although an association with tamoxifen use has been documented (16–18) and cases have arisen in endometriosis after low-dose estrogen use (19). Patients usually present with abnormal vaginal bleeding or less commonly with abdomino-pelvic pain.

Gross Pathology (Figs. 1 and 2)

The uterus is usually enlarged with a nodule resembling a leiomyoma within the uterine wall. Sometimes there may be several intramural masses associated with polyp-like protrusions into the uterine cavity. The tumor is seen as worm-like plugs in the myometrium or parametrial veins. The tumor is typically soft and fleshy, tan to yellow in color.

Microscopic Pathology

The tumor cells infiltrate the myometrium in "tongue-like" masses with a blunt, pushing margin. The cells resemble those seen in the stroma of proliferative-phase endometrium and are typically bland, oval to spindled cells with little cytoplasm, and scarce mitoses (0–3/10 HPF). The mitotic rate is no longer used to separate low- from high-grade tumors, therefore mitoses in excess of 10 MF/ 10 HPF may be seen and the diagnosis of low-grade stromal sarcoma remains

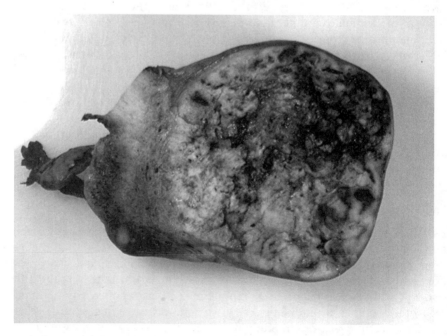

Figure 1 Leiomyosarcoma demonstrating a variegated cut surface with extensive areas of hemorrhage and necrosis.

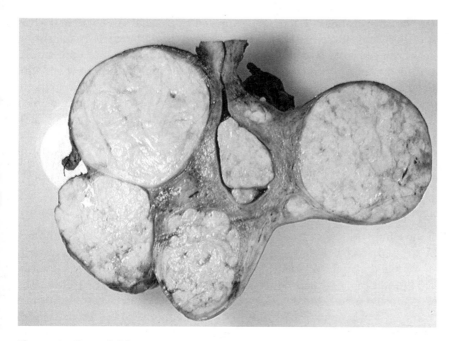

Figure 2 Several leiomyomata exhibiting well circumscribed, gray-white masses with a whorled cut surface.

acceptable as long as the other criteria are met. Reticulin surrounds the individual stromal cells. Hyalinization of collagen is also a feature, which is seen in an intercellular location. This may be a helpful feature when considering the differential diagnosis of a tumor with small cells, and prominent hyalinization in an extrauterine site, in particular the abdomen or lung.

Smooth muscle differentiation can be seen in a small proportion of endometrial stromal neoplasms (20,21). Some authors have used the term "stromomyoma" to characterize these tumors but the preferred terminology is a descriptive one, endometrial stromal tumor with smooth muscle differentiation. If the margin is irregular with evidence of invasion, then the tumor is labeled as endometrial stromal sarcoma with smooth muscle differentiation. The smooth muscle component should account for at least 30% of the tumor cells (22). The smooth muscle component is seen as irregular, discrete islands, or nodules with central hyalinization, producing a so-called "star-burst" pattern. It is thought that smooth muscle forms as a metaplastic event, as stromal cells are able to differentiate along smooth muscle lines, but the opposite is not recognized.

Foam cells may be seen in endometrial stromal sarcoma. These are morphologically identical to those seen in endometrial hyperplasia and carcinoma and are a useful diagnostic feature when distinguishing a stromal lesion from a highly cellular smooth muscle neoplasm.

The other features that may be exhibited by stromal sarcoma are fibrosis and at times myxoid change (23). Focal sex cord-like differentiation consisting of cells arranged in nests, trabeculae, cords, or tubules may also be present. In some tumors, positive immunoreactivity for vimentin, muscle-specific actin, desmin, cytokeratin, inhibin, and CD 99 may be noted. The latter two markers suggest true sex cord elements (24,25). Foci of rhabdoid-like cells may be seen and these are not thought to have an effect on the prognosis of the tumor (26,27).

Endometrial stromal tumors can show glandular differentiation; in the three reported cases these comprised benign endometrioid glands in two and malignant endometrioid glands in the third (28).

Diagnosis of Endometrial Stromal Sarcoma on Curettage Material

The morphological features of an endometrial stromal nodule and endometrial stromal sarcoma are identical except that in a nodule a largely well-circumscribed margin is evident. Minor degrees of irregularity have also been noted but not thought to be of clinical significance (29,30). In a sarcoma, the presence of lymphovascular space permeation or myometrial infiltration is identified. Clearly, in curettage material this diagnosis cannot be made with confidence as it is unlikely that the entire lesion would be visualized. The diagnosis of a stromal nodule can only be made in those rare instances where the entire nodule with its margins intact is seen. In most instances, a hysterectomy will be required in order to assess the margins and exclude vascular invasion. The other major problem area of diagnosis lies in the distinction of a stromal lesion from a highly cellular leiomyoma. This is a very important distinction because the former can behave in an aggressive fashion while the latter is entirely benign. Again, morphology and immunohistochemistry are used in tandem to establish this diagnosis.

IMMUNOHISTOCHEMISTRY OF UTERINE SARCOMAS

Immunohistochemistry is of value in the distinction of endometrial stromal from smooth muscle lesions, in particular when the latter may be "highly" cellular with diminished cytoplasm and therefore mimic endometrial stromal cells.

Immunohistochemistry is best used as a panel of markers with CD10, Vimentin, actin, desmin, and h-caldesmon used together. CD10 initially described as a tumor-specific antigen in acute lymphoblastic leukemia was found to be a useful marker in the distinction of endometrial stromal cells from smooth muscle cells (31–33). It is now recognized to be positive in several other mesenchymal tumors (34), but its usefulness in the diagnosis of endometrial stromal tumors remains, if used as part of a comprehensive panel of markers and if uniform strong staining is looked for.

The h-caldesmon is a calcium, calmodulin, and actin-binding protein widely distributed in smooth and nonsmooth muscle cells and is thought to regulate cellular contraction. Its isoform, high molecular weight caldesmon, is specific for smooth muscle cells and smooth muscle tumors (35–37) and, therefore, the antibody is now used increasingly to confirm smooth muscle differentiation in uterine tumors.

Smooth muscle actin, muscle specific actin, and vimentin have been shown to be positive in both smooth muscle and endometrial stromal lesions and there are conflicting results with regard to the usefulness of desmin. In their study, (38) demonstrated positive immunoreactivity for desmin in all highly cellular leiomyomas and negative immunoreactivity in all their stromal nodules and stromal sarcomas (ESS). Farhood and Abrams found that 7 of 23 endometrial stromal sarcomas were positive for desmin (39). Franquemont et al. also identified positive desmin immunoreactivity in normal endometrial stromal cells as well as in neoplastic stromal cells (seven ESSs and two stromal nodules) (40). It is likely that there is some degree of variability in desmin immunoreactivity dependent on individual cases and laboratory staining protocols.

CD 34, a myeloid progenitor cell antigen present in endothelial cells, may be a useful marker in the distinction of metastatic endometrial stromal tumors from gastro-intestinal stromal tumor (GIST), where on rare occasions this may be a diagnostic problem. Up to 70% of GISTs show positive immunoreactivity with CD34.

C-kit is a proto-oncogene that codes for a transmembrane tyrosine kinase receptor (CD117). The gene product is overexpressed in mastocytosis GIST. While diffuse positivity of GIST for c-kit is of diagnostic value in the distinction of GI stromal tumors from metastatic Mullerian sarcomas, it opens up therapeutic options in the form of imatinib mesylate, a tyrosine kinase inhibitor. Uterine sarcomas express KIT protein as detected by immunohistochemistry but they lack KIT-activating mutations in exon 11 or 17 of c-kit. These tumors are therefore unlikely to respond to imatinib mesylate (41–44).

Inhibin positivity has only been demonstrated in those endometrial stromal sarcomas that exhibit sex cord stromal differentiation. This is seen in 15–60% of endometrial stromal sarcomas (45).

HORMONAL ASPECTS OF STROMAL SARCOMAS

Total abdominal hysterectomy with bilateral salpingo-oophorectomy is the mainstay of primary treatment of uterine sarcoma. The role of chemotherapy, radiation therapy, and hormonal therapy is poorly defined. In a large number of publications, estrogen and progesterone receptor positivity has been consistently demonstrated in uterine endometrial stromal sarcomas of low grade (46–50). Chu et al., in their study, found that four of five patients with low-grade endometrial stromal sarcoma who were given estrogen replacement therapy recurred. They also found a lack of estrogen receptors β (ERβ) expression in endometrial stromal sarcomas compared with normal endometrial stromal cells suggesting that the loss of ERβ expression may be a marker for malignancy (51). Progesterone treatment has been employed with benefit. In many centers, it is now routine to establish the ER and progesterone receptors (PR) status of a stromal sarcoma when resected, in order to predict its likely outcome to hormonal treatment. Hormonal therapy is of particular benefit in high stage disease. There are further isolated case reports of treatment with Depo-Lupron and Megace (52), where treatment achieved significant reduction in tumor bulk to render a patient previously found to be inoperable amenable to surgical resection. There may also be a role for aromatase inhibitors in the management of patients with metastatic endometrial stromal sarcoma (53).

In uterine leiomyosarcomas, estrogen and progesterone receptors are frequently expressed but their receptor status does not appear to correlate with clinical stage, disease recurrence, or overall disease-free survival (54). The data are scarce and further work remains to be done to determine if ER and PR status in leiomyosarcomas have any clinical utility.

Leiomyosarcoma

This is the commonest pure sarcoma to occur within the uterus. It is a malignant tumor showing smooth muscle differentiation. It is a tumor of adult women distributed evenly through adult life after the age of 30 years. The median age of occurrence is early 50s. It is rare in women in their third decade (55). It accounts for between 25% and 45% of uterine sarcomas and up to 1% of all uterine malignancies (56).

Leiomyosarcomas arise de novo with examples of malignant change in leiomyomas being extremely rare (57). Presentation is with abnormal uterine bleeding, pain, prolapse, or the effects of metastases. A history of a rapidly enlarging smooth muscle tumor in an elderly patient or the presence of degenerative changes on imaging in an enlarged "fibroid" in an elderly patient should be treated with suspicion for malignancy. Definitive diagnosis is usually made at the time of hysterectomy.

Gross Appearance

These are typically solitary masses, which are large, and if present in association with other uterine leiomyomas they tend to be the largest mass and are conspicuously different from the well-circumscribed, gray-white masses with a whorled appearance of the usual leiomyomata. The maximum diameter is often more than 10 cm. It is a fleshy, soft tumor, which is poorly circumscribed, and has a variegated cut surface characterized by extensive areas of hemorrhage and necrosis. In advanced cases, extension beyond the uterus will be evident (Figs. 1, 2).

Histological Features

Leiomyosarcomas exhibiting usual smooth muscle differentiation are typically cellular (58,59) smooth muscle tumors characterized by interlacing fascicles of oval to spindled cells with blunt-ended, cigar-shaped nuclei. They exhibit marked cytological atypia and the formation of multi-nucleated giant cells is often. Mitoses are frequent, usually in excess of 20 MF/10 HPF with numerous atypical forms. The borders of the tumor with the surrounding myometrium are irregular and infiltrative with lymphovascular space permeation. Coagulative tumor cell necrosis and areas of hemorrhage are often seen.

In other cases, the diagnosis of leiomyosarcoma can be very difficult and the most useful diagnostic criteria at present are those of Bell, Hendrickson, and Kempson based on their study of 213 problematic smooth muscle tumors (60). They advocate the diagnosis of leiomyosarcoma in any tumor demonstrating coagulative tumor cell necrosis in the presence of cytological atypia and any mitotic activity, as well as in those tumors with an excess of 10 MF/10 HPF and coagulative tumor cell necrosis, in the absence of cytological atypia.

MYXOID LEIOMYOSARCOMA

Myxoid smooth muscle tumors are rare; about 20 cases of myxoid leiomyosarcoma have been reported in the literature (61–63). The age ranges from 20 to 76 years. Recently, a case of myxoid leiomyosarcoma of the uterus has been reported in a 20-year-old female who developed recurrent disease after initial laparotomy; the recurrent tumor was resected. Two years following the second operation, she became pregnant and a healthy baby was delivered following Caesarean section at which time further recurrent tumor masses were resected. She remains well a year later with no evidence of recurrent disease (64).

They have an unpredictable outcome either resulting in death a few years after diagnosis or long-term survival despite recurrent disease.

Gross examination usually reveals a large gelatinous intramural mass that may appear well-circumscribed, but on histological examination the typical paucicellular appearance characterized by spindled, stellate, or epithelioid cells is seen. Cytological atypia is minimal and mitoses are difficult to find, usually less than 2 MF/10 HPF are present. The low mitotic rate is due to the overall poor cellularity of the tumor with cells separated by large amounts of myxoid matrix. Thorough sampling usually reveals some areas of leiomyosarcoma of usual differentiation and at the periphery an infiltrative margin with evidence of lymphatic space permeation is further evidence of its malignant nature. In this tumor, it is mandatory to extensively sample the periphery of the tumor with the adjacent myometrium, as it is this feature that most often establishes the diagnosis. The main differential diagnosis is from a leiomyoma showing hydropic degeneration. The latter is a focal finding and often associated with hyalinization.

EPITHELIOID LEIOMYOSARCOMA

Epithelioid smooth muscle tumors are also unusual tumors. This term suggests that the tumor cells adopt a more rounded appearance resembling epithelial cells rather than the typical spindled, smooth muscle morphology seen in the usual cases. Approximately 50% of the tumors do contain admixed, intermingled spindled cells. The cells have copious amounts of cytoplasm, which may be esinophilic or clear. These tumors tend to be hypercellular with marked nuclear atypia and mitotic activity in the range of 3–4 MF/ 10 HPF and microscopic evidence of tumor cell necrosis is seen. Necrosis is an important predictor of malignant behavior; Hendrickson and Kempson in their unpublished series found that epithelioid tumors with necrosis behaved in a malignant fashion (65). Rhabdoid differentiation in an epithelioid leiomyosarcoma of the uterus has recently been described; its clinical importance being that the rhabdoid phenotype is prone to aggressive behavior (66).

CARCINOSARCOMA: A METAPLASTIC CARCINOMA OR SARCOMA?

Historically carcinosarcomas have been regarded as a subtype of uterine sarcoma and have been managed as such. The pathogenesis of carcinosarcoma is still controversial, although the fact that the vast majority are now believed to be metaplastic carcinomas and, therefore, monoclonal, is gaining favor supported by molecular evidence. The behavior of these neoplasms is indeed aggressive but resembles that of high-grade endometrioid type of endometrial carcinoma (67). The vast majority of these tumors are monoclonal (68). In a study by Wada et al., three carcinosarcomas showed different patterns of chromosome-X inactivation between the carcinomatous and sarcomatous components. This suggests that these are true collision tumors. In 21 tumors, the patterns of chromosome-X inactivation, K-ras sequence, and *p53* sequences were identical in both the carcinomatous and sarcomatous components suggesting that these are combination tumors (69). Approximately 8% of these tumors are collision tumors in which the endometrial carcinosarcomas have arisen because of malignant transformation of the epithelial component within or in the endometrium adjacent to an adenosarcoma (70).

PURE SARCOMAS

Overgrowth of a sarcomatous component in a carcinosarcoma or adenosarcoma can occur and thereby become the dominant component of the uterine tumor. Usually thorough sampling excludes epithelial elements or foci of more usual adenosarcoma that may be present. In those rare instances where an underlying mixed uterine tumor has not been identified, then the tumor probably represents a pure heterologous sarcoma manifested as rhabdomyosarcoma of adult type, which may even acquire a spindle cell phenotype (71) or may resemble similar tumors seen at other sites (72–74).

Occasional cases of osteosarcoma, liposarcoma (75), and chondrosarcoma have also been described (76,77).

TAMOXIFEN AND ITS ROLE IN UTERINE SARCOMA

The United States Food and Drug Administration issued a new warning last year on the dangers of tamoxifen. The warning was related to the association of uterine sarcoma and tamoxifen and was not directed at women who already had invasive breast carcinoma and were maintained on tamoxifen to prevent recurrent carcinoma, in whom the benefits were thought to outweigh risks. It was directed at those women who were considered a high-risk group for developing breast carcinoma and those who had noninvasive breast carcinoma ductal carcinoma in situ (DCIS), in whom the benefits and risks must be carefully considered.

Uterine sarcoma is estimated to occur in 0.17 cases per 1000 women a year who take tamoxifen and in women not taking tamoxifen only 0.01–0.02 cases per 1000 women. Apparently since 1978 when tamoxifen was first marketed, there have been an additional 159 cases of uterine sarcoma globally that could be attributable to the drug (78).

REFERENCES

1. Hannigan E, Curtin JP, Silverberg SG, Thigpn JT, Spanos WJ. Corpus: mesenchymal tumors. In: Hoskins WJ, Perez CA, YoungRC, eds. Principles and Practice Of Gynaecologic Oncology. Philadelphia: Lippincott, 1992:695–714.
2. Koss LG, Spiro RH, Brunschwig A. Endometrial stromal sarcoma. Surg Obstet Gynaecol 1965; 121:531–537.
3. Aaro LA, Symonds RE, Dockerty MD. Sarcoma of the uterus: a clinical and pathologic study of 177 cases. Am J Obstet Gynaecol 1966; 94:101–109.
4. Kahanpaa KV, Wahlstrom T, Grohn P, Heinonen E, Nieminen U, Widholm O. Sarcomas of the uterus: a clinicopathologic study of 119 patients. Obstet Gynaecol 1986; 67:417–424.
5. Silverberg SG, Kurman RJ. Smooth muscle and other mesenchymal tumors. In: Rosai J, Sobin LH, eds. AFIP Atlas of Tumor Pathology. Tumors of the Uterine Corpus and Gestational Trophoblastic Disease. Washington: Armed Forces Institute of Pathology, 1992:113–151.

6. Norris HJ, Taylor HB. Mesenchymal tumors of the uterus.1. A clinical and pathological study of 53 endometrial stromal tumors. Cancer 1966; 19: 755–766.
7. Evans HL. Endometrial stromal sarcoma and poorly differentiated endometrial endometrial sarcoma. Cancer 1982 ; 50:2170–2182.
8. Cheung AN, Ng WF, Chung LP, Khoo US. Mixed low grade and high grade endometrial stromal sarcoma of uterus: differences on immunohistochemistry and chromosome in situ hybridisation. J Clin Pathol 1996; 49:604–607.
9. Chang KL, Crabtree GS, Lim-Tan SK, Kempson RL, Hendrickson MR. Primary uterine endometrial stromal neoplasms. A clinicopathologic study of 117 cases. Am J Surg Pathol 1990; 14(5):415–438.
10. Silverberg SG, Kurman RJ. Smooth muscle and other mesenchymal tumors. In: Rosai J, Sobin LH, eds. AFIP Atlas of Tumor Pathology. Tumors of the Uterine Corpus and Gestational Trophoblastic Disease. Washington: Armed Forces Institute of Pathology, 1992:113–151.
11. Zaloudek CJ, Norris HJ. Mesenchymal tumors of the uterus. In: Fenoglio CM, Wolff M, eds. Progress in Surgical Pathology. New York: Masson Publishing USA Inc, 1981:1–35.
12. Fekete PS, Vellios F. The clinical and histological spectrum of endometrial stromal neoplasms: a report of 41 cases. Int J Gynaecol Pathol 1984; 3:198–212.
13. Berchuck A, Rubin SC, Hoskins WJ, Saigo PE, Pierce VK, Lewis JL Jr. Treatment of endometrial stromal tumors. Gynecol Oncol 1990; 36:60–65.
14. Rabczynski J, Rzeszutko W, Kornafel J. Stromal sarcoma of the uterine body in an 18-year-old girl. Ginekol Polska 1997; 68:641–645.
15. Yilmaz A, Rush DS, Soslow RA. Endometrial stromal sarcoma with unusual histologic features a report of 24 primary and metastatic tumors emphasizing fibroblastic and smooth muscle differentiation. Am J Surg Pathol 2002; 26(9):1142–1150.
16. Eddy GL, Mazur MT. Endolymphatic stromal myosis associated with Tamoxifen use. Gynecol Oncol 1997; 64:262–264.
17. Pang LC. Endometrial stromal sarcoma with sex cord-like differentiation associated with Tamoxifen therapy. South Med J 1998; 91:592–594.
18. Kennedy MM, Baigrie CF, Manek S. Tamoxifen and the endometrium: review of 102 cases and comparison with HRT-related and non-HRT-related endometrial pathology. Int J Gynecol Pathol 1999; 18:130–137.
19. McGluggage WG, Bailie C, Weir P, Barucha H. Endometrial stromal sarcoma arising in pelvic endometriosis in a patient receiving unopposed oestrogen therapy. Br J Obstet Gynaecol 1996; 103:1252–1254.
20. Oliva E, Clement PB, Young RH, Scully RE. Mixed endometrial stromal and smooth muscle tumors of the uterus: a clinico-pathologic study of 15 cases. Am J Surg Pathol 1998; 22:997–1005.
21. Schammel DP, Silver SA, Tavassoli FA. Combined endometrial stromal/ smooth muscle neoplasms. A clinicopathologic study of 38 cases [abstract]. Mod Pathol 1999; 12:124A.
22. Oliva E, Clement PB, Young RH. Endometrial stromal tumors: an update on a group of tumors with a protean phenotype. Adv Anat Pathol 2000; 5:257–281.

23. Oliva E, Young RH, Clement PB, Scully RE. Myxoid and fibrous endometrial stromal tumors of the uterus: a report of 10 cases. Int J Gynecol Pathol 1999; 18:310–319.
24. Baker RJ, Hildebrandt RH, Rouse RV, Hendrickson MR, Longacre TA. Inhibin and CD99 (Mic 2) expression in uterine stromal neoplasms with sex-cord-like elements. Hum Pathol 1999; 30:671–679.
25. Ohta Y, Suzuki T, Kojima M, Shiokawa A, Mitsuya T. Low-grade endometrial stromal sarcoma with an extensive epithelial-like element. Pathol Int 2003; 53(4): 246–251.
26. McGluggage WG, Date A, Bharucha H, Toner PG. Endometrial stromal sarcoma with sex cord-like areas and focal rhabdoid differentiation. Histopathology 1996; 29:369–374.
27. Tanimoto A, Sasaguri T, Arima N, Hashimoto H, Hamada T, Sasaguri Y. Endometrial stromal sarcoma of the uterus with rhabdoid features. Pathol Int 1996; 46:231–237.
28. Clement PB, Scully RE. Endometrial stromal sarcomas of the uterus with extensive endometrioid glandular differentiation: a report of three cases that caused problems in differential diagnosis. Int J Gynecol Pathol 1992; 11: 163–173.
29. Tavassoli FA, Norris HJ. Mesenchymal tumors of the uterus. VII. A clinicopathological study of 60 endometrial stromal nodules. Histopathology 1981; 5:1–10.
30. Dionigi A, Oliva E, Clement PB, Young RH. Endometrial stromal nodules and endometrial stromal tumors with limited infiltration: a clinicopathologic study of 50 cases. Am J Surg Pathol 2002; 26:567–581.
31. Chu P, Arber DA. Paraffin-section detection of CD10 in 505 nonhematopoietic neoplasms. Frequent expression in renal cell carcinoma and endometrial stromal sarcoma. Am J Clin Pathol 2000; 113:374–382.
32. Toki T, Shimizu M, Takagi Y, Ashida T, Konishi I. CD10 is a marker for normal and neoplastic endometrial stromal cells. Int J Gynecol Pathol 2002; 21: 41–47.
33. McGluggage WG, Sumathi VP, Maxwell P. CD10 is a sensitive and diagnostically useful immunohistochemical marker of normal endometrial stroma and of endometrial stromal neoplasms. Histopathology 2001; 39:273–278.
34. Mikami Y, Hata S, Kiyokawa T, Manabe T. Expression of CD10 in malignant mullerian mixed tumors and adenosarcomas: an immunohistochemical study. Mod Pathol 2002; 15:923–930.
35. Watanabe K, Tajino T, Sekiguchi M, Suzuki T. h-Caldesmon as a specific marker for smooth muscletumors. Comparison with other smooth muscle markers in bone tumors. Am J Clin Pathol 2000; 113:663–668.
36. Nucci MR, O'Connell JT, Huettner PC, Cviko A, Sun D, Quade BJ. h-Caldesmon expression effectively distinguishes endometrial stromal tumors from uterine smooth muscle tumors. Am J Surg Pathol 2001; 25:455–463.
37. Rush DS, Tan J, Baergen RN, Soslow RA. h-Caldesmon, a novel smooth muscle-specific antibody, distinguishes between cellular leiomyoma endometrial stromal sarcoma. Am J surg Path 2001; 25:253–258.

38. Oliva E, Young RH, Clement PB, Bhan AK, Scully RE. Cellular benign mese-chymal tumors of the uterus. A comparative morphologic and immunohisto-chemical analysis of 33 highly cellular leiomyomas and six endometrial stromal nodules, two frequently confused tumors. Am J Surg Pathol 1995; 19: 757–768.

39. Farhood AI, Abrams J. Immunohistochemistry of endometrial stromal sarcoma. Hum Pathol 1991; 22:224–230.

40. Franquemont DW, Frierson HF Jr, Mills SE. An immunohistochemical study of normal endometrial stroma and endometrial neoplasms. Evidence for smooth muscle differentiation. Am J Surg Pathol 1991; 15:861–870.

41. Rushing RS, Shajahan S, Chendil D, Wilder JL, Pulliam J, Lee EY, Ueland FR, van Nagell JR, Ahmed MM, Lele SM. Uterine sarcomas express KIT protein but lack mutation(s) exon 11 or 17 of c-KIT. Gynecol Oncol 2003; 1:9–14.

42. Miettinen M, Lasota J. Gastro-intestinal stromal tumors—definition, clinical, histological, immunohistochemical, and molecular genetic features and differ-ential diagnosis. Virchows Arch 2001; 438:1–12.

43. Wang L, Felix JC, Lee JL, Tan PY, Tourgeman DE, O'Meara AT, Amezcua CA. The proto-oncogene c-kit is expressed in Leiomyosarcomas of Uterus. Gynecol Oncol 2003; 2:402–406.

44. Klein WM, Kurman RJ. Lack of expression of c-kit protein (CD117) in mesenchymal tumors of the uterus and ovary. Int J Gynecol Pathol 2003; 2:181–184.

45. Baker RJ, Hildebrandt H, Rouse RV, Hendrikson MR, Longacre TA. Inhibin and CD 99 (MIC 2) expression in uterine stromal neoplasms with sex cord-like elements. Hum Pathol 1999; 30:671–679.

46. Lantta M, Kahanpaa K, Karkkainen J, Lehtovirta P, Wahlstrom T, Widholm O. Estradiol and progesterone receptors in two cases of endometrial stromal sarcoma. Gynecol Oncol 1984; 18:233–239.

47. Katz L, Merino MJ, Sakamoto H, Schwartz PE. Endometrial stromal sarcoma: a clinicopathologic study of 11 cases with determination of estrogen and proges-tin receptor levels in three tumors. Gynecol Oncol 1987; 26:87–97.

48. Sabini G, Chumas JC, Mann WJ. Steroid hormone receptors in endometrial stromal sarcomas. Biochemical and immunohistochemical study. Am J Clin Pathol 1992; 97:381–386.

49. Navarro D, Cabrera JJ, Leon L, Chirino R, Fernandez L, Lopez A, Rivero JF, Fernandez P, Falcon O, Jimenez P, et al. Endometrial stromal sarcoma expres-sion of estrogen receptor, progesterone receptors and estrogen-induced srp27 (24K) suggests hormone responsiveness. J Steroid Biochem Mol Biol 1992; 41:589–596.

50. Reich O, Regauer S, Urdl W, Lahousen M, Winter R. Expression of oestrogen and progesterone receptors in low grade endometrial stromal sarcomas Br J Cancer 2000; 82:1030–1034.

51. Chu MC, Mor G, Lim C, Zheng W, Parkash V, Schwartz PE. Low-grade endometrial stromal sarcoma: hormonal aspects. Gynecol Oncol 2003; 90: 170–176.

52. Scribner DR Jr, Walker JL. Low grade endometrial stromal sarcoma preoperative treatment with Depo-Lupron and Megace. Gynecol Oncol 1998; 71: 458–460.
53. Spano JP, Soria JC, Kambouchner M, Piperno-Neuman S, Morin F, Morere JF, Martin A, Breau JL. Long-term survival of patients given hormonal therapy for metastatic endometrial stromal sarcoma. Med Oncol 2003; 20:87–93.
54. Bodner K, Bodner-Adler B, Kimberger O, Czerwenka K, Leodolter S, Mayerhofer K. Estrogen and progesterone receptor expression in patients with uterine leiomyosarcoma and correlation with different clinicopathological parameters. Anticancer Res 2003; 23:729–732.
55. Harlow BL, Weiss NS, Lofton S. The epidemiology of sarcomas of the uterus. J Natl Cancer Inst 1986; 76:399–402.
56. Echt G, Jepson J, Steel J, Longholz B, Luxton G, Hernandez W, Astrahan M, Petrovich Z. Treatment of uterine sarcomas. Cancer 1990; 66:35–39.
57. Scurry J, Hack M. Leiomyosarcoma arising in a lipoleiomyoma. Gynecol Oncol 1990; 39:381–383.
58. Evans HL, Chawla SP, Simpson C, Finn KP. Smooth muscle neoplasms of the uterus other than ordinary leiomyoma. A study of 46 cases with emphasis on diagnostic criteria and prognostic factors. Cancer 1988; 62:2239–2247.
59. Kempson RL, Hendrickson MR. Pure mesenchymal neoplasms of the uterine corpus. In: Fox H, ed. Haines and Taylor Obstetrical and Gynaecological Pathology. 3rd ed. Edinburgh: Churchill Livingstone. 1987:411–456.
60. Bell S, Kempson RL, Hendrickson MR. Problematic uterine smooth muscle neoplasms: a clinicopathologic study of 213 cases. Am J Surg Pathol 1994; 18:535–558.
61. King ME, Dickersin GR, Scully RE. Myxoid leiomyosarcoma of the uterus. A report of six cases. Am J Surg Pathol 1982; 6:589–598.
62. Peacock G, Archer S. Myxoid leiomyosarcoma of the uterus. Am J Obstet Gynecol 1989; 160:1515–1519.
63. Chen KTK. Myxoid leiomyosarcoma of the uterus. Int J Gynecol Pathol 1984; 3:389–392.
64. Kagami S, Kashimura M, Toki N, Katuhata Y. Myxoid leiomyosarcoma of the uterus with subsequent pregnancy and delivery. Gynecol Oncol 2002; 85: 538–542.
65. Hendrickson MR, Kempson RL. A diagnostic approach to smooth muscle tumors of the uterus. Curr Diagn Pathol 2000; 6:21–30.
66. Levine PH, Mittal K. Rhabdoid epithelioid leiomyosarcoma of the uterine corpus: a case report and literature review. Int J Surg Pathol 2002; 10:231–236.
67. McCluggage WG. Uterine carcinosarcomas (malignant mixed Mullerian tumors) are metaplastic carcinomas. Int J Gynecol Cancer 2002; 12:687–690.
68. Jin Z, Ogata S, Tamura G, Katayama Y, Fukase M, Yajima M, Motoyama T. Carcinosarcomas (malignant mullerian mixed tumors of the uterus and ovary: a genetic study with special reference to histogenesis). Int J Gynecol Pathol 2003; 22:368–373.
69. Wada H, Enomoto T, Fujita M, Yoshino K, Nakashima R, Kurachi H, Haba T, Wakasa K, Shroyer KR, Tsujimoto M, Hongyo T, Nomura T, Muarata Y.

Molecular evidence that most but not all carcinosarcomas of the uterus are combination tumors. Cancer Res 1997; 57:5379–5385.

70. Seidman JD, Chauhan S. Evaluation of the relationship between adenosarcoma and carcinosarcoma and a hypothesis of the histogenesis of uterine sarcomas. Int J Gynecol Pathol 2003; 22:75–82.

71. McCluggage WG, Lioe TF, McClelland HR, Lamki H. Rhabdomyosarcoma of the uterus: report of two cases, including one of the spindle cell variant. Int J Gynecol Cancer 2002; 12:128–132.

72. Chiarle R, Godio L, Fusi D, Soldati T, Palestro G. Pure alveolar rhabdomyosacoma of the corpus uteri: description of a case with increased serum level of CA-125. Gynecol Oncol 1997; 66:320–323.

73. Siegal GP, Taylor LL III, Nelson KG, Reddick RL, Frazelle M, Siegfried JM, Walton LA, Kaufman DG. Characterization of a pure heterologous sarcoma of the uterus: rhabdomyosarcoma of the corpus. Int J Gynecol Pathol 1983; 2:303–315.

74. Zhonghua Yi, Xue Za Zhi. Pure rhabdomyosarcoma of the corpus uteri in a postpartum patient: rep of a case and review of the literature. (Taipei) 1992; 50(1):73–76 (review).

75. Levine PH, Wei XJ, Gagner JP, Flax H, Mittal K, Blank SV. Pleomorphic liposarcoma of the uterus: case report and literature review. Int J Gynecol Pathol 2003; 4:407–411.

76. Lin JW, Ko SF, Ng SH, Eng HL, Changchien CC, Huang CC. Primary osteosarcoma of the uterus with peritoneal osteosarcomatosis: C features. Br J Radiol 2002; 75(897):772–774.

77. Rollason TP, Wilkinson N. Non-neoplastic conditions of the myometrium and pure mesenchymal tumors of the uterus. In: Fox H, Wells M, eds. Haines and Taylor Obstetrical and Gynaecological Pathology. 5th ed. 2003; 538–539.

78. Gottlieb S. Tamoxifen may increase risk of uterine sarcoma. BMJ 2002; 325:7.

5

The Molecular Genetics of Endometrial Cancer

G. Larry Maxwell

Division of Gynecologic Oncology, Walter Reed Army Medical Center, Washington, D.C., U.S.A.

John I. Risinger and J. Carl Barrett

Laboratory of Biosystems and Cancer, National Cancer Institute, Bethesda, Maryland, U.S.A.

Andrew Berchuck

Division of Gynecologic Oncology, Duke University Medical Center, Durham, North Carolina, U.S.A.

INTRODUCTION

Endometrial cancer is the most common gynecological malignancy in the United States. It is the fourth most common cancer in females, and the seventh leading cause of cancer-related deaths. The American Cancer Society estimates that 39,300 cases occured in 2002 and approximately 6600 women died from this disease (1). Endometrial cancer is primarily a disease of the postmenopausal female. However, 25% of cases occur in premenopausal women, with 5% occurring in women younger than 40 years of age (2).

Epidemiologic and clinical studies of endometrial cancer have suggested that there are two distinct types of endometrial cancer. Type I endometrial cancers, which account for approximately 75% of endometrial cancer cases, are usually endometrioid in histology, well-differentiated, and present with early stage disease. These tumors are frequently associated with

Table 1 Clinical Phenotypes of Endometrial Cancer

	Type I	Type II
Race	Caucasian > African-American	Caucasian = African-American
Grade	Well differentiated	Poorly differentiated
Histology	Endometrioid	Non-endometrioid
Stage	I/II	III/IV
Prognosis	Favorable	Unfavorable
Precursor	Atypical hyperplasia	Endometrial intraepithelial carcinoma

a history of unopposed estrogen exposure or other hyperestrogenic risk factors such as obesity. Patients with type I endometrial cancer typically have a favorable prognosis with appropriate therapy. In contrast, type II endometrial cancers are more often moderately to poorly differentiated and non-endometrioid in histology. These tumors are usually metastatic at presentation, and are more likely to recur despite aggressive surgical and medical management (Table 1). In practice, not all cancers can be neatly characterized as either pure type I or II lesions and endometrial cancers can also be viewed as a continuous spectrum with respect to etiology and clinical behavior. However, as the genetic events involved in the development of endometrial cancer have been elucidated, it has been found that specific alterations often, but not always, are seen primarily in either type I or II cases.

In search of genetic alterations characteristic of types I and II endometrial cancers, our group and others have utilized a candidate gene-based approach in combination with allelotyping, functional chromosomal transfer analysis, comparative genomic hybridization, and conventional cytogenetic data to focus on specific genes and/or regions of chromosomes which might be involved in endometrial carcinogenesis. This approach has been highly successful in identifying critical target genes and suggests that distinct molecular alterations may be characteristic of type I versus II endometrial cancers.

SOMATIC GENETIC ALTERATIONS

Oncogenes

It has been convincingly demonstrated that alterations in genes that stimulate cellular growth (oncogenes) can cause malignant transformation. Oncogenes can be activated via several mechanisms. In some cancers, amplification of oncogenes with resultant overexpression of the corresponding protein has been noted. Some oncogenes may become overactive when affected by point mutations. Finally, oncogenes may be translocated from one chromosomal location to another and then come under the influence of promoter sequences that cause overexpression of the gene.

RAS Genes

The retrovirus associated sequence (RAS) gene family consists of three genes: Harvey RAS (HRAS) located on chromosome 11; Kirsten RAS (*KRAS2*) located on chromosome 12; and neuroblastoma RAS (*NRAS*), located on chromosome 1. Each of the genes encodes for a similar 21 kDa transmembrane protein (p-21), which is functionally and structurally similar to the G-proteins involved in adenylate cyclase activation. It is believed that the RAS proteins are involved in transference of external stimuli to the cell through second messenger activation. Amplification or mutation of RAS may lead to hyperstimulation of second messengers and subsequent transformation.

The *KRAS2* oncogene undergoes point mutations in codons 12, 13, or 61 that result in constitutively activated molecules in many types of cancers. Initially, these codons of the *KRAS2*, *NRAS*, and *HRAS1* genes were examined in 11 immortalized endometrial cancer cell lines. Mutations in codon 12 of *KRAS2* were seen in four cell lines whereas three had mutations in codon 61 of *HRAS* (3). Subsequent studies of primary endometrial adenocarcinomas have confirmed that codon 12 of *KRAS2* is mutated in about 10% of American cases (3–5) and 20% of Japanese cases (6–9) but there does not appear to be a strong relationship between *KRAS2* mutation and clinical features or survival of endometrial cancers. The *KRAS2* mutations also have been identified in some endometrial hyperplasias (10,11) however, which suggests that this may be a relatively early event in the development of some type I endometrial cancers.

ERBB2

The erythroblastic leukemia viral oncogene homolog (ERBB2) proto-oncogene encodes a transmembrane glycoprotein receptor tyrosinase (HER-2/*neu*) that is structurally similar to the human epidermal growth factor. The mechanism by which increased HER-2/*neu* activation results in transformation is presently unknown but may reflect an increased protein tyrosine kinase (PTK) mediated phosphorylation of intracellular proteins. Mutation of the ERBB2 proto-oncogene has resulted in augmentation of tyrosinase activity and subsequent transformation within certain cell lines (12).

Overexpression of the HER-2/*neu* receptor tyrosine kinase has been noted in 10–15% of endometrial cancer (13–17) and is associated with advanced stage and poor outcome. In a study of HER-2/*neu* expression in 247 endometrial cancers, expression was scored as high in 15% of cases, moderate in 58%, and absent in 27%; disease-free survival was 56%, 83%, and 95% in these groups, respectively. Among stage I cases, 13% had high expression of HER-2/*neu* and progression-free survival was 62% compared to 97% in cases with lesser expression. The incidence of overexpression was higher in advanced stage cases (25%). Multivariate analysis revealed that high expression was an independent variable associated with poor survival (18).

Papillary serous (PS) endometrial cancers most frequently overexpress HER-2/*neu* and it has been suggested that this might provide a therapeutic opportunity (19). The levels of HER-2/*neu* overexpression in endometrial cancers are much less striking than in breast cancers, however, and thus far there is no evidence that Herceptin (anti-HER-2/*neu* antibody) is of therapeutic benefit in endometrial cancer.

β-Catenin

β-catenin is a multifunctional protein that acts as a regulator of cellular adhesion when coupled with E-cadherin and signal transduction. However, β-catenin also functions as an oncogene in the Wnt signal transduction pathway. Normally, cytoplasmic pools of β-catenin are phophorylated by glycogen synthase kinase (GSK) and associate with the adenomatous polyposis coli (APC) tumor suppressor genes, AXIN 1 and AXIN 2. Formation of the GSK-APC-β-catenin complex facilitates the binding of more β-catenin, which is subsequently ubiquinated and degraded. Increased β-catenin can form complexes with Tcf/Lef that activate transcription. Constitutive transcriptional activation is associated with tumorigenesis and can be achieved either by mutation of the APC tumor suppressor protein or by activating mutations within the *CTNNB1* gene encoding β-catenin. These alterations occur at key serine and threonine residues present in exon 3 and like alterations in *KRAS2* act in a constitutive manner without disruption of the remaining wild type allele. Alteration of these residues impedes the degradation of β-catenin by GSK-3β (20). Either of these events can lead to protein stabilization and ultimately cellular proliferation. In colon cancer, activation of the β-catenin/Tcf pathway is mediated through mutation of APC in approximately 50% of cases while β-catenin mutation substitutes for APC alterations in the remaining cases (21). Because mutation and/or loss of heterozygosity (LOH) are uncommon at the APC locus in endometrial carcinomas (22), multiple investigators have focused on mutational analysis of β-catenin in the investigation of the Tcf/Lef pathway. Our group (23) and others (24–27) have determined that mutation of β-catenin is an infrequent event in endometrial cancers, occurring in approximately 3–14% of cases. However, as many as 25% of endometrial cancers have nuclear accumulation of β-catenin despite an absence of β-catenin mutations (28) suggesting that other mechanisms are responsible for overexpression of β-catenin in endometrial carcinogenesis.

Tumor Suppressor Genes

Loss of tumor suppressor gene function plays a significant role in the development of endometrial cancer. This usually involves a two-step process in which both copies of a tumor suppressor gene are inactivated. In most cases, there is mutation of one copy of a tumor suppressor gene and loss of the other remaining wild type copy due to deletion of a large segment of the chromosome where the gene resides. There is also evidence that some tumor suppressor genes may be inactivated through epigenetic silencing often associated with methylation of CpG-rich sequences in promoter regions.

Allelotype analysis has been performed to identify chromosomal regions of LOH present in endometrial cancers. Through these analyses, regions of chromosomes 1, 3, 6, 10, 14, 17, and 18 have been identified as having regions of LOH (29). Such regions may be indicative of the presence of a tumor suppressor gene(s). In addition, functional studies using chromosome transfer into human endometrial cancer cell lines supported the existence of tumor suppressing loci on human chromosomes 1, 6, 9, 11, and 18 (30–32).

p53

The *TP53* tumor suppressor gene on chromosome 17q encodes a 393 amino acid protein that plays a role in the regulation of both proliferation and apoptosis. In normal cells, *p53* exerts its tumor suppressor activity by binding to transcriptional regulatory elements of genes such as the cdk inhibitor p21 that act to arrest cells in G1. In addition, wild type *p53* may play a role in preventing cancer by stimulating apoptosis of cells that have undergone excessive genetic damage.

Overexpression of mutant *p53* protein occurs in about 20% of endometrial adenocarcinomas and is associated with several known prognostic factors including advanced stage, poor grade, and non-endometrioid histology (33,34). In one early study, overexpression was seen in 9% of stage I/II and 41% of stage III/IV cancers (34). Additional studies have confirmed the strong association between *p53* overexpression and poor prognostic factors and decreased survival (35–37). In some of these studies, *p53* overexpression has been associated with worse survival even after controlling for stage. This suggests that loss of *p53* tumor suppressor function confers a particularly virulent phenotype. Carcinomas with *p53* mutations often are typically type II non-endometrioid cancers, often of the serous type but also occurring in advanced cases of endometrioid endometrial cancer. Overexpression of *p53* has not been found in atypical endometrial hyperplasia (38), the precursor lesion for endometrioid carcinoma. In contrast, increased *p53* expression associated with mutation has been detected in as many as 78% of endometrial intraepithelial carcinomas (EIC), the suspected precursor of some type II tumors serous cancers (39). These studies implicate *p53* mutation as an important component of type II non-endometrioid tumors and as an infrequent late stage alteration in type I endometrioid endometrial carcinoma progression.

PTEN

Phosphatase and tensin homolog (*PTEN*) (mutated in multiple advanced cancers 1) normally acts as a phosphatidylinositol phosphatase directly opposing the activity of the PI3' kinase. Loss of *PTEN* results in an increased phosphorylation state of the phophainosotide lipid as a result of PI3' kinase activity. Without the lipid phosphatase activity of the *PTEN* enzyme this pathway remains activated. Activation of this signal cascade can result in many endpoints of which phosphorylated and activated AKT/PKB plays a key role (40). Activated AKT/PKB is associated with proliferative and antiapoptotic pathways dependent on PI3' kinase signaling. In this regard restoration of mutant *PTEN* to *PTEN* wild type endometrial carcinoma cells results in the onset of apoptosis (41).

Allele loss studies of endometrial cancer indicated that one or more tumor suppressor genes may be located on chromosome 10 with one focus of LOH centered around 10q22–23 and another more distally at 10q25–26 (42–45). Others and we identified the *PTEN* gene as the tumor suppressor gene present at the 10q23 locus in endometrial cancer (46–48). In an analysis of 70 endometrial carcinomas, we detected somatic mutations in 24 cases (34%) including 21 cases that resulted in premature truncation of the protein, two tumors with missense alterations in the conserved phosphatase domain, and one tumor with a large insertion (Fig. 1) (48). These data indicated that *PTEN* is more commonly mutated than any other known gene in endometrial cancer.

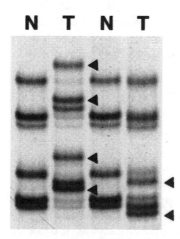

Figure 1 Demonstration of *PTEN* mutation using single-stranded conformation analysis of PCR products amplified from endometrial cancers. The lanes labeled N depict normal mobility bands associated with endometrial cancer specimens. The lanes labeled T illustrate altered mobility bands (*arrows*), consistent with a mutation of the *PTEN* gene.

   PTEN mutation was subsequently evaluated in endometrial hyperplasia to determine whether *PTEN* alterations occur early in endometrial carcinogenesis (49). In a mutation analysis of 51 hyperplasias, we found that 20% had mutations in the *PTEN* gene. The spectrum of *PTEN* mutations in endometrial hyperplasias was similar to those seen in our analysis of invasive endometrial cancer. Most of the mutations resulted in truncated protein products. Although many of the mutations directly involve the highly conserved central phosphatase domain, more distal mutations also were observed.

   Loss of the tumor suppressor gene *PTEN* is associated with favorable pathologic features such as low grade and lack of myometrial invasion. The frequency of *PTEN* mutations in PS and clear cell (CC) cancers (5/21, 5%) is significantly lower than that seen in endometrioid cancers (43/115, 38%). The highest frequency of *PTEN* mutations is seen in stage IA endometrioid cases that were confined to the endometrium without evidence of myometrial invasion or other spread of disease (6/11, 55%). Cases with *PTEN* mutations have a lower recurrence rate than those lacking mutations (50).

   Correlation of *PTEN* mutation with other molecular features in endometrial cancer has suggested that *PTEN* alterations occur in the majority of tumors with microsatellite instability (MI) (51,52). Cells with MI lack mismatch repair (MMR) activity and subsequently display somatic allele length variation in simple sequence repeat sequences (microsatellites). The disruption of DNA MMR results in elevated mutation rates in endoglandular cells leading to the acquisition of additional mutations in growth regulatory or other cancer disposition genes such as *PTEN*. The *PTEN* gene may be a target for mutations in endometrial cancers that have deficiencies in DNA-MMR.

DNA Repair Genes

Microsatellites are repetitive DNA sequences that are widely dispersed throughout the genome. Because of their repetitive structure, microsatellites are particularly susceptible to slippage errors by DNA polymerase during replication, resulting in either insertion or deletion mutations. The proteins encoded by MMR genes normally recognize and repair these genetic mutations. Alterations in MMR genes such as *MLH1, MLH6, MSH2, MSH3*, and *PMS2* lead to accumulation of mutations in microsatellite sequences throughout the genome, a phenomenon known as MI. The MI initially was noted in colorectal cancers of patients with hereditary nonpolyposis Colorectal cancer (HNPCC) syndrome (52,53). Endometrial cancer is the second most common malignancy observed in HNPCC families and genetic analysis of these tumors revealed MI in 75% of cases (54).

   The MI occurs in approximately 20% of sporadic endometrial cancers (55). The MI phenotype was associated with type I cancers and has a more favorable clinical outcome than endometrial carcinomas without MI. In a multivariate analysis of 131 patients with endometrioid endometrial cancer, MI remained predictive of survival ($p = 0.03$) after controlling for stage and grade (56). The MI was present in a subset of atypical endometrial hyperplasias. Like *PTEN* mutation, MI occurs early in endometrial carcinogenesis.

HEREDITARY ENDOMETRIAL CANCER

The MI initially was noted in colorectal cancers of patients with HNPCC, also known as Lynch syndrome type II (52,53). Endometrial cancer is the second most common malignancy observed in these families, but ovarian, gastrointestinal and upper urinary tract malignancies also occur. Subsequently, it was shown that affected individuals in HNPCC families carry germline mutations in one of a family of DNA repair genes. Alterations of *MSH2* gene on chromosome 2p, the *MLH1* gene on chromosome 3p, and the *MSH6* on chromosome 2 accounts for most HNPCC families, but at least two other DNA repair genes (*PMS1* and *PMS2*) also have been implicated (57–62). In bacteria and yeast, mutations in these DNA repair enzymes also lead to MI, confirming the cause and effect relationship between these events.

In families in which early onset colon cancer occurs along with other cancers including endometrial cancer, genetic testing for mutations in DNA repair genes is appropriate. In one study of several kindreds in which MSH2 or MLH1 mutations had been identified, the lifetime risk in women of endometrial cancer (42%) exceeded the risk of colon cancer (30%) (59). Early diagnosis and prevention of colon, endometrial, and other associated cancers is an important issue in families with germline mutations in DNA repair genes. The role of colonoscopy versus prophylatic colectomy remains controversial. An annual endometrial biopsy or vaginal probe ultrasound have been advocated for screening in patients with HNPCC. Hysterectomy should be performed in female carriers in whom colectomy is undertaken. In view of the increased risk of ovarian cancer in HNPCC syndrome, concomitant prophylactic oophorectomy should be strongly considered.

EPIGENETICS IN ENDOMETRIAL CARCINOMA

Several studies have addressed the molecular genetic features of endometrial carcinomas by global survey methodologies such as allelotyping and comparative genomic hybridization. One observation in these studies by our group and others is the existence of cancers without evidence of genetic alterations (i.e., no detectable LOH, chromosomal gain or loss, or mutation in genes such as *PTEN, KRAS2, CTNNB1* or *TP53*). In view of this, we hypothesize that epigenetic mechanisms may play a significant role in endometrial carcinogenesis. These epigenetic changes probably are the result of multiple mechanisms including loss of imprinting and gene promoter silencing associated with CpG hypermethylation.

MLH1 Methylation

Most sporadic endometrial carcinomas with MI do not contain mutations of the MMR genes, *hMLH1* or *hMSH2* (63,64), but instead lack normal expression of the *hMLH1* gene. Hypermethylation of the *hMLH1* promoter and subsequent lack of normal mRNA expression is an underlying cause of MI in the majority of endometrial cancer (65). Our group has confirmed that hypermethylation of the *hMLH1* promoter occurs in approximately 20% of sporadic endometrial cancers (unpublished data) (Fig. 2). These data also demonstrate that the MI phenotype and this specific epigenetic mechanism are specific for type I endometrioid endometrial cancers. The epigenetic silencing of MLH1 has been observed in endometrial hyerplasias suggesting that this event may occur early in the development of endometrial cancer (66).

APC Methylation

Accumulation of β-catenin and activation of the Tcf/Lef pathway is a feature of some endometrial cancers. Although β-catenin overexpression is not

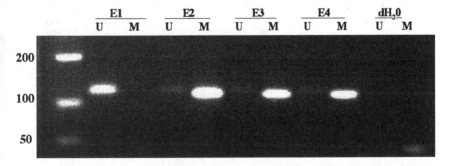

Figure 2 Methylation specific PCR of the *hMLH1* promoter in endometrial carcinomas. U represents unmethylated and M represents PCR products specific for unmethylated or methylated promoter sequence. Endometrial carcinoma case E1 has unmethylated *hMLH1* promoter sequences based on the presence of a strong PCR product in the unmethylated PCR reaction and absence of any product in the methylation specific reaction. Cases E3–E4 all have strong PCR product in the methylation specific PCR assay indicating the presence of methylated sequence in the *hMLH1* promoter. These cases also depict weak amplification in the unmethylated reactions presumably due to amplification from non-tumor DNA components of the biopsy (i.e., stromal cells or infiltrating lymphocytes). Microsatellite analysis of these cases indicates that case E1 has stable microsatellites and E2–E4 have microsatellite instability (data not depicted).

mediated through mutation of APC or β-catenin in a majority of cases (22,28) hypermethylation of the APC promoter can result in a loss of APC expression and subsequent β-catenin accumulation. A preliminary analysis (unpublished) by our group has revealed hypermethylation of the APC promoter in 70% of endometrial cancer cell lines and in 30% of primary endometrial cancers. Others have found hypermethylation of the APC promoter in 46% of endometrial cancers, and determined that this alteration is more commonly found in association with type I cancers with endometrioid histology and MI (67,68). Methylation of the APC promoter has not yet been demonstated to result in reduced levels of APC protein in endometrial cancers.

Methylation Epigenetic Silencing of Other Genes

Global hypermethylation of genes involved in cell cycle control, apoptosis, cell adhesion and other regulatory cellular functions has been implicated in gene silencing and resultant carcinogenesis (69). Gene promotor regions rich in CpG pairs are particularly susceptible to methylation and cancers characterized by global hypermethylation are noted as having a CpG island methylator phenotype (70). In an assessment of HOXA11, THBS-1 and 2, MLH1, CTNNB1, VDR, and CDKN2A, investigators have observed that endometrioid endometrial cancers are characterized by a methylator phenotype. Hypermethylation of HOXA11 was found in over 70% of endometrioid endometrial cancers and was found to be associated with poor outcome (71). Our group similarly performed promoter methylation analysis on a panel of 64 endometrial cancers that typify type I (endometrioid) and type II (serous or CC) lesions. The genes chosen for analysis (*MLH1, MGMT, APC, P14, P15, P16, P73, RASSF1A, DAPK, GSTPI,* and *BRCA1*) have been previously noted to have promoter methylation in various cancer types. Promoter methylation was found in at least one cancer in 5:11 genes screened in type I endometrial cancers, while no evidence of hypermethylation was detected at any of the loci in the type II cancers (72).

Some endometrial cancers develop in the setting of a hyperestrogenic milieu and resultant endometrial hyperplasia. Progestin is protective against the tumorgenic effects of estrogen, and can decrease the growth of endometrial cancers that express progestin receptor. Investigators have evaluated the promoter methylation status of the genes encoding the various isoforms of the estrogen and progesterone receptors (73–76) in order to determine if epigenetic inactivation of hormone receptor genes is associated with endometrial carcinogenesis. A recent report revealed a high incidence of methylation of the progesterone receptor B isoform in endometrial cancers suggesting that a hyperestrogenic state might be induced by decreasing the effects of progestin. Immunohistochemical staining of primary endometrial cancers revealed decreased expression of progestin receptor B in those cases with methylated promoter. No significant changes in progestin receptor A protocol methylation or immunohistochemical expression were noted (76).

Hormones as an Epigenetic Phenomena

The synthetic non-steroidal estrogen, diethylstilbestrol (DES), was administered during pregnancy to over two million women during 1940–1960. Subsequently, the use of DES was banned by the U.S. Food and Drug Administration (FDA) due to teratogenic effects on limb bud development. Epidemiological studies later revealed that seemingly normal offspring of mothers who ingested DES prenatally developed CC adenocarcinomas of the vagina and cervix as young adults (77,78). In a laboratory setting, DES was found to induce gynecologic carcinomas in developmentally exposed rodents (79,80). Mice treated neonatally with DES on days one to five have a 90–95% incidence of endometrial carcinoma at 18 months of life (81). These data strongly implicate a direct role for estrogen exposure (even early in development) in gynecologic carcinogenesis. Although an increased incidence of vaginal and cervical CC cancers have been linked to antenatal DES exposure, an increased risk of endometrial carcinoma may be more difficult to detect because it is much more common in the population. In addition, since the cohort of DES exposed patients has not yet reached the median age of patients with endometrial cancer, the increased risk of this cancer type may not be currently apparent.

The increased incidence of gynecologic cancer associated with antenatal DES exposure would suggest that the developing fetus or neonate is particularly susceptible to the epigenetic effects of estrogen. Investigators recently evaluated the carcinogenic potential of neonatal exposure for another estrogen compound, genistein, and a naturally occurring phytoestrogen that is found in many soy products. In this study, treated mice received equivalent estrogenic doses of either DES, genistein, or control on days one to five. At 18 months, the incidence of uterine adenocarcinomas was 31% for DES and 35% for genistein, suggesting that estrogenic compounds other than DES may be carcinogenic if exposure occurs early during key developmental windows (81).

The mechanism by which DES induces cancers in the gynecologic tract is not well known. Some proposed mechanisms include hormonal induction of cell proliferation, the heritable reprogramming of gene expression, somatic induction of mutation by DES metabolites, and induction of chromosomal abnormalities by disruption of the spindle microtubule apparatus (82–87). Activation of specific regulatory genes also may occur secondary to DES exposure; widespread gene amplification has been demonstrated in DES-induced mouse uterine adenocarcinomas (88). Although mutations in specific oncogenes and tumor suppressor genes (i.e., *p53*, K-RAS, H-RAS, and WT1) have not been found in vaginal and cervical CC carcinomas from patients with a history of DES exposure, MI appears to be increased in the tumors from these DES exposed patients (89). The specific molecular alteration leading to the MI has not been elucidated but could be related to either mutation of an MMR gene or epigenetic modulation of an MMR gene promoter. Rodent studies have revealed that DES can affect the promoter methylation state leading to a remodeling of gene expression (90).

MICROARRAY

The ability to interrogate thousands of genes simultaneously using microarray technology has significantly changed our approach to the analysis of gene expression profiles in cancers and normal tissues. Such comprehensive technologies permit the assessment not of individual genes, but of clusters of genes that are coordinately expressed to generate fingerprints of specific cell types. Using this technique, mRNA is extracted from a tissue specimen and through reverse transcription cDNA or cRNA is made. Although hybridization has been used for decades to detect and quantify nucleic acids, the miniaturization of the process has facilitated the review of gene expression on a genomic scale.

The use of an oligonucleotide platform such as Affymetrix involves the synthesis of biotin-labeled cRNA that is used to hybridize to oligomers on the microarray chip. Approximately 11–16 probes are selected among all possible 25-mers to represent each transcript. For each probe designed to be perfectly complementary to a target sequence, a partner probe is generated that is identical except for a single base mismatch in its center. These probe pairs, called the Perfect Match probe (PM) and the Mismatch probe (MM), allow subtraction of signals caused by non-specific hybridization. The difference in hybridization signals between the partners, as well as their intensity ratios, serve as indicators of specific transcript abundance.

The use of a cDNA microarray chip requires both a tissue specimen cRNA and a "universal standard" cRNA, each of which is labeled with either cytochrome 3 (dark grey) or cytochrome 5 (light grey). Following hybridization of the mixture containing both the labeled specimen and universal standard cRNAs with the microchip containing cDNA probes, the microarray scanner determines whether known probes on the microchip bind to either or both of the cytochromes. Determination of the ratio of expression of the two cytochromes facilitates an estimation of target expression in the specimen.

To elucidate further the molecular pathogenesis of endometrial cancers, high through-put technologies such as microarray offer the opportunity to increase our understanding of the molecular pathogenesis of endometrial cancer and to enhance prediction of clinical phenotypes. The molecular pathogenesis of endometrial cancer is incompletely understood. Although alterations in several genes noted above have been described, none are present in the majority of cases and some endometrial cancers lack

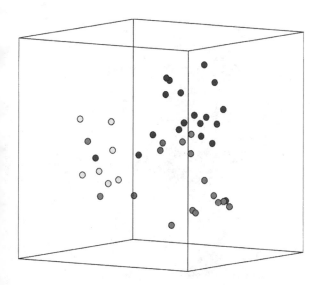

Figure 3 Multidimensional scaling model based on the overall gene expression in papillary serous, endometrioid, clear cell, and normal endometrium.

evidence of alterations in any of these genes. Recently, microarray pilot studies have confirmed that although both endometrioid and non-endometrioid endometrial cancers share some common genetic alterations when compared to normal endometrium, there are multiple genes that are differentially up-regulated and down-regulated among types I and II endometrial cancers (Fig. 3). In addition, expression profiles may be unique even for subgroups of type I endometrial cancers. Microarray experiments have provided additional unrecognized genes important in the development of endometrial cancer (Fig. 4) and suggest multiple avenues of investigation for targeted molecular therapies (91,92). Current studies are underway to define expression patterns associated with poor prognostic features.

SUMMARY OF THE MOLECULAR BIOLOGY OF ENDOMETRIAL CANCER

Type I endometrial cancers display a high incidence (37–82%) of mutation in the *PTEN* tumor suppressor gene. In addition, approximately 20% display MI with corresponding hypermethylation and lack of expression of the *hMLH1* DNA–MMR gene. In contrast type II tumors rarely if ever contain *PTEN* mutations or MI, but are more likely to be characterized by *p53* mutation, HER-2/*neu* overexpression, and widespread aneuploidy (Table 2). Despite these important characterizations distinguishing type I from type II endometrial cancers, little is known regarding the molecular events underlying the pathogenesis of endometrial cancer. In fact, many type I endometrial cancers

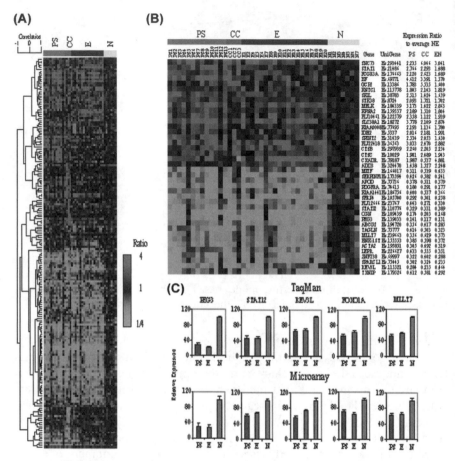

Figure 4 Molecular profiles of all 42 specimens: 13 papillary serous (PS), 19 endometrioid (E), three clear cell (CC), and seven normal endometrium (N). (**A**) Hierarchical clustering of the 20 most upregulated and the 20 most down-regulated genes in the comparison of the four groups (*p* < 0.001) using a threshold of twofold. The cluster is color-coded using white for up-regulation from normal endometrium, gray for down-regulation and black for median expression. Agglomerative clustering of genes was illustrated with dendrograms. The symbol for each gene is followed by the Unigene clone number of the corresponding DNA spotted on the array. Expression ratios comparing each of the two groups to normal endometrium as well as to each other are listed. (**B**) Quantitative PCR (TaqMan) and microarray expression analysis of five selected genes differentially expressed between papillary serous and endometrioid cancers with normal endometria.

present with no outward evidence of genetic disease as they have no mutations in *PTEN* or K-RAS, are microsatellite stable, have no detectable LOH, and have near-diploid karyotypes. Similarly, many type II endometrial cancers lack known mutations or deletions of important oncogenes and tumor suppressor genes. Recent evidence suggests that a significant proportion of endometrial

Table 2 Endometrial Cancer: Molecular Profiles of Clinical Phenotypes

	Type I	Type II
Ploidy	Near-diploid	Aneuploid
HER-2/*neu* overexpression	Infrequent	Frequent
p53 mutation	Infrequent	Frequent
K-ras activating mutation	Frequent	Infrequent
PTEN mutation	Frequent	Infrequent
Microsatellite instability	Frequent	Infrequent
β-Catenin mutation	Frequent	Infrequent

cancers may develop via epigenetic mechanisms (such as promoter methylation), particularly in type I endometrial cancers. Preliminary microarray experiments have revealed that the genomic expression profiles of various histologic subtypes are unique. Elucidation of these molecular expression signatures may be useful in predicting the clinical behavior of endometrial cancers as well as identifying candidate cellular pathways that can be targets for chemopreventive strategies.

REFERENCES

1. American Cancer Society: Cancer Facts and Figures 2002.
2. Gallup DG, Stock RJ. Adenocarcinoma of the endometrium in women 40 years of age or younger. Obstet Gynecol 1984; 64:417.
3. Boyd J, Risinger JI. Analysis of oncogene alterations in human endometrial carcinoma: prevalence of ras mutations. Mol Carcinog 1991; 4:189–195.
4. Ignar-Trowbridge D, Risinger JI, Dent GA, Kohler M, Berchuck A, McLachlan JA, Boyd J. Mutations of the Ki-ras oncogene in endometrial carcinoma. Am J Obstet Gynecol 1992; 167:227–232.
5. Lagarda H, Catasus L, Arguelles R, Matias-Guiu X, Prat J. K-ras mutations in endometrial carcinomas with microsatellite instability. J Pathol 2001; 193: 193–199.
6. Enomoto T, Fujita M, Inoue M, Rice JM, Nakajima R, Tanazawa O, Nomura, T. Alterations of the *p53* tumor suppressor gene and its association with activation of the c-K-*ras*-2 protooncogene in premalignant and malignant lesions of the human uterine endometrium. Cancer Res 1993; 53:1883–1888.
7. Enomoto T, Inoue M, Perantoni AO, Terakawa N, Tanizawa O, Rice JM. K-ras activation in neoplasms of the human female reproductive tract. Cancer Res 1990; 50:6139–6145.
8. Enomoto T, Inoue M, Perantoni AO, Buzard GS, Miki H, Tanizawa O, Rice JM. K-*ras* activation in premalignant and malignant epithelial lesions of the human uterus. Cancer Res 1991; 51:5308–5314.
9. Fujimoto I, Shimizu Y, Hirai Y, Chen J-T, Teshima H, Hasumi K, Masubuchi K, Takahashi M. Studies on *ras* oncogene activation in endometrial carcinoma. Cancer Res 1993; 48:196–202.

10. Duggan BD, Felix JC, Muderspach LI, Tsao JL, Shibata DK. Early mutational activation of the c-Ki-ras oncogene in endometrial carcinoma. Cancer Res 1994; 54:1604–1607.

11. Sasaki H, Nishii H, Tada A, Furusato M, Terashima Y, Siegal GP, Parker SL, Kohler MF, Berchuck A, Boyd J. Mutation of the Ki-*ras* protooncogene in human endometrial hyperplasia and carcinoma. Cancer Res 1993; 53:1906–1910.

12. Cirisano FD, Karlan BY. Role of Her-2/neu in gynecologic malignancies. Contemp Ob-Gyn 1996; 39:49–75.

13. Lukes AS, Kohler MF, Pieper CF, Kerns BJ, Bentley R, Rodriguez GC, Soper JT, Clarke-Pearson DL, Bast RC Jr, Berchuck A. Multivariable analysis of DNA ploidy, *p53*, and HER-2/neu as prognostic factors in endometrial cancer. Cancer 1994; 73:2380–2385.

14. Khalifa MA, Mannel RS, Haraway SD, Walker J, Min K-W. Expression of EGFR, HER-2/*neu*, *p53*, and PCNA in endometrioid, serous papillary, and clear cell endometrial adenocarcinomas. Cancer Res 1994; 53:84–92.

15. Berchuck A, Rodriguez G, Kinney RB, Soper JT, Dodge RK, Clarke-Pearson DL, Bast RC Jr. Overexpression of HER-2/neu in endometrial cancer is associated with advanced stage disease. Am J Obstet Gynecol 1991; 164:15–21.

16. Bigsby RM, Aixin L, Bomalaski J, Stehman FB, Look KY, Sutton GP. Immunohistochemical study of HER-2/*neu*, epidermal growth factor receptor, and steroid receptor expression in normal and malignant endometrium. Obstet Gynecol 1992; 79:95–100.

17. Monk BJ, Chapman JA, Johnson GA, Brightman BK, Wilczynski SP, Schell MJ, Fan H. Correlation of c-*myc* and HER-2/*neu* amplification and expression with histopathologic variables in uterine corpus cancer. Am J Obstet Gynecol 1994; 171:1193–1198.

18. Hetzel DJ, Wilson TO, Keeney GL, Roche PC, Cha SS, Podratz KC. HER-2/ *neu* expression: a major prognostic factor in endometrial cancer. Cancer Res 1992; 47:179–185.

19. Abulafia O, Ruiz JE, Holcomb K, Dimaio TM, Lee YC, Sherer DM. Angiogenesis in early-invasive and low-malignant-potential epithelial ovarian carcinoma. Obstet Gynecol 2000; 95:548–552.

20. Bullions LC, Levine AJ. The role of beta-catenin in cell adhesion, signal transduction, and cancer. Cancer Biol 1998; 10:81–87.

21. Sparks AB, Morin PJ, Vogelstein B, Kinzler KW. Mutational analysis of the APC/ β-Catenin/Tcf pathway in colorectal cancer. Cancer Res 1998; 58: 1130–1134.

22. Schlosshauer PW, Pirog EC, Levine RL, Elleson LH. Mutational analysis of the CTNNB1 and APC genes in uterine endometrioid carcinoma. Mod Pathol 2000; 13:1066–1071.

23. Maxwell GL, Risinger JI, Carney ME, Hayes K, Dodge R, Barrett JC, Berchuck A. Mutation in the *PTEN* and β-Catenin genes and in microsatellite sequences are features of some endometrioid endometrial cancers. Gynecol Oncol 1999; 72:467.

24. Kobayashi K, Sagae S, Nishioka Y, Tokino T, Kudo R. Mutations of the B-catenin gene in endometrial carcinomas. Jpn J Cancer Res 1999; 90:55–59.

25. Saegusa M, Hashimura M, Yoshida T, Okayasu I. Beta-Catenin mutations and aberrant nuclear expression during endometrial tumorigenesis. Br J Cancer 2001; 84:209–217.
26. Ikeda T, Yoshinaga K, SembaD, Kondo E, Ohmori H, Horii A. Mutational analysis of the CTNNB1 (beta-catenin) gene in human endometrial cancer: frequent mutations at codon 34 that cause nuclear accumulation. Oncol Rep 2000; 7:323–326.
27. Machin P, Catasus L, Pons C, Munoz J, Matias-Guiu X, Prat J. CTNNB1 mutations and beta-catenin expression in endometrial carcinomas. Hum Pathol 2002; 33:206–212.
28. Fukuchi T, Sakamoto M, Tsuda H, Maruyama K, Nozawa S, Hirohashi S. Beta-catenin mutation in carcinoma of the uterine endometrium. Cancer Res 1998; 58:3526–3528.
29. Fujino T, Risinger JI, Collins NK, Liu FS, Nishii H, Takahashi H, Westphal EM, Barrett JC, Sasaki H, Kohler MF, et al. Allelotype of endometrial carcinoma. Cancer Res 1994; 54:4294–4298.
30. Oshimura M, Kugoh H, Koi M, Shimizu M, Yamada H, Satoh H, Barrett JC. Transfer of a normal human chromosome 11 suppresses tumorigenicity of some but not all tumor cell lines. J Cell Biochem 1990; 42:135–142.
31. Yamada H, Wake N, Fujimoto S, Barrett JC, Oshimura M. Multiple chromosomes carrying tumor suppressor activity for a uterine endometrial carcinoma cell line identified by microcell-mediated chromosome transfer. Oncogene 1990; 5:1141–1147.
32. Yamada H, Sasaki M, Honda T, Wake N, Boyd J, Oshimura M, Barrett JC. Suppression of endometrial carcinoma cell tumorigenicity by human chromosome 18. Genes Chromosomes Cancer 1995; 13:18–24.
33. Lukes AS, Kohler MF, Pieper CF, Kerns BJ, Bentley R, Rodriguez GC, Soper JT, Clarke-Pearson DL, Bast RC Jr, Berchuck A. Multivariable analysis of DNA ploidy, *p53*, and HER-2/neu as prognostic factors in endometrial cancer. Cancer 1994; 73:2380–2385.
34. Kohler MF, Berchuck A, Davidoff AM, Humphrey PA, Dodge RK, Iglehart JD, Soper JT, Clarke-Pearson DL, Bast RC Jr, Marks JR. Overexpression and mutation of *p53* in endometrial carcinoma. Cancer Res 1992; 52:1622–1627.
35. Hachisuga T, Fukuda K, Uchiyama M, Matsuo N, Iwasaka T, Sugimore H. Immunohistochemical study of *p53* expression in endometrial carcinomas: correlation with markers of proliferating cells and clinicopathologic features. Int J Gynecol Cancer 1993; 3:363–368.
36. Boike GM, Petru E, Sevin BU, Averette HE, Chou TC, Penalver M, Donato D, Schiano M, Hilsenbeck SG, Perras I. Chemical enhancement of cisplatin cytotoxicity in a human ovarian and cervical cancer cell line. Cancer Res 1990; 38:315–322.
37. Bonneterre J, Peyrat JP, Beuscart R, Demaille A. Prognostic significance of insulin-like growth factor 1 receptors in human breast cancer. Cancer Res 1990; 50:6931–6935.
38. Kohler MF, Nishii H, Humphrey PA, Saski H, Marks J, Bast RC, Clarke-Pearson DL, Boyd J, Berchuck A. Mutation of the *p53* tumor-suppressor gene is not a feature of endometrial hyperplasias. Am J Obstet Gynecol 1993; 169:690–694.

39. Tashiro H, Isacson C, Levine R, Kurman RJ, Cho KR, Hedrick L. *p53* gene mutations are common in uterine serous carcinoma and occur early in their pathogenesis. Am J Pathol 1997; 150:177–185.
40. Simpson L, Parsons R. PTEN. life as a tumor suppressor. Exp Cell Res 2001; 264:29–41.
41. Sakurada A, Hamada H, Fukushige S, Yokoyama T, Yoshinaga K, Furukawa T, Sato S, Yajima A, Sato M, Fujimura S, Horii A. Adenovirus-mediated delivery of the PTEN gene inhibits cell growth by induction of apoptosis in endometrial cancer. Int J Oncol 1999; 15:1069–1074.
42. Nagase S, Sato S, Tezuka F, Wada Y, Yajima A, Horii A. Deletion mapping on chromosome 10q25-q26 in human endometrial cancer. Br J Cancer 1996; 74: 1979–1983.
43. Yamakawa H, Nagase S, Yuki M, Shiwaku HO, Furukawa T, Yoshinaga K, Soeda E, Hoshi M, Hayashi Y, Sato S, Yajima A, Horii A. Identification of a 100-kb region of common allelic loss on chromosome bands 10q25-q26 in human endometrial cancer. Genes Chromosomes Cancer 1998; 23:74–77.
44. Peiffer-Schneider S, Noonan FC, Mutch DG, Simpkins SB, Herzog T, Rader J, Elbendary A, Gersell DJ, Call K, Goodfellow PJ. Mapping an endometrial cancer tumor suppressor gene at 10q25 and development of a bacterial clone contig for the consensus deletion interval. Genomics 1998; 52:9–16.
45. Simpkins SB, Peiffer-Schneider S, Mutch DG, Gersell D, Goodfellow PJ. PTEN mutations in endometrial cancers with 10q LOH: additional evidence for the involvement of multiple tumor suppressors. Gynecol Oncol1998 1998; 71:391–395.
46. Risinger JI, Hayes AK, Berchuck A, Barrett JC. PTEN/MMAC1 mutations in endometrial cancers. Cancer Res 1997; 57:4736–4738.
47. Kong D, Suzuki A, Zou TT, Sakurada A, Kemp LW, Wakatsuki S, Yokoyama T, Yamakawa H, Furukawa T, Sato M, et al. PTEN1 is frequently mutated in primary endometrial carcinomas. Nat Genet 1997; 17:143–144.
48. Tashiro H, Blazes MS, Wu R, Cho KR, Bose S, Wang SI, Li J, Parsons R, Ellenson LH. Mutations in PTEN are frequent in endometrial carcinoma but rare in other common gynecological malignancies. Cancer Res 1997; 57:3935–3940.
49. Risinger JI, Hayes K, Maxwell GL, Carney ME, Dodge RK, Barrett JC, Berchuck A. PTEN mutation in endometrial cancers is associated with favorable clinical and pathologic characteristics. Clin Cancer Res 1998; 4:3005–3010.
50. Maxwell GL, Risinger JI, Gumbs C, Shaw H, Bentley RC, Barrett JC, Berchuck A, Futreal PA. Mutation of the PTEN tumor suppressor gene in endometrial hyperplasias. Cancer Res 1998; 58:2500–2503.
51. Maxwell GL, Risinger JI, Hayes KA, Alvarez AA, Dodge RK, Barrett JC, Berchuck A. Racial disparity in the frequency of PTEN mutations, but not microsatellite instability, in advanced endometrial cancers. Clin Cancer Res 2000; 6:2999–3005.
52. Munoz N, Bosch FX, de Sanjose S, Herrero R, Castellsague X, Shah KV, Snijders PJ, Meijer CJ. Epidemiologic classification of human papillomavirus types associated with cervical cancer. N Engl J Med 2003; 348:518–527.
53. Thibodeau SN, Bren G, Schaid D. Microsatellite instability in cancer of the proximal colon. Science 1993; 260:816–819.

54. Risinger JI, Berchuck A, Kohler MF, Watson P, Lynch HT, Boyd J. Genetic instability of microsatellites in endometrial carcinoma. Cancer Res 1993; 53: 5100–5133.
55. Risinger JI, Berchuck A, Kohler MF, Watson P, Lynch HT, Boyd J. Genetic instability of microsatellites in endometrial carcinoma. Cancer Res 1993; 53: 5100–5103.
56. Maxwell GL, Risinger JI, Alvarez AA, Barrett JC, Berchuck A. Favorable survival associated with microsatellite instability in endometrioid endometrial cancers. Obstet Gynecol 2001; 97:417–422.
57. Lynch HT, Lemon SJ, Karr B, Franklin B, Lynch JF, Watson P, Tinley S, Lerman C, Carter C. Etiology, natural history, management and molecular genetics of hereditary nonpolyposis colorectal cancer (Lynch syndromes): genetic counseling implications. Cancer Epidemiol Biomarkers Prev 1997; 6: 987–991.
58. Lynch HT, Smyrk T, Lynch J. An update of HNPCC (Lynch syndrome). Cancer Genet Cytogenet 1997; 93:84–99.
59. Bacus SS, Ruby SG, Weinberg DS, Chin D, Ortiz R, Bacus JW. Her-2/neu oncogene expression and proliferation in breast cancers. Am J Pathol 1990; 137:103–111.
60. Goodfellow PJ, Buttin BM, Herzog TJ, Rader JS, Gibb RK, Swisher E, Look K, Walls KC, Fan M-Y, Mutch DG. Prevalence of defective DNA mismatch repair and MSH6 mutation in an unselected series of endometrial cancers. PNAS 2003; 100:5908–5913.
61. Charames GS, Millar AL, Pal T, Narod S, Bapat B. Do MSH6 mutations contribute to double primary cancers of the colorectum and endometrium. Hum Genet 2000; 107:623–629.
62. Wijnen J, de Leeuw W, Vasen H, van der KH, Moller P, Stormorken A, Meijers-Heijboer H, Lindhout D, Menko F, Vossen S, Moslein G, Tops C, Brocker-Vriends A, Wn Y, Hofstra R, Sijmons R, Cornelisse C, Morrean H, Fodde R. Familial endometrial cancer in female carriers of MSH6 germline mutations. Nat Genet 1999; 23:142–144.
63. Akiyama T, Sudo C, Ogawara H, Toyoshima K, Yamamoto T. The product of the human o-erbB-2 gene: a 185-kilodalton glycoprotein with tyrosine kinase activity. Science 1986; 232:1644–1646.
64. Kowalski LD, Mutch DG, Herzog TJ, Rader JS, Goodfellow PJ. Mutational analysis of MLH1 and MSH2 in 25 prospectively- acquired RER+ endometrial cancers. Genes Chromosomes Cancer 1997; 18:219–227.
65. Esteller M, Levine R, Baylin SB, Ellenson LH, Herman JG. MLH1 promoter hypermethylation is associated with the microsatellite instability phenotype in sporadic endometrial carcinomas. Oncogene 1998; 17:2413–2417.
66. Esteller M, Catasus L, Matias-Guiu X, Mutter GL, Prat J, Baylin SB, Herman JG. hMLH1 promoter hypermethylation is an early event in human endometrial tumorigenesis. Am J Pathol 1999; 155:1762–1772.
67. Moreno-Bueno G, Hardisson D, Sanchez C, Sarrio D, Cassia R, Garcia-Rostan G, Prat J, Guo M, Herman JG, Matias-Guiu X, Esteller M, Palacios J. Abnormalities of the APC/beta-catenin pathway in endometrial cancer. Oncogene 2002; 21:7981–7990.

68. Zysman M, Saka A, Millar A, Knight J, Chapman W, Bapat B. Methylation of adenomatous polyposis coli in endometrial cancer occurs more frequently in tumors with microsatellite instability phenotype. Cancer Res 2002; 62: 3663–3666.
69. Herman JG, Baylin SB. Promotor-region hypermethylation and gene silencing in human cancer. Curr Top Microbiol Immunol 2000; 249:35–54.
70. Toyota M, Ahuja N, Ohe-Toyota M, Herman JG, Baylin SB, Issa JP. CpG island mthylator phenotype inncolorectal cancer. Proc Natl Acad Sci USA 1999; 96:8681–8686.
71. Whitcomb BP, Mutch DG, Herzog TJ, Rader JS, Gibb RK, Goodfellow PJ. Frequent HOXA11 and THBS2 promoter methylation, and a methylator phenotype in endometrial adenocarcinoma. Clin Cancer Res 2003; 9:2277–2287.
72. Risinger J, Maxwell GL, Berchuck A, Barrett C. Promoter hypermethylation as an epigenetic component in Type I and Type II Cancers. Ann N Y Acad Sci 2003; 983:209–212.
73. Hori M, Takechi Km Arai Y, Yomo H, Itabashi M, Shimazaki J, Inagawa S, Hori M. Assessment of hypermethylated DNA in two promoter regions of the estrogen receptor alpha gene in human endometrial diseases. Gynecol Oncol 2000; 76:89–96.
74. Navari JR, Roland PY, Keh P, Salvesen HB, Akslen LA, Iversen OE, Das S, Kothari R, Howy S, Phillips B. Loss of estrogen receptor (ER) expression in endometrial tumors is not associated with de novo methylation of the 5' end of the ER gene. Clin Cancer Res 2000; 6:4026–4032.
75. Shiozawa T, Ohara M, Itoh K, Shizawa T, Konishi I. Down-regulation of estrogen receptor by the methylation of the estrogen receptor gene in endometrial carcinoma. Anticancer Res 2002; 22:139–143.
76. Sasaki M, Dharia A, Oh BR, Tanaka Y, Fujimoto S, Dahiya R. Progesterone receptor B gene inactivation and CpG hypermethylation in human uterine endometrial cancer. Cancer Res 2001; 6:97–102.
77. Herbst AL, Ulfelder H, Poskanzer DC. Adenocarcinoma of the vagina. Association of maternal stilbestrol therapy with tumor appearance in young women. N Engl J Med 1971; 284:878–881.
78. Herbst AL, Cole P, Colton T, Robboy SJ, Scully RE. Age-incidence and risk of diethylstilbestrol-related clear cell adenocarcinoma of the vagina and cervix. Am J Obstet Gynecol 1977; 128:43–50.
79. McLachlan JA, Newbold RR, Bullock BC. Long-term effects on the female mouse genital tract associated with prenatal exposure to diethylstilbestrol. Cancer Res 1980; 40:3988–3999.
80. Newbold RR, Bullock BC, McLachlan JA. Uterine adenocarcinoma in mice following developmental treatment with estrogen: a model for hormonal carcinogenesis. Cancer Res 1990; 50:7677–7681.
81. Newbold RR, Banks EP, Bullock B, Jefferson WN. Uterine adenocarcinoma in mice treated neonatally with Genistein. Cancer Res 2001; 61: (In press) Still unpublished..
82. Barrett JC, Wong, A, McLachlan JA. Diethylstilbestrol induces neoplastic transformation without measurable gene mutation at two loci. Science 1981; 212:1402–1404.

83. Barrett JC, Hesterberg TW, Oshimura M, Tsutsui T. Role of chemically induced mutagenic events in neoplastic transformation of Syrian hamster embryo cells. Carcinog Compr Surv 1985; 9:123–137.
84. Barrett JC. Cell culture models of multistep carcinogenesis. IARC Sci Publ 1985; 58:181–202.
85. Barrett JC, Shelby MD. Mechanisms of multistep carcinogenesis: keys to developing in vitro approaches for assessing the carcinogenicity of chemicals. Food Chem Toxicol 1986; 24:657–61.
86. Tsutsui T, Suzuki N, Fukuda S, Sato M, Maizumi H, McLachlan JA, Barrett JC. 17beta-Estradiol-induced cell transformation and aneuploidy of Syrian hamster embryo cells in culture. Carcinogenesis 1987; 8:1715–1719.
87. Tsutsui T, Suzuki N, Maizumi H, Barrett JC. Aneuploidy induction in human fibroblasts: comparison with results in Syrian hamster fibroblasts. Mutat Res 1990; 240:241–249.
88. Risinger JI, Terry LA, Boyd J. Use of representational difference analysis for the identification of mdm2 oncogene amplification in diethylstilbestrol-induced murine uterine adenocarcinomas. Mol Carcinog 1994; 11:13–8.
89. Boyd J, Takahashi H, Waggoner SE, Jones LA, Hajek RA, Wharton JT, Liu FS, Fujino T, Barrett JC, McLachlan JA. Molecular genetic analysis of clear cell adenoarcinomas of the vagina and cervix associated and unassociated with diethylstilbestrol exposure in utero. Cancer 1996; 77:507–513.
90. Li S, Washburn KA, Moore R, Uno T, Teng C, Newbold RR, McLachlan JA, Negishi M. Developmental exposure to diethylstilbestrol elicits demethylation of estrogen-responsive lactoferrin gene in mouse uterus. Cancer Res 1997; 57: 4356–4359.
91. Risinger JI, Maxwell GL, Chandramouli GV, Jazaeri A, Aprelikova O, Patterson T, Berchuck A, Barrett JC. Microarray analysis reveals distinct gene expression profiles among different histologic types of endometrial cancer. Cancer Res 2003; 63:6–11.
92. Mutter GL, Baak JP, Fitzgerald JT, Gray R, Neuberg D, Kust GA, Gentleman R, Gullans SR, Wei LJ, Wilcox M. Global expression changes of constitutive and hormonally regulated genes during endometrial neoplasia. Gynecol Oncol 2001; 83:177–185.

6

Clinical Presentation and Investigation: The "One-Stop" Clinic, Endometrial Sampling, Hysteroscopy, Vaginal Ultrasound

Christopher Lee and Davor Jurkovic

Early Pregnancy and Gynaecology Assessment Unit, Kings College Hospital, London, U.K.

INTRODUCTION

Endometrial cancer typically presents with a history of postmenopausal bleeding. The reported incidence of malignancy in women presenting with bleeding after menopause is between 5% and 15% (1–3). All women presenting in this way, therefore, warrant further investigation; the primary aim of investigation being to differentiate benign from malignant causes of bleeding. Women experiencing irregular bleeding on hormone replacement therapy also require further investigation, although the risk of malignancy is significantly lower in this group (overall relative risk 1.3%) (4). It is now well established that women treated with the anti-breast cancer drug tamoxifen are at increased risk of developing endometrial cancer (5–7). The increase in incidence of endometrial cancer in women treated with tamoxifen was twofold (0.79 vs. 0.37) in the literature review of placebo-controlled trials by Assikis et al. (8). The worldwide overview on tamoxifen as an adjuvant for breast cancer therapy from the Early Breast Cancer Trialists' Collaborative (9) found that tamoxifen treatment in postmenopausal women reduced mortality by almost 25% and recurrence of breast cancer by 50% (9). Because of these beneficial effects in the treatment of breast cancer, tamoxifen usage is very widespread. Special consideration is required in planning investigation and endometrial surveillance in these women.

A thorough clinical history and examination remain vital components of the assessment of women with a history of abnormal bleeding. Factors associated with an increased incidence of endometrial cancer include advanced age, obesity, infertility, low parity, and family history (10,11). The nature of the bleeding should be ascertained; recurrent episodes of bleeding are more likely to be associated with endometrial pathology.

In this chapter, we will review the current evidence on outpatient investigation and management planning for women presenting with postmenopausal bleeding, as well as describe the key elements that need to be addressed in planning an accurate, cost-effective, clinic-based service for the triage and management of women presenting in this way.

INVESTIGATIONS

Blind Endometrial Biopsy

For many years, blind endometrial biopsy in the form of dilatation and curettage with histopathological analysis was considered the gold standard for investigation of postmenopausal bleeding. The procedure may be very uncomfortable when performed in the outpatient setting, and in the past, women were routinely admitted to hospital for dilatation and curettage performed under general anesthesia. However, it has been shown that blind dilatation and curettage alone is an inadequate technique for either the diagnosis or treatment of intrauterine lesions (12–15). The complication rate was 1.7% in the study of Grimes including uterine perforation (0.9%), infection (0.4%), and hemorrhage (0.4%) (16). For these reasons, this procedure is now considered obsolete for the investigation of abnormal uterine bleeding.

More recently, several manufacturers have designed devices to enable endometrial biopsy in the outpatient setting. The Pipelle de Cornier (Unimar, Wilton, Connecticut, U.S.) is a widely used device. This is a plastic catheter with an internal piston to generate negative pressure within the lumen of the catheter. The sensitivity of Pipelle to detect endometrial cancer has been assessed in a group of women with a histological diagnosis of uterine cancer following previous dilatation and curettage. The findings of Pipelle biopsy obtained in the outpatient clinic were compared with histological assessment of the hysterectomy specimen. The Pipelle device was reported to have a 97.5% sensitivity to detect endometrial cancer (17). However, these findings must be interpreted with caution. All women included in the study already had an established diagnosis of endometrial carcinoma, which left the study open to operator bias. In addition, all women probably had extensive disease, which was readily detected on blind dilatation and curettage. The study, therefore, probably overestimated the sensitivity of the Pipelle biopsy for the detection of endometrial cancer.

Guido et al. (18) performed another study of similar design, which showed lower sensitivity of Pipelle in the detection of endometrial cancer (83%); 11 of 65 (17%) patients had falsely reassuring results. Of these, five (8%) had tumors confined to an endometrial polyp, and three (5%) had disease localized to <5% of the surface area of the endometrium. The Pipelle missed none of the tumors in which more than 50% of the endometrium was involved (30 of 65 patients or 46%). Although Pipelle is accurate for detecting global processes in the endometrium, tumors localized to a polyp or small area of the endometrium may go undetected (18). This is supported in a further study which found that blind endometrial biopsy in the office setting will miss small lesions in up to 50% of cases (19). These studies provide a compelling argument against the use of blind endometrial sampling in the absence of imaging of the endometrium.

Transvaginal Ultrasound

The advent of ultrasound technology, originally by the transabdominal route and in more recent years transvaginal ultrasound, allowed visualization of the endometrial cavity in the outpatient setting. Endometrial thickness measured by transvaginal ultrasound can be used as a discriminatory parameter to distinguish those women who are at low risk of endometrial pathology ($\leq$4 mm) from those who are at high risk ($\geq$5 mm) and require further investigation (20–23).

In the detection of any intrauterine pathology, the specificity and sensitivity of transvaginal ultrasound alone varies considerably between different reports (24). While some reports suggested that it was an accurate test in more than 95% of cases (25,26), the reported sensitivity was between 60% and 77% in several studies (27–31).

The endometrial thickness may be more difficult to measure in postmenopausal women compared with women of reproductive age due to a more diffuse endometrial–myometrial border. In women in whom the endometrium is not measurable, the scan should be considered non-diagnostic and an alternative means of evaluation should be employed such as hysteroscopy or saline infusion sonohysterography (SIS) (32).

To measure endometrial thickness, the uterus should be visualized in longitudinal section with the endometrial echo visible from the fundus to the cervix. The endometrium is measured across the thickest part from anterior to posterior, perpendicular to the axis of the cavity. This point is usually 1–2 cm below the fundus. The hypoechoic layer of surrounding myometrium should not be included in the measurement. By convention, the endometrial thickness includes both anterior and posterior layers of the endometrium, as the endometrial–myometrial interface is often more easy to visualize than the interface between the anterior and posterior endometrial layers. If there is any fluid present within the uterine cavity, the thickness of the fluid layer should be subtracted from the total cavity diameter (33). Anechoic fluid within the cavity is a common finding in postmenopausal women, and in conjunction with a thin regular endometrium with no focal lesions, it may be considered a normal finding (32).

The reproducibility of endometrial thickness measurement by transvaginal ultrasound was tested in a study by Epstein and Valentin who found the reproducibility to be clinically acceptable. Interobserver agreement in classifying endometrial thickness as ≤ 4.4 mm or ≥ 4.5 mm was very good ($\kappa = 0.81$). They also concluded that in clinical practice, it is sufficient to take just one measurement of endometrial thickness (34).

Several studies have evaluated the reliability of ultrasound to exclude endometrial cancer in women presenting with postmenopausal bleeding (35–38). In a multicenter study, Karlsson et al. measured endometrial thickness using transvaginal ultrasound prior to curettage in 1168 women presenting with postmenopausal bleeding (39). They found no malignancies when the endometrium measured <5 mm. They concluded that in women with an endometrium ≤ 4 mm, it is justified to refrain from curettage.

Thus in patients presenting with postmenopausal bleeding, an endometrial thickness of ≤ 4 mm is sufficient to reassure the patient that a sinister cause for the bleeding is extremely unlikely. The patient may be discharged with no further investigations or follow-up. However, repeat assessment using transvaginal ultrasound is indicated should recurrent episodes of postmenopausal bleeding occur.

A study assessing the implications of rebleeding and endometrial growth in women with postmenopausal bleeding and endometrial thickness <5 mm was published in 2001 (40). This showed that rebleeding and endometrial growth are common during a 12-month follow-up period in women with postmenopausal bleeding and an endometrial thickness <5 mm whether or not dilatation and curettage is carried out. If women are managed expectantly with ultrasound follow-up, a histological diagnosis should be obtained by endometrial sampling if the endometrial thickness increases to >5 mm but not necessarily in the case of rebleeding without endometrial growth (40).

Saline Infusion Sonohysterography

A new technique of enhanced endometrial examination, termed "echohysteroscopy," was described in 1981 (41). Now commonly known as SIS or hydrosonography, this ultrasound technique involves instillation of sterile saline through the cervix into the uterine cavity during transvaginal ultrasound examination. SIS is simple to perform in the outpatient setting and allows enhanced visualization of the endometrium at the fluid–endometrial interface. This provides increased sensitivity compared with conventional transvaginal ultrasound for detection of uterine cavity abnormalities including endometrial polyps, submucous fibroids, and endometrial carcinoma

(27,31,42–45). This technique has some clear advantages over both hystero-salpingography (HSG) and hysteroscopy. Advantages compared with HSG include simplicity, cost, minimal invasiveness, absence of ionizing radiation, and a high level of diagnostic accuracy (46). The technique is less painful than outpatient hysteroscopy and better tolerated by patients. It is also less expensive, requiring minimal additional equipment, and can be performed as part of the transvaginal ultrasound examination (47–49).

The accuracy of SIS has been evaluated in several studies. Epstein et al. compared TVS, SIS, and hysteroscopy for the investigation of women with postmenopausal bleeding and an endometrial thickness >5 mm. They found almost perfect agreement (96%) between SIS and hysteroscopy in the diagnosis of focally growing lesions (50). This was supported by the findings of Krampl et al., who evaluated the diagnostic accuracy of TVS, SIS, and hysteroscopy in patients presenting with abnormal uterine bleeding. They found SIS to be significantly better than TVS in detecting focal intrauterine pathology. Direct visualization of the endometrium at hysteroscopy imparted no improvement to detection or exclusion of focal intrauterine pathology over SIS (31).

SIS is therefore indicated in patients in whom unenhanced TVS reveals a thickened endometrium but is inconclusive as to whether the thickening is focal or diffuse. A systematic approach to performing SIS is essential. One must explain the purpose and nature of the examination to the patient in detail, paying particular attention to benefits including increased diagnostic accuracy, and potential risks such as bleeding and infection. The risk of infection is small and has been reported to be <1% (51). Antibiotic prophy-axis may therefore be limited to women deemed to be at particular risk, such as those with a history of pelvic infection, unexplained pelvic tenderness, or immune suppression. Mild lower abdominal discomfort is commonly expe-rienced during the examination and this should be explained prior to com-mencing the procedure. Discomfort appears to be both more common and more severe in nulliparous compared to multiparous women.

Outpatient Hysteroscopy

Diagnostic hysteroscopy allows direct inspection of the uterine cavity in the outpatient setting. Kremer et al. found no difference in patient acceptability of outpatient hysteroscopy when compared with day case hysteroscopy (involving general anesthesia) and also found that recovery was significantly quicker in women who had outpatient hysteroscopy (52).

This technique has been employed both as a first- and second-line investigation in women presenting with abnormal uterine bleeding. How-ever, we would propose that diagnostic hysteroscopy is best used as a second-line investigative tool, in view of the invasive nature of the procedure when compared to TVS. Indications are similar to those for SIS; it may be used in patients for whom TVS does not demonstrate a thin regular endo-metrial echo, and the nature of the abnormality is not clearly delineated on scan. Recent studies have confirmed the diagnostic accuracy and high degree of feasibility of diagnostic hysteroscopy carried out as an outpatient procedure (52–56). Distension of the uterus is necessary for visual inspection of the uterine cavity (57). This is achieved either by the instillation of fluid such as saline, or insufflation with CO_2 gas (58). Although CO_2 gas is gene-rally well tolerated, uterine distension with saline has been shown to be more comfortable, more cost-effective, and to provide superior views in the presence of uterine bleeding (58).

Hysteroscopes broadly fall into two subtypes—rigid and flexible. Unfried et al. prospectively compared flexible with rigid hysteroscopy in the outpatient setting. They found that flexible hysteroscopy seemed to be less painful, but that rigid scopes provided superior views with lower opera-ting times and higher success rates at lower cost (59).

Outersheaths are available with an operating channel through which it is possible to perform minor surgical procedures such as polypectomies, directed biopsies, or removal of intrauterine contraceptive device (IUCDs) under direct vision (57,60,61). The ability to perform directed biopsies and polypectomies in the outpatient setting offers a distinct advantage over SIS. In addition to avoiding a day case procedure with the added cost impli-cations in women found on SIS to have focal pathology, outpatient hystero-scopy renders the "one-stop clinic" truly feasible. The nature of endometrial thickening is established, as well as providing a histological specimen and in some cases, definitive treatment all during a single clinic visit. There have, however, been reports of a lower sensitivity of hysteroscopy in the diagnosis of endometrial cancer. In their study looking at the role of outpatient diag-nostic hysteroscopy, Lo and Yuen found a low sensitivity and positive predictive value of 58.8% and 20.8%, respectively, in the detection of endo-metrial cancer (62). In addition, 0.9% of women who were diagnosed at hys-teroscopy with normal or atrophic endometrium were later found on biopsy to have endometrial hyperplasia. They, therefore, felt it necessary to per-form biopsy during hysteroscopy in all cases in order to facilitate accurate diagnosis of endometrial pathology. In addition, there have been reports of endometrial cancer being found incidentally at hysteroscopic endometrial resection, having been missed at diagnostic hysteroscopy (63,64). A further consideration is the possibility of dissemination of malignant cells from the uterine cavity into the peritoneal cavity as a result of hysteroscopy. Several studies have reported positive cytology for endometrial cells in peritoneal washings after hysteroscopy (65–67). However, the risk of peritoneal metas-tases by this route remains unclear.

When compared with SIS, diagnostic hysteroscopy is a relatively expensive procedure, which is more invasive, less well tolerated by patients, and carries higher complication rates. Potential complications include cervical laceration by the tenaculum, fluid overload, and uterine perforation (68). Furthermore, diagnostic hysteroscopy does not appear to improve diagnostic accuracy (31,50,69).

On balance, both SIS and outpatient hysteroscopy with directed biopsy are accurate and clinically acceptable second-line investigative tools for women presenting with abnormal uterine bleeding, who are found on TVS to have a thickened endometrium. The choice of investigation employed in a particular unit will depend on issues such as local expertise and training, and personal preference, as well as cost implications.

THE RAPID ACCESS CLINIC

In order to facilitate early diagnosis and treatment of gynecological cancers, rapid access clinics have been established throughout the United Kingdom. The main objective of these clinics is to shorten the diagnostic process in women with suspected gynecological cancers and to minimize the interval between presentation and initiation of appropriate treatment. In the United Kingdom, the current maximum waiting time for patients to attend for the initial assessment is two weeks. Therefore, it is important that the clinics are organized in a way that ensures rational use of resources. This can be achieved if the diagnostic process is completed on an outpatient basis using methods which enable reliable differentiation between benign gynecological conditions and cancer. A flow-chart outlining management of postmenopausal bleeding (PMB) is illustrated (Fig. 1). A full clinical history and examination should precede investigations. Particular attention should be paid to risk factors for endometrial cancer as discussed previously. It has been reported that 0.8–1.8% of women with postmenopausal bleeding (PMP) have cervical carcinoma (39,70). The speculum examination with cervical smear test, if indicated, are therefore essential components of the investigation of women presenting with postmenopausal bleeding.

According to current evidence, transvaginal ultrasound scanning is the method of choice for the initial assessment of women presenting with postmenopausal bleeding. Using an endometrial thickness of ≤ 4 mm as the discrimatory parameter, 40–50% of women presenting with postmenopausal bleeding can be reassured that their risk of endometrial cancer is low, without undergoing an invasive test (20). This approach ensures that the resources are used effectively by avoiding unnecessary interventions in women with no uterine pathology. However, this approach is less suitable for women with a history of vaginal bleeding on tamoxifcn treatment as almost 90% of them will have increased endometrial thickness on ultrasound scan. Many of these women will have tamoxifen-induced polyps, and therefore hysteroscopy may be a more appropriate first-line investigation for this group of women.

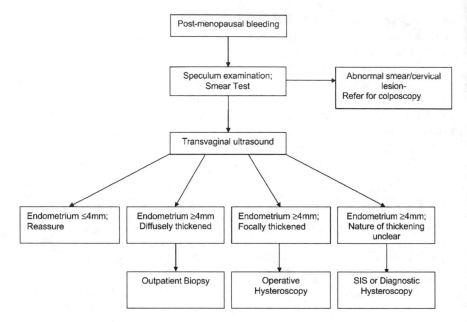

Figure 1 A strategy for the triage of women presenting to the rapid access clinic with postmenopausal bleeding.

In women demonstrated on TVS to have a uniformly thickened endometrium (Fig. 2), the secondary test may be either outpatient endometrial sampling with a device such as the Pipelle or hysteroscopy. Van den Bosch et al. advocated the combined use of TVS with outpatient endometrial sampling. They found a sensitivity of 100% in the detection of endometrial carcinoma by Pipelle endometrial sampling after TVS. They suggested that endometrial sampling is indicated in patients with an endometrial thickness >4 mm (71). For women with focal endometrial lesions, however, hysteroscopy is indicated (Fig. 3). This may be performed in the outpatient setting, as a day case procedure, or if necessary the patient may be admitted for an inpatient operation. The choice of the method will depend on several factors including the size of the lesion, degree of vaginal and cervical atrophy, and availability of the methods.

In women in whom the TVS is inconclusive regarding the nature of the endometrial thickening, the choice of secondary investigation is either SIS or hysteroscopy. With saline infusion into the uterine cavity, the sensitivity of transvaginal ultrasound to detect subtle focal pathology within the uterine cavity can be enhanced to a level comparable with hysteroscopy (47,48,50,69,72). This allows triage into those requiring an operative procedure and directed biopsy, and those for whom an endometrial biopsy in the outpatient clinic is likely to provide information accurate enough to inform management decisions.

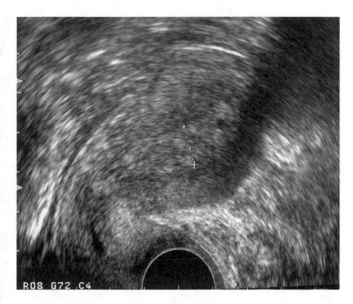

Figure 2 Diffusely thickened and cystic endometrium.

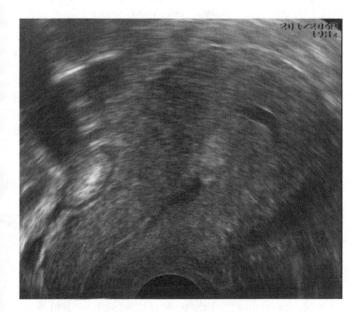

Figure 3 A longitudinal view of the uterine cavity obtained on transvaginal ultrasound scan, showing a well-defined hyperechoic lesion surrounded by a small amount of hypoehoic fluid. These features are typical of an endometrial polyp.

SIS has been found to be more acceptable to the patients and less costly with lower complication rates (73). de Kroon et al. commented that diagnostic hysteroscopy can be restricted to patients in whom SIS is inconclusive or fails (74). Again, the choice between these methods will depend on the level of ultrasound expertise available locally.

Hysteroscopy may be used as the primary test when ultrasound is not available. However, this approach is more expensive and carries the risk of surgical and anesthetic complications. Women who are most likely to suffer complications are those with bleeding as a result of atrophic changes of the genital organs. This population of women is less likely to harbor endometrial disease.

Although hysteroscopy is a widely accepted method for the diagnosis of endometrial cancer, it is important to note that this method is not without failures, both technical and diagnostic. Endometrial biopsies should be performed routinely during hysteroscopy to reduce the risk of missing endometrial cancer. After the triage process and secondary investigations, those women with a histological diagnosis of endometrial cancer should be referred directly to the regional cancer center for further expert management.

CONCLUSION

Recent developments in ultrasound and hysteroscopy have facilitated the rapid diagnosis of endometrial cancer in the outpatient setting. The ability to discriminate between women with a normal endometrium and those with pathological lesions, thus avoiding the need for operative intervention, has significantly improved the quality of care provided to women presenting with postmenopausal bleeding. The facility to establish the diagnosis of cancer by noninvasive investigative modalities is particularly important in postmenopausal women, many of whom have additional medical problems and in whom both surgical and anesthetic complications are more likely to occur. Addressing the importance of shortened waiting times for clinic appointments and increasing the accessibility of the service are likely to result in improved long-term cure rates of this common disease.

REFERENCES

1. Lidor A, Ismajovich B, Confino E, David MP. Histopathological findings in 226 women with post-menopausal uterine bleeding. Acta Obstet Gynecol Scand 1986; 65:41–43.
2. Danero S, Ricci MG, La Rosa R, et al. Critical review of dilatation and curettage in the diagnosis of malignant pathology of the endometrium. Eur J Gyaecol Oncol 1986; 7:162–165.
3. O'Connell LP, Fries MH, Zeringue E, Brehm W. Triage of abnormal postmenopausal bleeding: a comparison of endometrial biopsy and transvaginal sonohysterography versus fractional curettage with hysteroscopy. Am J Obstet Gynecol 1998; 178:956–961.

4. Beral V, Banks E, Reeves G, Appleby P. Use of HRT and the subsequent risk of cancer. J Epidemiol Biostat 1999; 4:191–210; discussion 210–215.
5. Fornander T, Rutqvist LE, Cedermark B, et al. Adjuvant tamoxifen in early breast cancer: occurrence of new primary cancers. Lancet 1989; 1:117–120.
6. Andersson M, Storm HH, Mouridsen HT. Incidence of new primary cancers after adjuvant tamoxifen therapy and radiotherapy for early breast cancer. J Natl Cancer Inst 1991; 83:1013–1017.
7. Fisher B, Constantino JP, Redmond CK, Fisher ER, Wickerham DL, Cronin WM. Endometrial cancer in tamoxifen-treated breast cancer patients: findings from the National Surgical Adjuvant Breast and Bowel Project (NSABP) B-14. J Natl Cancer Inst 1994; 86:527–537.
8. Assikis VJ, Neven P, Jordan VC, Vergote I. A realistic clinical perspective of tamoxifen and endometrial carcinogenesis. Eur J Cancer 1996; 32A: 1464–1476.
9. Early Breast Cancer Trialists' Collaborative Group. Tamoxifen for early breast cancer: an overview of the randomised trials. Lancet 1998; 351:1451–1467.
10. Bristow R. Endometrial cancer. Curr Opin Oncol 1999; 11:388–393.
11. Farquhar CM, Lethaby A, Sowter M, Verry J, Baranyai J. An evaluation of risk factors for endometrial hyperplasia in premenopausal women with abnormal menstrual bleeding. Am J Obstet Gynecol 1999; 181:525–529.
12. Bettocchi S, Ceci O, Vicino M, Marello F, Impedovo L, Selvaggi L. Diagnostic inadequacy of dilatation and curettage. Fertil Steril 2001; 75:803–805.
13. Emanuel MH, Wamsteker K, Lammes FB. Is dilatation and curettage obsolete for diagnosing intrauterine disorders in premenopausal patients with persistent abnormal uterine bleeding? Acta Obstet Gynecol Scand 1997; 76:65–68.
14. Stock RJ, Kanbour. Prehysterectomy curettage. Acta Obstet Gynecol Scand 1975; 45:537–541.
15. Lerner HM. Lack of efficacy of prehysterectomy curettage as a diagnostic procedure. Am J Obstet Gynecol 1984; 148:1055–1056.
16. Grimes DA. Diagnostic dilatation and curettage: a reappraisal. Am J Obstet Gynecol 1982; 142:1–6.
17. Stovall TG, Photopulus GJ, Poston WM, Ling FW, Sandles LG. Pipelle endometrial sampling in patients with known endometrial carcinoma. Obstet Gynecol 1991; 77:954–956.
18. Guido RS, Kanbour-Shakir A, Rulin MC, Christopherson WA. Pipelle endometrial sampling. Sensitivity in the detection of endometrial cancer. J Reprod Med 1995; 40:553–555.
19. Pal L, Lapensee L, Toth TL, Isaacson KB. Comparison of office hysteroscopy, transvaginal ultrasonography and endometrial biopsy in evaluation of abnormal uterine bleeding. J Soc Laparoendosc Surg 1997; 1:125–130.
20. Karlsson B, Granberg S, Wikland M, et al. Transvaginal ultrasonography of the endometrium in women with postmenopausal bleeding—a Nordic multicenter study. Am J Obstet Gynecol 1995; 172:1488–1494.
21. Gupta JK, Chien PF, Voit D, Clark TJ, Khan KS. Ultrasonographic endometrial thickness for diagnosing endometrial pathology in women with postmenopausal bleeding: a meta-analysis. Acta Obstet Gynecol Scand 2002; 81:799–816.

22. Goldstein RB, Bree RL, Benson CB, et al. Evaluation of the woman with post-menopausal bleeding: Society of Radiologists in Ultrasound-Sponsored Consensus Conference statement. J Ultrasound Med 2001; 20:1025–1036.
23. Smith-Bindman R, Kerlikowske K, Feldstein VA, et al. Endovaginal ultrasound to exclude endometrial cancer and other endometrial abnormalities. JAMA 1998; 280:1510–1517.
24. Farquhar C, Ekeroma A, Furness S, Arroll B. A systematic review of transvaginal ultrasonography, sonohysterography and hysteroscopy for the investigation of abnormal uterine bleeding in premenopausal women. Acta Obstet Gynecol Scand 2003; 82:493–504.
25. Fedele L, Bianchi S, Dorta M, Brioschi D, Zanotti F, Vercellini P. Transvaginal ultrasonography versus hysteroscopy in the diagnosis of uterine submucous myomas. Obstet Gynecol 1991; 77:745–748.
26. Vercellini P, Cortesi I, Oldani S, et al. The role of transvaginal ultrasonography and outpatient diagnostic hysteroscopy in the evaluation of patients with menorrhagia. Hum Reprod 1997; 12:1768–1771.
27. Bronz L, Suter T, Rusca T. The value of transvaginal sonography with and without saline instillation in the diagnosis of uterine pathology in pre- and post-menopausal women with abnormal bleeding or suspect sonographic findings. Ultrasound Obstet Gynecol 1997; 9:53–58.
28. De Vries L, Dijkhuizen FP, Mol BW, Brölmann HA, Moret E, Heintz AP. Comparison of transvaginal sonography, saline infusion sonography and hysteroscopy in premenopausal women with abnormal uterine bleeding. J Clin Ultrasound 2000; 28:217–213.
29. Dijkhuizen FP, Brölmann HA, Potters AE, Bongers MY, Heintz AP. The accuracy of transvaginal ultrasound in the diagnosis of endometrial abnormalities. Obstet Gynecol 1996; 87:345–349.
30. Dijkhuizen FP, De Vries LD, Mol BW, et al. Comparison of transvaginal ultrasonography and saline infusion sonography for the detection of intracavitary abnormalities in premenopausal women. Ultrasound Obstet Gynecol 2000; 15:372–376.
31. Krampl E, Bourne T, Hurlen-Solbakken H, Istre O. Transvaginal ultrasonography sonohysterography and operative hysteroscopy for the evaluation of abnormal uterine bleeding. Acta Obstet Gynecol Scand 2001; 80:616–622.
32. Epstein E, Valentin L. Managing women with post-menopausal bleeding. Best Prac Res Clin Obstet Gynaecol 2004; 18:125–143.
33. Fleischer AC, Kalemeris GC, Entman SS. Sonographic depiction of the endometrium during normal cycles. Ultrasound Med Biol 1986; 12:271–277.
34. Epstein E, Valentin L. Intraobserver and interobserver reproducibility of ultrasound measurements of endometrial thickness in postmenopausal women. Ultrasound Obstet Gynecol 2002; 20:486–491.
35. Nasri MN, Coast GJ. Correlation of ultrasound findings and endometrial histopathology in postmenopausal women. Br J Obstet Gynaecol 1989; 96:1333–1338.
36. Osmers R, Volksen M, Schauer A. Vaginosonography for early detection of endometrial carcinoma? Lancet 1990; 335:1569–1571.

37. Goldstein SR, Nachtigall M, Snyder JR, Nachtigall L. Endometrial assessment by vaginal ultrasonography before endometrial sampling in patients with postmenopausal bleeding. Am J Obstet Gynecol 1990; 163:119–123.
38. Granberg S, Wikland M, Karlsson B, Norstrom A, Friberg LG. Endometrial thickness as measured by endovaginal ultrasonography for identifying endometrial abnormality. Am J Obstet Gynecol 1991; 164:47–52.
39. Karlsson B, Granberg S, Wikland M, et al. Transvaginal ultrasonography of the endometrium in women with postmenopausal bleeding-a Nordic multicenter study. Am J Obstet Gynecol 1995; 172:1488–1494.
40. Epstein E, Valentin L. Rebleeding and endometrial growth in women with postmenopausal bleeding and endometrial thickness <5 mm managed by dilatation and curettage or ultrasound follow-up: a randomized controlled study. Ultrasound Obstet Gynecol 2001; 18:499–504.
41. Nannini R, Chelo E, Branconi F, Tantini C, Scarselli GF. Dynamic echo-hysteroscopy: a new diagnostic technique in the study of female infertility. Acta Eur Fertil 1981; 12:165–171.
42. Lindheim SR, Adsuar N, Kushner DM, Pritts EA, Olive DL. Sonohysterography: A valuable tool in evaluating the female pelvis. Obstet Gynecol Survey 2003; 58:770–784.
43. Dueholm M, Forman A, Jensen ML, Laursen H, Kracht P. Transvaginal sonography combined with saline contrast sonohysterography in evaluating the uterine cavity in premenopausal patients with abnormal uterine bleeding. Ultrasound Obstet Gynecol 2001; 18:54–61.
44. Nanda S, Chadha N, Sen J, Sangwan K. Transvaginal sonography and saline infusion sonohysterogrphy in the evaluation of abnormal uterine bleeding. Aust N Z J Obstet Gynaecol 2002; 42:530–534.
45. Valenzano M, Costantini S, Cucuccio S, Dugnani MC, Paoletti R, Ragni N. Use of hysterosonography in women with abnormal postmenopausal bleeding. Eur J Gynaec Oncol 1999; 20:217–222.
46. Parsons AK, Lense JJ. Sonohysterography for endometrial abnormalities: preliminary results. J Clin Ultrasound 1993; 21:87–95.
47. Widrich T, Bradley LD, Mitchinson AR, Collins RL. Comparison of saline infusion sonography with office hysteroscopy for the evaluation of the endometrium. Am J Obstet Gynecol 1996; 174:1327–1334.
48. Bernard JP, Lécuru F, Darles C, Robin F, de Bievre P, Taurelle R. Saline contrast sonohysterography as first-line investigation for women with uterine bleeding. Ultrasound Obstet Gynecol 1997; 10:121–125.
49. Rogerson L, Bates J, Weston M, Duffy S. A comparison of outpatient hysteroscopy with saline infusion hysterosonography. Br J Obstet Gynaecol 2002; 109:800–804.
50. Epstein E, Ramirez A, Skoog L, Valentin L. Transvaginal sonography, saline contrast sonohysterography and hysteroscopy for the investigation of women with postmenopausal bleeding and endometrium >5mm. Ultrasound Obstet Gynecol 2001; 18:157–162.
51. Bonnamy L, Marret H, Perrotin F, Body G, Berger C, Lansac J. Sonohysterography: a prospective survery of results and complications in 81 patients. Eur J Obstet Gynecol Reprod Biol 2002; 102:42–47.

52. Kremer C, Duffy S, Moroney M. Patient satisfaction with outpatient hysteroscopy versus day case hysteroscopy: randomised controlled trial. BMJ 2000; 320:279–282.
53. Downes E, al-Azzawi F. The predictive value of outpatient hysteroscopy in a menopause clinic. Br J Obstet Gynaecol 1993; 100:1148–1149.
54. Nagele F, O'Connor H, Davies A, Badawy A, Mohamed H, Magos A. Two thousand five hundred outpatient diagnostic hysteroscopies. Obstet Gynecol 1996; 88:87–92.
55. Cicinelli E, Didonna T, Ambrosi G, Schonauer LM, Fiore G, Matteo MG. Topical anaesthesia for diagnostic hysteroscopy and endometrial biopsy in postmenopausal women: a randomised placebo-controlled double-blind study. Br J Obstet Gynaecol 1997; 104:316–319.
56. Tahir MM, Bigrigg MA, Browning JJ, Brookes ST, Smith PA. A randomized controlled trial comparing transvaginal ultrasound, outpatient hysteroscopy and endometrial biopsy with inpatient hysteroscopy and curettage. Br J Obstet Gynaecol 1999; 106:1259–1264.
57. Wieser F, Tempfer C, Kurz C, Nagele F. Hysteroscopy in 2001: a comprehensive review. Acta Obstet Gynecol Scand 2001; 80:773–783.
58. Nagele F, Bournas N, O'Connor H, Broadbent M, Richardson R, Magos AL. A comparison of carbon dioxide and normal saline for uterine distension in outpatient hysteroscopy. Fertil Steril 1996; 65:305–309.
59. Unfried G, Wieser F, Albrecht A, Kaider A, Nagele F. Flexible versus rigid endoscopes for outpatient hysteroscopy: a prospective randomized clinical trial. Hum Reprod 2001; 16:168–171.
60. Campo R, Van Belle Y, Rombauts L, Brosens I, Gordts S. Office mini-hysteroscopy. Hum Reprod Update 1999; 5:73–81.
61. Gimpelson RJ. Office hysteroscopy. Clin Obstet Gynecol 1992; 35:270–281.
62. Lo KWK, Yuen PM. The role of outpatient diagnostic hysteroscopy in identifying anatomic pathology and histopathology in the endometrial cavity. J Am Assoc Gynecol Laparosc 2000; 7:381–385.
63. Dwyer NA, Stirrat GM. Early endometrial carcinoma: an incidental finding after endometrial resection. Case report. Br J Obstet Gynaecol 1991; 98: 733–734.
64. Colafranceschi M, Bettochi S, Mencaglia L, van Herendael BJ. Missed hysteroscopic detection of uterine carcinoma before endometrial resection: report of three cases. Gynecol Oncol 1996; 62:298–300.
65. Ranta H, Aine R, Oksanen H, Heinonen PK. Dissemination of endometrial cells during carbon dioxide hysteroscopy and chromotubation among infertile patients. Fertil Steril 1990; 53:751–753.
66. Egarter C, Krestan C, Kurz C. Abdominal dissemination of malignant cells with hysteroscopy. Gynecol Oncol 1996; 63:143–144.
67. Leveque J, Goyat F, Dugast J, Loeillet L, Grall JY, Le Bars S. Value of peritoneal cytology after hysteroscopy in surgical stage I adenocarcinoma of the endometrium. Oncol Reports 1998; 5:713–715.
68. Jansen FW, Vredevoogd CB, van Ulzen K, Hermans J, Trimbos JB, Trimbos-Kemper TC. Complications of hysteroscopy: a prospective, multicenter study. Obstet Gynecol 2000; 96:266–270.

69. Williams CD, Marshburn PB. A prospective study of transvaginal hydrosono-graphy in the evaluation of abnormal uterine bleeding. Am J Obstet Gynecol 1998; 179:292–298.
70. Gredmark T, Kvint S, Havel G, Mattson LA. Histopathological findings in women with postmenopausal bleeding. BJOG 1995; 102:133–136.
71. Van den Bosch T, Vandendael A, Van Schoubroeck D, Wranz PAB, Lombard CJ. Combining vaginal ultrasonography and office endometrial sampling in the diagnosis of endometrial disease in postmenopausal women. Obstet Gynecol 1995; 85:349–352.
72. Kamel HS, Darwish AM, Mohamed SA. Comparison of transvaginal ultra-sonography and vaginal sonohysterography in the detection of endometrial polyps. Acta Obstet Gynecol Scand 2000; 79:60–64.
73. Timmerman D, Deprest J, Bourne T, Van den Berghe I, Collins WP, Vergote I. A randomized trial on the use of ultrasonography or office hysteroscopy for endometrial assessment in postmenopausal patients with breast cancer who were treated with tamoxifen. Am J Obstet Gynecol 1998; 179:62–70.
74. de Kroon CD, Jansen FW, Louwé LA, Dieben SWM, van Houwelingen HC, Trimbos JB. Technology assessment of saline contrast hysterosonography. Am J Obstet Gynecol 2003; 188:945–949.

7

Imaging Endometrial Cancer

Moji Balogun

Department of Radiology, Birmingham Women's Hospital, Birmingham, U.K.

Julie Olliff

Department of Radiology, University Hospital NHS Trust, Birmingham, U.K.

Ultrasound (US), computed tomography (CT), and magnetic resonance imaging (MRI) are the most common imaging modalities used in the evaluation of patients with suspected endometrial cancer. Most women with endometrial cancer will have surgery for staging and initial treatment, but imaging can be invaluable in the pretreatment assessment of patients with suspected endometrial cancer—first to identify patients who require more invasive investigations to establish the diagnosis and second to identify those patients who would not benefit from primary surgery because of the presence of extensive disease.

Ultrasound, particularly transvaginal ultrasound (TVS), is used for the initial evaluation of patients with suspected endometrial cancer. Postmenopausal bleeding is a common presentation and has been shown to incur a 64-fold risk for endometrial cancer (1), but abnormal vaginal bleeding may be caused by a number of gynecological or nongynecological disorders. Endometrial atrophy is reported to be the most common cause of postmenopausal bleeding (2). Other conditions such as endometrial hyperplasia, endometrial polyps, and submucosal leiomyomas may cause endometrial postmenopausal bleeding in addition to endometrial carcinoma. Dilatation and curettage may fail to detect focal lesions in the uterine cavity in women with postmenopausal bleeding (3). Transvaginal US has evolved as an imaging technique that allows identification of abnormal endometrial thickening (Fig. 1). Large trials

(A)

(B)

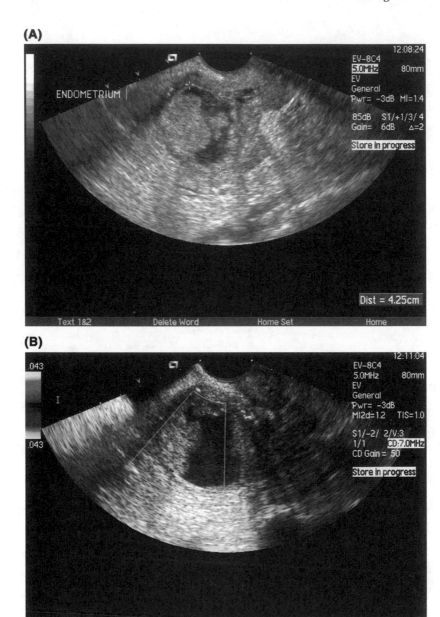

Figure 1 (A) Transvaginal ultrasound demonstrating abnormal thickening of the endometrium (*between cursors*). The uterus is enlarged with a distended cavity. (B) Abnormal vascularity within the thickened endometrium is shown on color doppler.

have been performed to define an endometrial thickness that can be used as a cut-off to exclude underlying pathology in order to use TVS as a screening tool in postmenopausal women with abnormal uterine bleeding (4–9). Cut-off values ranging from 4 to 10 mm (double layer endometrial thickness) have been proposed. The technique most often used to measure the endometrial thickness is measurement of the maximum thickness of the anterior and posterior layers of the endometrium in a sagittal scan. A meta-analysis of the 35 articles published between 1966 and 1996 (10) including 5892 women, showed that using a threshold value of greater than 5 mm to define abnormal endometrial thickness had a sensitivity of 96% [95% confidence interval (CI) 94–98%] (96% of women with cancer had an abnormal endovaginal US), whereas 92% (95% CI colon 90–93%) of women with endometrial pathology had an abnormal test result. The corresponding specificities were 61% (95% CI 59–63%) and 81% (95% CI 79–83%), respectively. There was a false-negative rate of 8%. This study concluded that endovaginal sonography is highly sensitive for detecting endometrial cancer and can identify patients who are at low risk and who therefore do not need endometrial sampling. Women taking hormone replacement therapy (HRT) had a significantly higher false-positive rate (specificity 77%; 95% CI 75–79%) compared with patients who are not taking HRT (specificity 92%; 95% CI 90–94%). This is because endometrial thickness is known to increase under the influence of HRT. Some authors therefore suggest that a higher threshold value for endometrial thickness be taken for patients who are postmenopausal taking HRT perhaps using 8 mm versus 5 mm (11–13).

In a prospective study of 1110 women with postmenopausal bleeding (PMB), no endometrial cancers were found in women with an endometrial thickness of 4 mm or less (14) and endometrial pathology was found most often with a thickness of more than 8 mm. Another study of 419 women with PMB found a sensitivity of 95.1%, specificity 54.8% if 4 mm was used as the cut-off and sensitivity of 83.8% and specificity of 81.3% if 8 mm was used (15). A further study of 182 women using a threshold of 5 mm or less missed no cases of endometrial cancer but three patients had endometrial hyperplasia (16). Bakour et al. concluded that a cut-off of 4 mm or less could reliably exclude cancer in patients with PMB (17). A more recent series following a cohort of 339 patients for more than 10 years found that no endometrial cancer was missed when the endometrial thickness measurement cut-off value greater than or equal to 4 mm was used and these authors concluded that TVS is an excellent tool for determining whether further investigation with curettage or some form of endometrial biopsy is needed, if it is necessary (1). A cut-off of 13 mm has been suggested in patients with irregular perimenopausal uterine bleeding (18). In a larger study of 1,286 women with peri- and postmenopausal women using a cut-off of 5 mm, endometrial cancers were missed by TVS and by hysteroscopy and the authors concluded that neither modality could be used as a single diagnostic tool to exclude endometrial cancer (19). Several authors suggest that an endometrial thickness of greater than 15 mm is highly suggestive of the diagnosis of cancer (20).

The use of TVS measuring diffuse or focal endometrial thickening as an initial test in the investigation of women with peri- or postmenopausal bleeding has been found to be cost-effective. There has been prediction of substantial cost savings if this is used rather than a biopsy-based algorithm (21).

Other US findings in patients with endometrial cancer include a distended or fluid-filled endometrial cavity, and an enlarged or lobular uterus (Fig. 1). There may be poor definition of the junctional zone and heterogeneity of the reflectivity of the endometrium. Endometrial thickness may be used as the sole criterion in the US assessment of the endometrium in postmenopausal women, but there is discussion in the literature whether assessment of the morphological appearances of the endometrium on US can improve the positive predictive value of TVS, if used in addition to measuring the endometrial thickness. Some authors (22–25) have concluded that using morphological features with endometrial thickness will improve the overall accuracy or raise threshold values of endometrial thickness before further evaluation becomes necessary. Other authors are less certain of the role of endometrial morphology in the identification of patients with endometrial cancer (14,26). Cystic spaces (Fig. 2) have been said to be predictive of endometrial polyps and that endometrial hyperplasia leads to an increase in the reflectivity of the endometrium on US (27). The fibrous core of an endometrial polyp is seen as central low signal intensity on the T2-weighted scans on MRI and the cystic spaces may also be recognized (28).

Doppler US has not been conclusively found to be of assistance in the diagnosis of uterine cancer (29), but it can be used to assess blood flow to a mass with a benign polyp having a single feeding vessel with endometrial cancers (Fig. 1B) being more likely to be broad based with multiple feeding vessels (30). Intratumor blood flow was seen in 72% of patients with endometrial cancer but in only one patient with endometrial hyperplasia (complicated with a pyometra) in a group of 71 patients (31). Endometrial cancer may, however, be hypovascular. US can also help decide whether the abnormality is diffuse or focal allowing a decision to be made with regard to method of endometrial sampling—blind or under direct hysteroscopic visualization.

US may have a role in the staging of endometrial cancers. This can be achieved by assessing the depth of invasion with reported accuracies of 77–84.6% (32–34). The reliability of TVS to determine myometrial invasion and to predict cervical or lymph node involvement has been questioned (33,35,36). MRI performs best in the pretreatment evaluation of myometrial or cervical invasion (37–41) compared to either US or CT (Fig. 3), but surgery with histopathology remains the gold standard (42). Distant metastases and lymph node involvement are better imaged with CT and MRI than US. MRI is overall the best imaging modality for staging pretreatment endometrial cancer with reported overall staging accuracies of 83–92% (41).

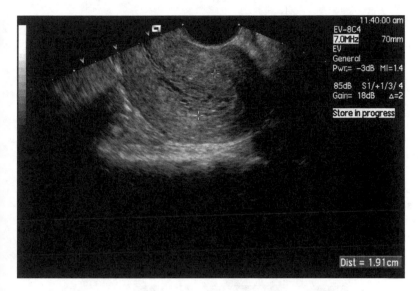

Figure 2 Transvaginal ultrasound showing a thickened endometrium containing at least one cystic space.

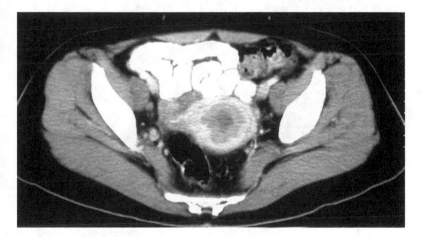

Figure 3 Contrast-enhanced axial CT scan of the pelvis demonstrates an enlarged uterus. There is distension of the endometrial cavity with abnormal intermediate attenuation tumor extending out into the deep myometrium but not extending to the serosa.

MAGNETIC RESONANCE IMAGING

The zonal anatomy of the uterus is best seen on T2-weighted magnetic resonance (MR) sequences (Fig. 4). The normal postmenopausal endometrium is seen as a thin hyperintense structure relative to normal myometrium. The endometrium is usually iso-intense to myometrium on unenhanced T1-weighted images, becoming hypo-intense on early postcontrast images, and then iso- or hyperintense on delayed contrast-enhanced scans. The junctional zone lies between the high-signal endometrium and more intermediate signal myometrium and is of lower signal intensity than the myometrium on T2-weighted scans. It will not be appreciated on unenhanced T1-weighted MR scans. It is seen in premenopausal women but may be absent in normal postmenopausal women. Contrast-enhanced MR imaging has been found to be helpful in cases of absence of a visible junctional zone on T2-weighted MR scans (43).

Endometrial cancer most commonly presents as focal (Fig. 5) or diffuse endometrial thickening of the endometrium on MRI. A large tumor

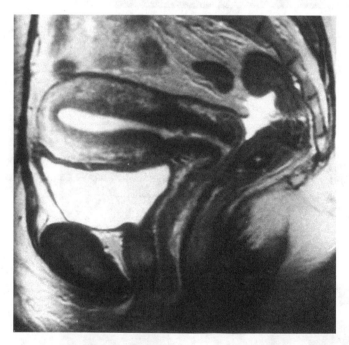

Figure 4 Sagittal T2-weighted MR scans demonstrating normal anatomy. The high signal endometrium is seen as a white "stripe" centrally. The lower signal junctional zone, which correlates to the inner myometrium, is seen lying between this and the more intermediate signal intensity myometrium. The cervix is well seen as an anterior and posterior lip predominantly of low signal intensity due to the presence of fibrous-cervical stroma, but with a central thin stripe of mucous within the endocervical centrally and less high signal plicae between this and the fibro-cervical stroma.

(A)

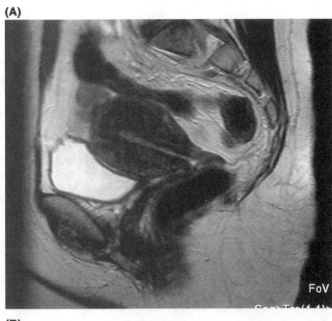

(B)

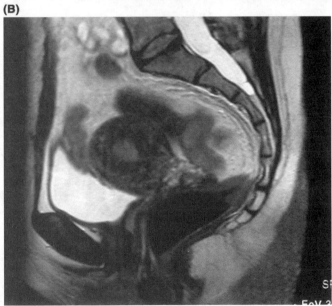

Figure 5 (**A**) Sagittal T2-weighted scan shows a normal appearing endometrial stripe in the mid-line. (**B**) Para sagittal T2 weighted scans show intermediate signal material widening the endometrial stripe towards the right cornua of the uterus. (**C**) Angled axial T2-weighted scan shows a focal area of abnormal intermediate signal intensity widening the endometrial canal in the region of the right cornu.

(Continued next page)

(C)

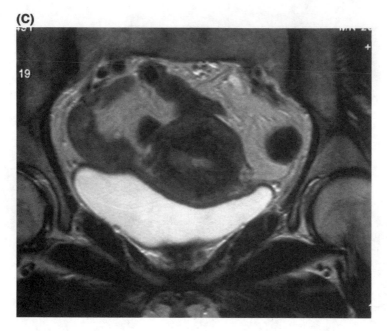

Figure 5 (*Continued*)

may be seen as an irregular mass distending the cavity (Fig. 6). Myometrial invasion causes loss of definition of the junctional zone with irregularity of the interface between the endometrium and the junctional zone (Fig. 7). This cannot be appreciated on T1-weighted images and is seen on the T2-weighted scans. Endometrial cancers enhance less than the myometrium on dynamic contrast-enhanced T1-weighted MR scans (Fig. 8), but the difference in enhancement becomes less marked on delayed scans.

Stage I tumors (tumor confined to the endometrium, stage Ia) may appear on MRI scan as a normal or thickened endometrium and the thickening may be focal or diffuse. The junctional zone will be preserved on T2-weighted sequences (Fig. 6) and normal subendometrial enhancement will be seen on dynamic scans (Fig. 8). The low-signal intensity zone of the inner myometrium will also be preserved on delayed contrast-enhanced T1-weighted scans. The interface between the tumor and the myometrium will be well defined and smooth. Stage IB tumors (tumor extending less than 50% into the myometrium) will be associated with disruption or irregularity of the junctional zone (Fig. 9A,B). There will be focal or diffuse absence of subendometrial enhancement on early contrast-enhanced scans and disruption of the low-signal intensity zone of the inner myometrium on delayed contrast-enhanced T1-weighted scans. A diagnosis of stage Ib tumor is also suggested by an irregular tumor–myometrial interface. In stage Ic disease (tumor involving deep myometrium), tumor will be seen to extend into the

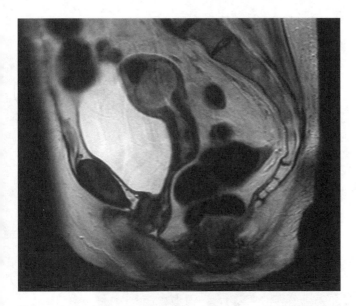

Figure 6 Sagittal T2-weighted scans show a small postmenopausal uterus but an intermediate signal intensity mass distending the endometrial cavity. A small fibroid is noted at the fundus of the uterus but the junctional zone is preserved despite the marked thinning of the myometrium.

myometrium for a depth greater than 50% (Fig. 10). There will, however, be intact normal outer myometrial tissue beyond the tumor. MRI has been found to be a reliable method for the preoperative assessment of myometrial invasion (41,44). MRI is 74–91% accurate for differentiating superficial from deep invasion in stage I tumors (41).

T2-weighted spin echo sequences can be used to determine depth of myometrial invasion and some have found use of this technique superior to contrast-enhanced MRI (45). Other authors have found that gadolinium enhancement will improve staging accuracy for myometrial invasion over non-enhanced scans (37,46–49) (Fig. 11). The inner muscle layer shows more rapid enhancement than the outer muscle layer on gradient echo T1-weighted contrast-enhanced scans even after menopause. In addition, contrast to noise ratio between the inner muscle layer and endometrial cancer has been shown to be maximum at approximately 50 seconds after administration of intravenous gadolinium (50). One study found this to be true in postmenopausal patients but that T2-weighted scans were more accurate in premenopausal patients (51). A meta-analysis correlated mean pretest probabilities for myometrial invasion with tumor grade from seven articles (1870 patients) and from 125 institutional pathology reports. The authors found that post-test probabilities of deep myometrial invasion increased for grade 1 cancer from 13% to 60%, for grade 2 cancer from 35% to 84%

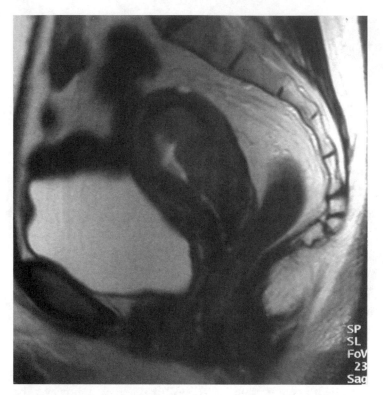

Figure 7 Sagittal T2-weighted scan shows loss of definition of the junctional zone and irregularity in the posterior myometrium. Note the endometrial cavity is distended by an intermediate, signal intensity irregular mass with some fluid seen centrally.

and for grade 3 cancer from 54% to 92% with positive contrast-enhanced MR imaging. MRI negative for myometrial invasion decreased the pretest probability to 1%, 5%, and 10%, respectively. The authors concluded that contrast-enhanced MRI significantly alters the post-test probability of deep myometrial invasion in patients with all grades of endometrial cancer and could be used to select patients for specialist referral (52).

A thickened or indistinct junctional zone can cause problems when staging endometrial cancer (Fig. 12A,B). Tanaka et al. (53) studied this phenomenon on T2-weighted MR images in patients with endometrial cancer. In addition they studied the enhancement of the junctional zone during dynamic contrast MRI and related this to histology. Thickening or an indistict junctional zone was found in 31 patients. Of these only 22% had evidence of invasive cancer. The authors found, however, that the sensitivity of a poor early enhancement pattern on dynamic enhanced images for detecting myometrial invasion was 71%, but with a specificity of 100% and overall accuracy of 92.5%. The authors found that the arteriole density

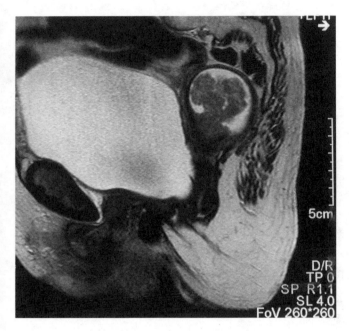

Figure 8 Sagittal T2-weighted scan shows a distended uterine cavity filled with fluid outlining a polypoid mass. The junctional zone appears preserved but there is marked thinning of the myometrium.

within the junctional zone with invasive cancer was significantly decreased. Poor enhancement of the junctional zone in the early dynamic phase was correlated with a decreased density of arterioles within the myometrium that was invaded by endometrial cancer. The authors concluded that dynamic contrast studies should be performed in staging endometrial cancer especially when the junctional zone is thickened or indistinct.

The depth of myometrial invasion may be difficult to establish in women with adenomyosis (Fig. 11). This is because the normal endometrial-myometrial interface in these women is irregular. This may cause either under- or overstaging in these patients. It must also be noted that a normal junctional zone may be absent in normal postmenopausal patients on T2-weighted MRI scans. A recent study (54) was performed on 11 patients who had a total of 12 lesions of endometrial cancer within adenomyosis. These authors compared T2-weighted and contrast-enhanced dynamic T1-weighted image with histological findings. They classed the depth of myometrial invasion as stage S (superficial invasion) and stage D (deep invasion) or undetectable. Deep myometrial invasion was confirmed histologically in 7 of 12 lesions. The depth of invasion was underestimated on T2-weighted images in two lesions and impossible to determine in five lesions. On dynamic T1-weighted images, the depth of invasion was

(A)

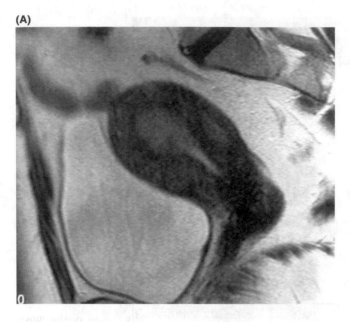

(B)

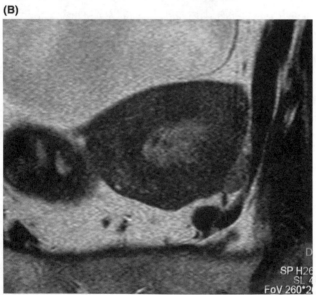

Figure 9 (**A**) Sagittal T2-weighted scan shows distension of the endometrial cavity by an intermediate signal intensity mass. There is focal disruption of the junctional zone but abnormal tissue extends into the myometrium for less than 50% of the thickness. (**B**) Angled axial T2-weighted scan shows irregularity of the junctional zone onto the left of the midline when comparison is made with the right.

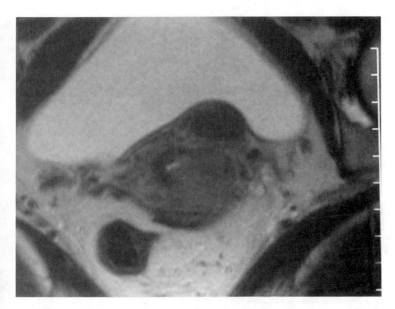

Figure 10 Thin angled T2-weighted scans demonstrate preservation of the junctional zone to the right and anterolaterally there is a large intermediate signal mass disrupting the junctional zone to the left and posteriorly extending to involve the outer half of the myometrium.

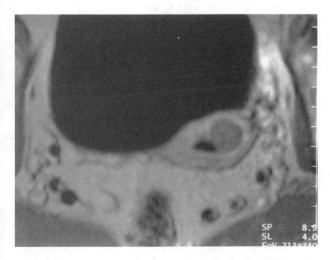

Figure 11 Dynamic Gadolinium enhanced gradient echo T1-weighted angled axial scan of the uterus showing an endometrial tumor to the left of the uterus with preservation of the early enhancement of the inner myometrium around the tumor indicating absense of myometrial invasion.

(A)

(B)

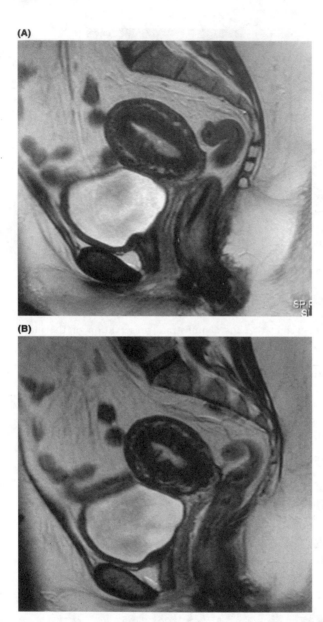

Figure 12 (A) Sagittal T2-weighted scan demonstrates an abnormal uterus with a thickened junctional zone but also widened endometrial stripe with an area of intermediate signal intensity. (B) The next sagittal section on the same patient demonstrates a cleft within the junctional zone that is filled with intermediate signal intensity material. At surgery this was proved to be stage-IB with invasion into the superficial myometrium.

overestimated in one lesion and underestimated in one lesion. Staging accuracy on dynamic gadolinium enhanced T1-weighted images was found to be 83% with an accuracy of 42% on T2-weighted scans. These authors concluded that dynamic T1-weighted images improve the accuracy of staging of endometrial cancer in patients with adenomyosis.

Tumor extension beyond the uterine corpus into the cervix can be identified reliably on MRI (Fig. 13) (38,44,55–57). Stage IIa disease (invasion of the endocervix) appears as widening of the internal os and endocervical canal but with preservation of the normal low signal (on T2-weighted scans) fibrocervical stroma. Potential overstaging may occur if there is polypoid extension of an endometrial cancer, debris, or a coexisting cervical polyp. The normal low signal fibrostroma of the cervix will be disrupted in stage IIb disease (Fig. 13). One study (58) concluded that pretreatment evaluation based on dilation and curettage was not accurate in a group of 29 patients, who underwent radical hysterectomy for suspected International Federation of Gynecology and Obstetrics (FIGO) stage II disease. Of these patients two had primary cervical cancer and of the remaining 27 only eight (29.6%) had cervical involvement. In one of this group with cervical involvement, extrau-

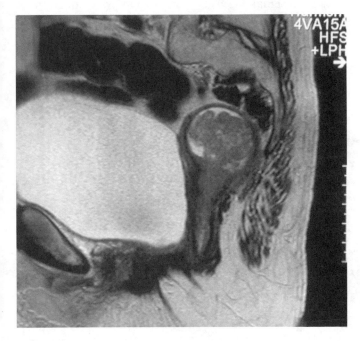

Figure 13 Sagittal T2-weighted scan demonstrates an expanded uterine cavity with abnormal intermediate signal intensity extending to the lower segment of the uterus and into the cervical canal. Early cervical stromal invasion was a concern on histopathology.

terine disease including ovarian spread was found. These authors had not taken account of preoperative imaging and suggested that a greater reliability on cross-sectional imaging with US, MRI, and CT would occur in the future. Another group (56) concluded that cervical cytology and MRI were useful to exclude cervical involvement. Endocervical curettage was useful for a positive diagnosis and that MRI may be useful for cervical stromal invasion.

Stage III endometrial cancer extends outside the uterus but not beyond the true pelvis. Full thickness tumor involvement will be seen on T2-weighted MR scans and contrast-enhanced scans. The integrity of the outer myometrium is usually irregular and/or disrupted (Fig. 14). Tumors that involve the cornua of the uterus (Fig. 15) may extend to involve the ovary. The ovaries may also be involved by metastatic disease. Involvement of the parametrial tissues is seen as disruption of the serosa with direct extension of intermediate signal intensity tumor into the surrounding high-signal parametrial fat (Fig. 14). There will be loss of the normal low-signal intensity vaginal wall (Fig. 16), if the tumor has extended into the upper vagina (stage IIIB disease).

US performs poorly for the detection of abnormal pelvic lymph nodes (59). Pathological lymph nodes are diagnosed on MRI and CT by size criteria (Fig. 17). MR signal intensity does not allow distinction of hyperplastic/inflammatory nodes from lymph nodes involved by metastatic

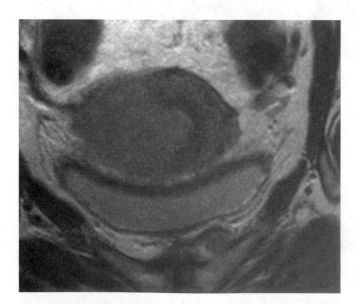

Figure 14 Angled axial T2-weighted scan shows full thickness involvement of the myometrium anteriorly and posteriorly to the right of the midline with loss of the serosa and irregularity of the margin between tumor and parametrial fat.

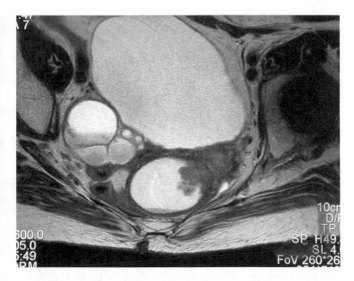

Figure 15 Axial T2-weighted scan shows abnormal intermediate signal intensity tumor extending out to the left cornu. Note is also made of an obstructed right fallopian tube and tumor was present within the tube on histopathology.

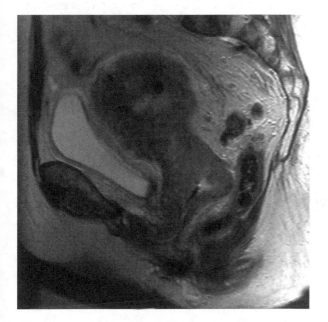

Figure 16 Sagittal T2-weighted scan demonstrates an endometrial carcinoma invading the cervix and extending into the vagina. The normal thin, low signal vaginal wall is replaced by intermediate signal tumor anteriorly and posteriorly.

disease. Stage IIIc disease (associated lymphadenopathy) is diagnosed when the short axis of the regional lymph nodes is larger than 1 cm although other authors have suggested that the acceptable short axis will vary depending upon the anatomical site within the pelvis (60). The ability of MRI to determine depth of myometrial invasion can be used in conjunction with the histological grading of the tumor to select patients at high risk of nodal involvement (61). A study carried out on 214 patients with endometrial cancer combined MRI, CA125 level, histological type, and grade to predict lymph node metastasis (62). These authors found that histological type, volume index, histological grade, and serum CA125 level were independent risk factors for pelvic lymph node metastasis; serum CA125 level and volume index were found to be independent risk factors for para-aortic lymph node metastases; 3.6% of patients with no risk factors had pelvic node disease while 0.7% of patients with no risk factors had para-aortic disease. Another study compared the cost of MRI and its ability to direct the use of lymph node dissection with the cost and ability of conventional surgery for the staging of endometrial cancer (63). When MR was utilized, all patients who needed lymph node dissection received it and 86% of these lymph node dissections were necessary. In the actual scenario one necessary lymph node dissection was not performed and 31% of the lymph node dissections were necessary. The authors concluded that staging with MR imaging has costs and accuracy similar to those of the current method of staging with intra-operative gross dissection of the uterus. In addition, MR imaging decreases the number of unnecessary lymph node dissections.

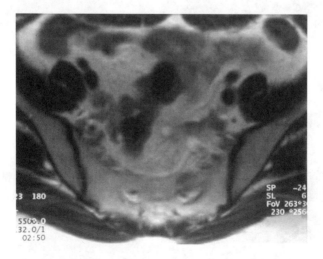

Figure 17 Axial T1-weighted scan demonstrating an enlarged right pelvic mode close to the external iliac vessels.

There are recognized indications for retroperitoneal lymph node sampling: deep myometrial invasion, isthmus-cervix extension, extrauterine spread, unfavorable histologies, and lymph node enlargement. As discussed above, deep myometrial invasion can be reliably excluded in patients with grades 1 and 2 disease (52) and MRI can identify cervical involvement. With this knowledge lymph node surgery is unnecessary in these patients.

(A)

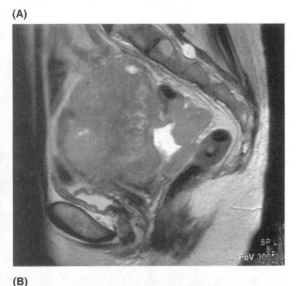

(B)

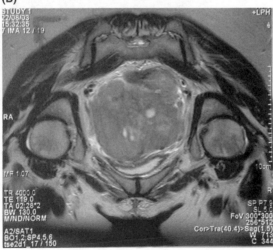

Figure 18 Sagittal (A) and angled axial (B) T2-weighted scans demonstrate a large abnormal tumor mass replacing the entire uterine corpus with involvement of the rectal wall posteriorly.

Stage IV tumor is recognized when disease extends beyond the true pelvis or there is evidence of invasion of the bladder or rectum (Fig. 18). Adjacent organ invasion can be recognized on MRI when there is focal loss of the low-signal intensity wall of the bladder or rectum and tumor is seen in continuity with these structures. Stage IVb disease (distant metastases) can be assessed on cross-sectional imaging. Peritoneal disease is best seen on fat-suppressed gadolinium enhanced T1-weighted imaging and in the presence of ascites. Neither MR nor CT are reliable in excluding peritoneal deposits measuring less than 1 cm in diameter.

In conclusion, transvaginal US has been shown to be reliable for the investigation of dysfunctional uterine bleeding. MRI should be used to stage proven endometrial cancer in those patients in whom assessment of myometrial invasion, or cervical and lymph node involvement is needed prior to surgery. Findings at MRI change the likelihood ratios for myometrial invasion and thus the need for lymph node dissection. This in turn may determine whether the patient can be treated at a cancer unit or center. Imaging findings of advanced disease may change patient management from potentially curative to that with palliative intent.

REFERENCES

1. Gull B, Karlsson B, Milson I, Granberg S. Can ultrasound replace dilatation curettage a longitudanal evaluation of post menopausal bleeding and trans vaginal sonographic measurement of the endometrium as predictive of endometrial cancer. Am J Obstet Gynaecol 2003; 188:401–408.
2. Brenner PF. Differential diagnosis of abnormal uterine bleeding. Am J Obstet Gynecol 1996; 175:766–769.
3. Epstein E, Ramirez A, Skoog L, Valentin L. Dilatation and curettage fails to detect most focal lesions in the uterine cavity in women with post menopausal bleeding. Acta Obstet Gynaecol Scand 2001; 80:1131–1136.
4. Karlsson B, Granberg S, Wikland M, Ylostalo P, Torvik K, Marsal K, Valentin L. Trans vaginal ultrasonography of the endometrium in women with post menopausal bleeding: a nordic multi centre study. Am J Obstet Gynecol 1995; 172:1488–1494.
5. Granberg S, Wikland M, Karlsson B, Norstrom A, Friberg LG. Endometrial thickness as measured by endovaginal ultrasonography for identifying endometrial abnormality. Am J Obstet Gynecol 1991; 164:47–52.
6. Guner H, Tiras MB, Karabacak O, Sarikaya H, Erden M, Yldririm M. Endometrial assessment by vaginal ultrasonography might reduce endomedtrial sampling in patients with post menopausal bleeding: a prospective study. Aust N Z J Obstet Gynecol 1996; 36:175–178.
7. Haller H, Matejcic N, Rukavina B, Krasevic M, Rupcic S, Mozetic D. Trans vaginal sonography and Hysteroscopy in women with post menopausal bleeding. Int J Gynecol Obstet 1996; 54:155–159.

8. Karlsson B, Granberg S, Wikland M, Ryd W, Norstrom A. Endovaginal scanning of the endometrium compared to cytology and histology in women with post menopausal bleeding. Gynecol Oncol 1993; 50:173–178.
9. Malanova M, Pehlivanov B. Trans vaginal sonography and progesterone challenge for identifying pathology in post menopausal women. Int J Gynecol Obstet 1996; 52:49–53.
10. Smith-Bindman R, Kerlikowske K, Feldstein VA, Subak L, Scheidler J, Segal M, Brand R, Grady D. Endovaginal ultrasound to exclude endometrial cancer and other endometrial abnormalities. JAMA 1998; 280:1510–1517.
11. Doren M, Suselbeck B, Schneider HP, Holzgreve W. Uterine perfusion and endometrial thickness in post menopausal women on long term continuous combined oestrogen and progesterone replacement. Ultrasound Obstet Gynecol 1997; 9:113–119.
12. Lin MC, Grosink BB, Wolf SI, Feldesman MR, Stuenkel CA, Braly PS, Pretorius DH. Endometrial thickness after menopause: effect of hormone replacement. Radiology 1991; 180:427–432.
13. Van den Bosch T, Van Shoubrouck D, Ameye L, De Brababantr A, Van Hussel S, Timmerman D. Ultrasound assessment of endometrial thickness and endometrial polyps in women on hormonal replacement therapy. Am J Obstet Gyaencol 2003; 188:1249–1253.
14. Graberg S, Ylostalo P, Wikland M, Karlsson B. Endometrial sonographic and hystologic findings in women with and without hormone replacement therapy suffering from post menopausal bleeding. Maturitas 1997; 27:35–40.
15. Garuti G, Sambruni I, Cellani F, Garzia D, Alleva P, Lueti M. Hysterscopy and transvaginal ultrasonography in postmenopausal women with uterine bleeding. Int J Gynaecol Obstet 1999; 65:25–33.
16. Briley M, Lindsell DR. The role of transvaginal ultrasound in the investigation of women with postmenopausal bleeding. Clin Rad 1998; 53:502–505.
17. Bakour SH, Dwarankanath LS, Khan KS, Newton JR, Gupta JK. The diagnostic accuracy of ultrasound scan in predicting endometrial hyperplasia and cancer in post-menopausal bleeding. Acta Obstet Gynecol Scand 1999; 78: 447–451.
18. Praskevaidis E, Kalantaridou SM, Papadimitirou B, Pappa L, Malamou-mitsi V, Zikopoulos K, Kazantzis E, Lolis BD, Agnantis M. Trans vaginal uterine ultrasonography compared with endometrial biopsy for the detection of endometrial disease in peri menopausal women with uterine bleeding. Anticancer Res 2002; 22:189–132.
19. Deckardt R, Lueken RP, Gallinat A, Moller CP, Busche D, Mugent W, Salfelder A, Dohnke H, Hoffmeister U, Dewitt E, Hennefrund J, Hasskamp T, Krichbaum M, Maucher A, Auweier U, Brokelmann J, Facf M, Fuger T. Comparison of trans vaginal ultrasound hysteroscopy and dilatation curettage in the diagnosis of abnormal vaginal bleeding and intra uterine pathology in peri menopausal and post menopausal women. J Am Assoc Gynaecol Laparosc 2002; 9:277–282.
20. Loverro G, Bettochi S, Cormio G, Nicolardi V, Greco P, Vimercati A, Selvaggi L. Transvaginal sonography and hysteroscopy in postmenopausal uterine bleeding. Maturitas 1999; 33:139–144.

21. Medverd JR, Dubinsky TJ. Cost analysis modelled: US versus endometrial biopsy in evaluation of peri and post menopausal abnormal vaginal bleeding. Radiology 2002; 222:619–627.
22. Weigel M, Friese K, Strittmatter HJ, Melchert F. Measuring the thickness; is that all we have to do for sonographic assessment of endometrium in post menopausal women? Ultrasound Obstet Gydecol 1995; 6:97–102.
23. Brandner P, Gnirs J, Neice KJ, Hetterbach A, Schmidt W. Vaginosonography in the non invasive evaluation of the endometrium of the post menopausal uterus. Geburtsh Frauenheik 1991; 51:734–740.
24. Sheikh M, Sawhnui S, Khurana A, Al-Uatma M. Alteration of sonographic texture of the endometrium in post menopausal bleeding a guide to further management. Acta Obstet Gynacol Scand 2000; 79:1006–1010.
25. Randelzhofer B, Prompeler HJ, Sauerbrei W, Madjar H, Emons G. Value of sonomorphological criteria of the endometrium in women with post menopausal bleeding a multi variate analysis. Ultrasound Obstet Gynaecol 2002; 19:62–68.
26. Atri M, Nazarnia S, Aldis AE, Reinhold C, Bret PM, Kintzen G. Transvaginal US appearance of endometrial abnormalities. Radiographics 1994; 14(3):483–92.
27. Hulka CA, Hall DA, McCarthy K, Simeone JF. Endometrial polyps, hyperplasiaand carcinoma in post-menopausal women: differentiation with endovaginal sonography. Radiology 1994; 191:755–758.
28. Grasel RP, Outwater EK, Siegelman ES, Capuzzi D, Parker L, Hussan SM. Endometrial polyps MR imaging features and distiction from endometrial carcinoma. Radiology 2000; 21:47–52.
29. Reinhold C, Khalili I. Postmenopausal bleeding: value of imaging. Rad Clin N Am 2002; 40:527–562.
30. Alcazar JL, Castillo G, Minguez JA, Galan MJ. Endometrial blood flow mapping using trans vaginal power doppler sonography in women with post menopausal bleeding and thickened endometrium. Ultrasound Obstet Gynacol 2003; 21:583–588.
31. Emoto M, Tamura R, Shirota K, Hacaisuga T, Kawarabayashi T. Clinical usefulness of colour dot ultrasound in patients with endometrial hyperplasia and carcinoma. Cancer 2002; 1(94):700–706.
32. Olaya FJ, Dualde D, Garcia E, Vidal P, Labrador T, Martiniez F, Gom G. Trans vaginal sonography in endometrial carcinoma: pre operative assessment of depth of myometrial invasion in 50 cases. EurJ Radiol 1998; 26:279–279.
33. Fishman A, Altarasm, Bernheim J, Cohen I, Beyth Y, Tepper R. The value of trans vaginal sonography in the pre operative assessment of myometrial invasion in high and low grade endometrial cancer and in comparison to frozen section in grade 1 disease. Eur J Gynaecol Oncol 2000; 21:128–130.
34. Szantho A, Szabo I, Csapo ZS, Balega J, Demeter A, Papp Z. Assessment of myometrial and cervical invasion of endometrial cancer by trans vaginal sonography. Eur J Gynaecol Oncol 2001; 22:209–212.
35. Van Doorn HC, Van der zee AG, Peeters PH, Kroeks MV, Van Eijkeren MA. Preoperative selection of patients with low-stage endometrial cancer at high risk of pelvic lymph mode metastases. Int J Gynaecol Cancer 2002; 12(2):144–8.

36. Kose G, Aka M, Api M. Pre operative assessment of myometrial invasion and cervical involvement of endometrial cancer by trans vaginal ultrasonography. Gynacol Obstet Invest 2003; 56:70–76.
37. Kinkel K, Kaji Y, Yu KK, Segal MR, Lu Y, Powell CB, Hricak H. Radiologic staging in patients with endometrial cancer: a met analysis. Radiology 1999; 21:711–718.
38. Frie KA, Kinkel K. Staging endometrial cancer: role of magnetic resonance imaging. J Magn Reson Imaging 2001; 13:850–855.
39. Hardesty LA, Sumkin JH, Haakim C, Johns C, Nath M. The ability of helical CT to pre operatively stage endometrial carcinoma. AJR 2001; 176(3):603–6.
40. Zarbo G, Caruso G, Caruso S, Mangano V, Zarbo R. Endometrial cancer: preoperative evaluation of myometrial infiltration magnetic resonance imaging versus transvaginal ultrasonography. Eur J Gynaecol Oncol 2000; 21(1):95–7.
41. Ascher SN, Reinhold C. Imaging cancer of the endometrium. Radiol Clin North Am 2002; 40(3):95–76.
42. Fleischer AC. Transvaginal sonography of endometrial disorders: on overview. Radiographics 1998; 18(4):293–30.
43. Savci G, Ozyaman T, Tutar M, Bilgin T, Erol O, Tuncel E. Assessment of depth of myometrial invasion by endometrial carcinoma: comparison of T2 weighted SE and contrast enhanced dynamic GRE MR imaging. Eur Radiol 1998; 8: 218–223.
44. Cunha TM, Fellix A, Cabral I. Pre operative assessment of deep myometrial and cervical invasion in endometrial carcinoma comparison of magnetic resonance imaging and gross visual inspection. Int J Gynacol Cancer 2001; 11: 130–136.
45. Takahashi S, Murakami T, Narymi Y, Kurach H, Tsuda K, Kim T, Enomoto T, Tomoda K, Miyake A, Murata Y, Nakamuri H. Pre operative staging of endometrial carcinoma diagnostic efficocy of T2 weighted fast spin echo MR imaging. Radiology 1998; 206:539–547.
46. Seki H, Kimura M, Sakai K. Myometrial invasion of endometrial carcinoma assessment with dynamic MR and contrast enhanced T1 weighted images. Clin Radiol 1997; 52:18–23.
47. Joja I, Asakawa T, Shiraiwa M, Shibutani O, Okuno K, Akaki S, Togami I, Kudo T, Hiraki Y. Endometrial carcinoma multi section dynamic MR Imaging using a 3 dimensional FLASH technique during breath holding. Radiat Med 1999; 17:211–218.
48. Saez S, Urresola A, Larena JA, Martin JI, Pijuan JI, Scheneidr J, Ibanez E. Endometrial carcinoma assessment of myometrial invasion with plain and gadolinium enhanced MR imaging. J Magn Reson Imaging 2000; 12:460–466.
49. Frei KA, Kinkel K, Bonel HM, Lu Y, Zaloudek C, Hricak H. Prediction of deep myometrial invasion in patients with endometrial cancer: clinical utility of contrast enhanced MR imaging—a meta- analysis and bayesian analysis. Radiology 2000; 216:449–449.
50. Joja I, Asakawa M, Asakawa T, Nakagawa T, Kanazawa S, Kuroda, Togami I, Hiraki Y, Akamatsu M, Kudo T. Endometrial carcinoma dynamic MRI with turbo SLASH technique. J Comput Assist Tomoger 1996: 20:878–887.

51. Lee EJ, Byun JY, Kim BS, Koong SE, Shinn KS. Staging of early endometrial carcinoma assessment with T2 weighted and gadolinium enhanced T1 weighted MR imaging. Radiographics 1999; 19:937–945.
52. Frei KA, Kinkel K, Bonel HM, Lu Y, Zaloudek C, Hricak H. Prediction of deep myometrial invasion in patients with endometrial cancer: clinical utility of contrast-enhanced MR imaging- a meta-analysis and Bayesian analysis. Radiology 2000; 216(2):444–9.
53. Tanaka YO, Nishida M, Tsunoda H, Ichikawa Y, Saida Y, Itiai Y. A thickened or indistinct junctional zone on t2 weighted mr images in patients with endometrial carcinoma: pathologic consideration based on micro circulation. Eur Radiol 2003; 13:2038–2045.
54. Utsunomiya D, Notsute S, Hayashaida Y, Lwakatare S, Katabuchi H, Okamura H, Awi K, Yamashita Y. Endometrial carcinoma in adenomyosis: assessment of myometrial invasion on T2 weighted spin echo and gadolinium enhanced T1 weighted images. AJR 2004; 182:399–404.
55. Toki T, Oka K, Nakayama K, Oguchi O, Fujii S. A comparative study of pre operative procedures to assess cervical invasion by endometrial carcinoma. Br J Obstet Gynacol 1998; 105:512–516.
56. Morimura Y, Soeda S, Hashimoto T, Takano Y, Ohwada M, Yamada, Yanagida K, Sato A, Fukushima J. The value of Pre-Operative diagnostic procedures for cervical involvement in uterine corpus carcinoma. Med Sci 2000; 46:1–11.
57. Seki H, Takano T, Sakai K. Value of dynamic MR imaging in assessing endometrial carcinoma involvement of the cervix. AJR 2000; 175:171–176.
58. Pete I, Godeny M, Toth E, Rado J, Pete B, Pulay T. Prediction of cervical infiltration in stage 2 endometrial cancer by different pre operative evaluation techniques (D&C, ultrasound, CT, and MRI). Eur J Gynacol Oncol 2003; 24: 517–522.
59. Sawicki W, Spiewankiewicz B, Stelmachw J, Cendrowski K. The value of ultrasonograpy in pre operative assessment of selective prognostic factors in endometrial cancer. Eur J Gynacol Oncol 2003; 24:293–298.
60. Grubnic S, Vinnicombe SJ, Normal AR, Husband JE. MR evaluation of normal retroperitoneal and pelvic lymph nodes. Clin Radiol 2000; 57(3):201–2.
61. Minderhoud-Bassie W, Trerriet FE, Koops W, Chadha-Ajwani S, Hage JC, Huikeshoven FJ. Magnetic resonance imaging (MRI) in endometrial carcinoma:preoperative estimation of depth of myometrial invasion. Acta Obstet Gynaecol Scand 1995; 74(10):827–31.
62. Todo Y, Sakuragi M, Nishiva R, Yamada T, Ebina Y, Yamanoto R, Fujimoto S. Combined use of magnetic resonance imaging Ca 124 histologic type and histologic grade in the prediction of lymph node metastasis in endometrial carcinoma. Am J Obstet Gynaecol 2003; 188:1265–1272.
63. Hardesty LA, Sumkin JH, Nath ME, Edwards RP, Price FV, Chang, Johns CM, Kelley JL. Use of pre operative MR imaging in the management of endometrial carcinoma: cost analysis. Radiology 2000; 215:45–49.

8

Surgery for Uterine Cancer

Neville F. Hacker and Donald E. Marsden
Gynaecological Cancer Centre, Royal Hospital for Women, Randwick, and School of Obstetrics and Gynaecology, University of New South Wales, New South Wales, Australia

Surgery is the mainstay of the treatment of malignant disease involving the uterine corpus. The nature of the surgery and its extent are the subject of ongoing debate, and there are still areas of significant controversy, which will be addressed in this chapter. Malignant disease of the uterine corpus falls into two major categories, namely endometrial carcinoma and uterine sarcomas, and these conditions will be addressed separately.

ENDOMETRIAL CANCER

For some time the potential seriousness of endometrial cancer was underestimated. In 1956, Peel commented that as a resident in the 1930s he had been taught that endometrial cancer was "a benign form of neoplasm with a very good prognosis from not very radical surgery" but that attitudes to the disease had "undergone a slow but radical change" (1). There was little evidence of that change when Stallworthy in 1973 expressed concern about the generally optimistic view of endometrial cancer, the actual reported survival figures, and about the poor approach of the occasional surgeon (2). The justification for this concern was clearly demonstrated by Jones, who in 1975 reported that despite the fact that the majority of women with endometrial cancer had early stage disease clinically, the worldwide five-year survival figures averaged only 68% (3). Following this, Boronow in 1976, discussed "four prevalent myths" relating to endometrial cancer (4). The first, that endometrial cancer is a relatively benign disease, he refuted by showing that, stage for stage, the prognosis for endometrial cancer was the same as that for cervical cancer, and that the overall five-year survival rate in the United States was less than 70%. The other "myths" he exposed were that the best therapy was known, the prognostic factors defined, and that lymph node status was of little importance.

The significance of lymph node involvement in endometrial carcinoma was initially reported by the workers at Oxford in England under the direction of Stallworthy (5,6). They reported their results with 109 patients operated on by radical hysterectomy and lymph node dissection for early stage endometrial carcinoma, and demonstrated a 5.5% incidence of positive nodes with grade 1 tumors, 10% for grade 2, and 26% for grade 3. Even when postoperative external beam radiation was used, the five-year survival for node positive patients was only 36%. Following the publication of these data, a cooperative study was instituted involving three institutions in the United States to investigate the risk factors and recurrence patterns of stage I endometrial cancer and the pathological findings in such patients (7,8). The results essentially confirmed the findings of the Oxford group. The Gynecologic Oncology Group (GOG) then set up a further study, which examined the surgical pathological features of 621 patients with clinical stage I carcinoma of the endometrium, with all patients undergoing a total abdominal hysterectomy, bilateral salpingo-oophorectomy, selective pelvic and para-aortic lymphadenectomy, and peritoneal cytology (9). Pelvic nodes were positive in 9% of patients, and para-aortic nodes in 6%, while in 5% there was adnexal involvement. Tumor grade and depth of myometrial penetration were the main indicators of extrauterine spread.

On the basis of these and similar studies, International Federation of Gynecology and Obstetrics (FIGO) introduced a surgical staging system of endometrial cancer in 1988 (10). The 1971 FIGO clinical staging system is shown in Table 1, and the 1988 surgical staging system in Table 2. It was hoped that use of surgical staging would help to determine the true extent of the disease in individual patients, and thus to allow the planning of appropriate therapy and improve survival. However, as Boronow has pointed out, the staging was based solely on surgico-patho-logic features and their presumed prognostic implications, but not on outcome data (11). He acknowledged that surgical staging was better at defining prognostic groups, but objected to the implication that without surgical staging patients were at risk of being inadequately treated, emphasizing that the benefits of the staging procedure had to outweigh the risks for individual patients. Speaking of the use of the full surgical staging procedure, Morrow commented that those familiar with the management of endometrial cancer were aware that many patients "are only suited to the minimum procedure because of age, obesity, or frailty from complicating medical problems" (12). In the GOG study Morrow

Table 1 The FIGO Clinical Staging for Endometrial Cancer (1971)

Stage I	The carcinoma is confined to the corpus
Stage IA	The length of the uterine cavity is 8 cm or less
Stage IB	The length of the uterine cavity is greater than 8 cm

Stage I cases should be subgrouped with regard to the histologic grade of the adenocarcinoma as follows:

Grade 1	Highly differentiated adenomatous carcinoma
Grade 2	Moderately differentiated adenomatous carcinoma with partly solid areas
Grade 3	Predominantly solid or entirely undifferentiated carcinoma
Stage II	The carcinoma has involved the corpus and the cervix but has not extended outside the uterus
Stage III	The carcinoma has extended outside the uterus but not outside the true pelvis
Stage IV	The carcinoma has extended outside the true pelvis or has obviously the mucosa of the bladder or rectum. Bullous edema as such does not permit a case to be allocated to stage IV
Stage IVA	Spread of the growth to adjacent organs
Stage IVB	Spread to distant organs

was commenting on, where patients were treated in recognized gynecologic oncology units by subspecialists, significant surgical complications occurred in 19.4% of patients, with three of the patients dying as a result of surgery.

Given the risks of a full staging procedure in unfit patients and the fact that a significant proportion of patients will not have nodal involvement, it seems appropriate to try to develop a treatment approach that avoids unnecessary complications in low-risk patients, but offers the potential advantages of a full staging procedure to those most likely to benefit. An examination of the major prognostic factors for endometrial cancer can help inform decision making.

PROGNOSTIC FACTORS THAT MAY HELP DETERMINE THE APPROPRIATE SURGERY FOR ENDOMETRIAL CANCER

The surgical pathological stage of endometrial cancer is obviously the most important prognostic factor, but in considering how to treat patients, and in particular deciding which patients are likely to benefit from a full surgical staging procedure, a clear understanding of the factors which affect prognosis within a given stage, and the factors which increase the risk of lymph node metastasis, is essential.

Age

A GOG study of over 700 patients with clinical stage I or occult stage II disease indicated that, when compared to women with endometrial

Table 2 FIGO Surgical Staging for Endometrial Cancer (1998)

Stage IA G1,2,3	Tumor limited to endometrium
Stage IB G1,2,3	Invasion to less than one half of the myometrium
Stage IC G1,2,3	Invasion to more than one half of the myometrium
Stage IIA G1,2,3	Endocervical glandular involvement only
Stage IIB G1,2,3	Cervical stromal invasion
Stage IIIA G1,2,3	Tumor invades serosa and/or adnexa and/or positive peritoneal cytology
Stage IIIB G1,2,3	Vaginal metastases
Stage IIIC G1,2,3	Metastases to pelvic and/or para-aortic lymph glands
Stage IVA G1,2,3	Tumor invasion of bladder and/or bowel mucosa
Stage IVB G1,2,3	Distant metastases including intra-abdominal and/or inguinal lymph nodes

Histopathology: degree of differentiation
Cases of carcinoma of the corpus should be classified (graded) according to the
degree of histologic differentiation as follows:

G1	5% or less of a nonsquamous or nonmorular/growth pattern
G2	6–50% of a nonsquamous or nonmorular solid growth pattern
G3	More than 50% of a nonsquamous or nonmorular solid growth pattern

Notes on pathological grading: 1. Notable nuclear atypia, inappropriate for the architectural grade, raises the grade of a grade 1 or 2 tumor by 1. 2. In serous adenocarcinomas, clear cell adenocarcinomas, and squamous cell carcinomas, nuclear grading takes precedence. 3. Adenocarcinomas with squamous differentiation are graded according to the nuclear grade of the glandular component.

Rules related to staging:1. Because corpus cancer is now staged surgically, procedures previously used for determination of stages are no longer applicable, such as the findings from fractional dilatation and curettage to differentiate between stages I and II. 2. It is appreciated that there may be a small number of patients with corpus cancer who will be treated primarily with radiation therapy. If that is the case, the clinical staging adopted by FIGO in 1971 would still apply, but designation of that staging system would be noted. 3. Ideally, width of the myometrium should be measured along with the width of tumor invasion.

cancer aged 45 or younger, those aged 55–64 had a two-fold increased risk of death from the disease; those aged 65–74, a 3.4-fold increase; and those age 75-plus a 4.7-fold increase (13). As most patients with endometrial cancer are postmenopausal, and some of quite advanced age, these figures must be kept in mind to ensure that patients are not treated on the basis of age alone.

Histologic Type

The vast majority of endometrial cancers are of the endometrioid type. In a retrospective study of 388 cases from the Mayo Clinic, the 87% with endometrioid tumors had a 92% survival rate (14). The uncommon subtypes included 20 cases of adenosquamous carcinoma, 14 serous papillary tumors, 11 clear cell, and seven undifferentiated carcinomas. In this group, 62% had extrauterine spread at the time of surgical staging and their overall survival rate was 33%.

It has been demonstrated that the presence of benign or malignant squamous differentiation in an endometrioid carcinoma of the endometrium is of little prognostic significance, when compared to the histological grade and depth of myometrial penetration of the glandular elements of the tumor, making the terms adenoacanthoma and adenosquamous carcinoma redundant (15).

The two tumor types that carry very poor prognoses are the papillary serous tumors and clear cell carcinomas of the endometrium; they are not uncommonly seen together.

Papillary serous tumors have a very poor prognosis even in the absence of other factors such as deep myometrial invasion or lymph node metastases. In a study of 50 surgically staged patients with papillary serous carcinoma of the uterus, Goff et al. found that 72% of patients had extra-uterine disease (16). Nodal metastases were present in 36% with no myoinvasion, 50% with inner-half and 40% with outer-half involvement. There was a similarly high rate of lymph node metastasis regardless of whether or not there was lymph vascular space invasion. Widespread dissemination and recurrence in the upper abdomen are particular features of these tumors (17). The overall survival rates are very poor. In a study of 41 cases where at least 25% of the tumor consisted of papillary serous carcinoma, the tumor-free survival rate was less than 20% and was the same whether the tumor was pure, mixed with another type of carcinoma, or involving a polyp (18).

Clear cell carcinoma of the endometrium also has a very poor prognosis. In a series of 181 cases from the Norwegian Radium Institute, the five-year actuarial disease-free survival was 43% (19). For surgical stage I disease it was 54%, while for stage II it was 27%. Where there was no myometrial invasion, the survival rate was 90%, whereas with deep myoinvasion it was 15%. Recurrence in the upper abdomen, liver, or lungs occurred in over 60% of cases.

Tumor Grade and Depth of Myometrial Invasion

For endometrioid carcinomas of the endometrium, tumor grade and depth of myometrial penetration are important prognostic factors. The GOG reported that with grade 1 endometrial cancers confined to the inner third of the myometrium, pelvic nodes were involved in about 3% of cases and para-aortic nodes in 1%, but for grade 3 tumors involving the outer one-third of the myometrium, positive pelvic nodes were found in 34% of cases and para-aortic nodes in 23% (9). The incidence of distant metastases is also directly related to tumor grade and depth of myometrial invasion. It has long been recognized that positive nodes are a significant prognostic factor, but the routine use of radiotherapy in node-positive patients has made it difficult to assess the magnitude of the risk.

Tumor Size

Schink et al., in a study of 142 women with clinical stage I endometrial cancer, demonstrated that lymph node metastases were present in 4% of cases with tumors less than 2 cm in diameter, 15% greater than 2 cm in diameter, and 35% where the entire endometrial cavity was involved (20).

Peritoneal Cytology

While peritoneal cytology does not affect the type of surgery performed, it has been considered an important part of the surgery. Positive peritoneal cytology increases the relative risk of death by a factor of three (21). However, in the Gynecologic Oncology study, while disease recurred in 29% of patients with positive cytology compared to 11% with negative cytology, in two-thirds of the cases the recurrence was outside the peritoneal cavity (12). Another study of 269 patients with clinical stages I and II disease concluded that if the disease was otherwise confined to the uterine cavity, positive cytology did not affect the prognosis, but that if there was adnexal, nodal, or peritoneal involvement with positive peritoneal cytology, the survival was reduced from 73% to 13%, but with all recurrences at distal sites (22). Other studies support these findings (23,24).

Other Prognostic Factors

There are a number of other factors recognized to influence the outcome of endometrial cancer, including hormone receptor status, nuclear grade, DNA ploidy, and other biologic markers, but these are not usually relevant to the planning of the surgical approach to endometrial cancer.

DIAGNOSIS

The histological diagnosis of endometrial cancer can be made by either endometrial sampling as an office procedure, or dilation and curettage. Numerous devices are available for office endometrial biopsy. In about 8% of patients cervical stenosis prevents sampling, and in women over 70 years of age the figure is around 18% (25). In a recent meta-analysis the Pipelle appeared to be the best device, correctly identifying endometrial carcinoma in 91% of premenopausal women and 99.5% of postmenopausal women (26). A negative biopsy demands dilatation and curettage. Dilatation and curettage has been considered the "gold standard" for diagnosing endometrial cancer. Whether the addition of hysteroscopy offers any improvement in the accuracy of the diagnosis, or in the preoperative staging, is unclear (27). Fears that hysteroscopy might increase the incidence of disseminated intraperitoneal disease by washing malignant cells through the fallopian tubes have proven unfounded (28,29).

PREOPERATIVE WORK UP

Endocervical involvement by endometrial cancer has traditionally been determined by fractional curettage but false positive rates of up to 50% have been reported, probably because either endometrium was sampled accidentally or there was "carry over" of tumor from the endometrial cavity (30,31).

As the depth of myometrial penetration may help decide both the type of surgery required and the site at which it is conducted, a number of techniques have been investigated to assess this feature preoperatively. Prospective studies have compared ultrasound, computed tomography (CT) scans, and magnetic resonance imaging (MRI) in this context. Magnetic resonance imaging, though promising, is costly, limited in availability, and does not really offer advantages over intraoperative assessment (32). Occasionally cystoscopy or sigmoidoscopy may be indicated if advanced stage disease is suspected clinically.

Where there is clinical suspicion of extrauterine disease, CT scans of the abdomen and pelvis may be helpful, but the assessment of nodal status is usually best performed by palpation of nodes intraoperatively.

Routine electrolyte assays, full blood counts, and a chest X-ray are essential before surgery, and many patients will need a full medical work up by a physician because of the co-morbidities that are common in endometrial cancer patients.

THE SURGICAL PROCEDURE

Total abdominal hysterectomy and bilateral salpingo-oophorectomy is, in most cases, the essential feature of treatment for this disease. This removes the primary tumor and the ovaries, which may be a site of metastasis or concurrent malignancy.

FIGO staging procedure requires peritoneal cytology and lymph node dissection in order to assign a stage, but the nature and extent of the lymphadenectomy has not been defined. Given that many patients are obese or medically unfit, and that most will have early stage disease, some form of selection seems appropriate in deciding which patients should undergo lymphadenectomy, in order to avoid the morbidity of the procedure. While it is true that there is a relatively low morbidity for lymphadenectomy in experienced hands, it does increase operating time, the risk of intraoperative hemorrhage and postoperative lymphocyst formation, and very importantly, the incidence of lymphoedema. Lymphoedema has been an underreported result of pelvic lymph node dissection, but work in our department has indicated that it occurs in approximately 20% of patients (33). Not only is the swelling of the limbs a problem in itself, but episodes of lymphangitis commonly complicate the condition. Once present, lymphoedema is a lifelong affliction and its management a significant burden for both patient and carers. Hence lymph node dissection should be used only where it appears likely to improve the outlook for the patient.

The most important way in which systematic node dissection can help the management of patients is by obviating the need for external beam radiotherapy. High-risk disease in the presence of negative pelvic nodes is generally believed to require only vaginal brachytherapy, which is a much less morbid procedure than external beam therapy. Nodal status determines the appropriate fields for external beam therapy: involvement of common iliac or low para-aortic nodes will require extended field radiotherapy to ensure tumor control.

For clinically early stage disease, we determine the need for systematic lymphadenectomy on the basis of the tumor type and grade as determined preoperatively, the size of the tumor and the apparent depth of myometrial invasion determined by bisecting the uterus in the operating theater, and on the basis of palpation of pelvic and para-aortic nodes at the time of laparotomy. Our indications for complete surgical staging are shown in Table 3.

The correlation between preoperative tumor grading and that found in the hysterectomy specimen is far from perfect, most likely due to heterogeneity of the tumor. Between 20% and 40% of tumors thought to be grade 1 on curettage will in fact be upgraded but the correlation is better for grade 2, and grade 3 tumors (34,35). In practice these differences are seldom of clinical significance, and in our belief do not justify routine lymphadenectomy for apparent grade 1 or grade 2 tumors.

The intraoperative inspection of the opened uterus allows a reasonably accurate assessment of tumor size and depth of invasion. In one study, macroscopic examination of the opened specimen accurately predicted the depth of invasion in 87% of grade 1 tumors, 65% of grade 2, and 31% of grade 3 tumors (36). In another study, the accuracy of intraoperative visual assessment was 85% if the decision was between less than 50% invasion or greater (37).

Table 3 Patients with Stage I and Occult Stage II Endometrial Cancer Who Require Surgical Staging

Patients with grade 3 lesions
Patients with grade 2 tumors over 2 cm in diameter
Patients with clear cell or papillary serous carcinomas
Patients with over 50% myometrial penetration
Patients with cervical extension of tumor

The tumor size assessed by examination of the opened specimen is particularly useful where a grade 2 tumor is present, as in one study no patients with grade 2 tumors less than 2 cm in diameter had nodal metastases compared to 22% where the tumor was greater than 2 cm (38).

Where there are palpably enlarged pelvic or para-aortic nodes, they should be resected and subjected to frozen section. In the presence of macroscopically positive nodes, radiation will be indicated and so a full lymphadenectomy is not appropriate. Where nodes are not macroscopically enlarged, we restrict lymph node dissection to patients with endometrioid carcinomas with penetration to the outer half of the myometrium, extension to the cervix, grade 3 histology, or bulky grade 2 disease. All patients with papillary serous clear cell carcinoma undergo pelvic lymphadenectomy, unless grossly enlarged nodes are present, in which case they are treated as already discussed.

The benefits of routine systematic lymphadenectomy have never been the subject of a randomized controlled trial, and are still controversial. Kilgore compared the outcomes for 212 patients undergoing multi-site pelvic node sampling with those of 205 with limited site sampling, and 208 who had no node sampling (39). The multi-site sampling group had a mean of 11 nodes removed, compared to four in the limited site group. Lymph node sampling was at the discretion of the surgeon. Risk factors for nodal metastasis were the same in each group. All patients received adjuvant radiation according to standard prognostic factors. With a mean three-year follow up, the group undergoing the more extensive lymphadenectomy had a significantly better overall survival, and better survival for both low- and high-risk groups. While the authors of the study conclude that these results indicate a therapeutic benefit for lymphadenectomy, it seems more likely to be due to the removal of enlarged nodes, which are less likely to be sterilized by radiation.

On the other hand, for patients with high-risk disease, the knowledge that the pelvic lymph nodes are negative may allow the patient to avoid external beam radiation with its accompanying morbidity. A number of studies, none of which were randomized, support this view (40–44).

We do not advocate routine para-aortic lymphadenectomy, as the incidence of aortic node metastasis is very low in the absence of pelvic-node involvement. We would, however, remove any grossly enlarged aortic nodes. Patients at greatest risk of para-aortic metastases are those with grossly positive pelvic nodes, grossly positive adnexae, or grade 2 or grade 3 lesions with outer third myometrial invasion (12). Omental biopsy is usually performed as the omentum may contain occult malignancy, especially in high-risk tumors, such as papillary serous or clear cell carcinomas, and those with grade 3 or deeply invasive tumors (45). It is accepted that this approach differs from surgical practice in many countries, especially in North America and some parts of Europe, where para-aortic lymphadenectomy is more commonly advocated.

Stage II Endometrial Cancer

Where the tumor is known to involve the endocervical canal (stage II disease), a type 2 radical hysterectomy and pelvic lymph node dissection to the level of the aortic bifurcation is performed, with peritoneal washings, omental biopsy, and resection of any bulky aortic nodes. There are no randomized controlled trials to justify such an approach but several retrospective studies provide support for it. Investigators in Italy reported their results in 203 patients with stage II endometrial cancer, 66% of whom had simple hysterectomies and 43% radical hysterectomies (46). Radiation was given to 59% of patients with stage IIA disease and 73% of patients with stage IIB. The five-year survival rates were 79% in the group undergoing simple hysterectomy and 94% for radical hysterectomy, and were essentially the same at 10 years. Loco-regional recurrence rates were lower in the radiation group but survival was not improved.

Examination of Surveillance, Epidemiology and End Results (SEER) data from 1988 to 1994 revealed 555 patients who underwent simple hysterectomy for stage II endometrial cancer and 377 who had radical hysterectomy (47). The five-year survival for patients undergoing simple hysterectomy was 84% compared to 93% for those having radical hysterectomy. Adjuvant radiation did not appear to improve survival in either arm. The conclusion was that radical hysterectomy was associated with better survival. Mariani et al. examined the results of radical hysterectomy and pelvic node dissection in stage II endometrial cancer and concluded that the results were excellent in cases with negative nodes, with no added benefit from adjuvant radiotherapy (48).

Clinical Stage III Disease

In the now superseded clinical staging system for endometrial carcinoma, apparent parametrial, adnexal, or sidewall disease was classified as stage III. When subjected to laparotomy many of these patients were found to have benign adnexal lesions. But by the same token, between 5% and 10% of women with no clinical evidence of extrauterine spread will have occult tumor metastases in the adnexal structures. These facts make interpretation of results of series of clinical stage III disease difficult. In one study the five-year survival for surgical stage III disease was 40% and for clinical stage III 16% (49). The prognosis in surgical stage III disease also is affected by the pelvic structures involved: in one study when the ovary and/or fallopian tube were involved, the five-year survival was 80% while when other extrauterine pelvic structures were involved it was 15% (50).

Where patients are thought to have extrauterine disease confined to the pelvis, a laparotomy is usually indicated to identify the nature and extent of pelvic extension. If possible a total abdominal hysterectomy and bilateral salpingo-oophorectomy should be performed to remove the primary tumor. The nature of clinically detectable adnexal masses can also be determined at that time. Other aspects of the treatment are individualized, but the aim is to remove, if possible, all gross disease from the pelvis. Where hysterectomy is precluded by parametrial infiltration, neoadjuvant radiation can be utilized with consideration of a completion hysterectomy at a later date.

The presence of vaginal metastases at the time of diagnosis of endometrial cancer is rare. In a review of 1940 patients treated for endometrial cancer in a single Australian institution, only 14 patients with apparently isolated vaginal metastases (FIGO stage IIIB) were identified (51). None of these women had node dissections, which could well have upstaged them to stage IIIC, and their survival was similar to patients with that stage of disease. Treatment should involve the surgical removal of vaginal metastases if feasible, together with the standard laparotomy, total abdominal hysterectomy and bilateral salpingo-oophorectomy, peritoneal washings, and omental biopsy. If the vaginal metastasis cannot be surgically removed and hysterectomy is feasible, it should be done as for other endometrial cancers and the vaginal metastasis treated with radiation. Enlarged pelvic and para-aortic nodes should be resected in either case.

Stage IV Endometrial Cancer

Stage IV endometrial cancer may involve the mucosa of the bladder or bowel (stage IVA) or distant metastases, most frequently to the lungs or upper abdomen. The prognosis in either case is guarded. Nevertheless, it is important to try to achieve control of pelvic disease, which, if untreated, can lead to a foul vaginal discharge or bleeding or fistulae, often together with severe pain. Hence a total abdominal hysterectomy and bilateral salpingo-oophorectomy should be performed if possible, even in the presence of distant metastases. Where advanced pelvic disease precludes hysterectomy, the occasional patient may benefit from pelvic exenteration.

In patients with stage IVB disease there may be a role for cytoreductive surgery. In a study of 65 patients undergoing surgery for stage IVB disease, in the 55% of patients in whom residual disease was 1 cm or less, the median survival was 34 months, compared to 11 months in the remainder (52). Whether this represents a difference in the aggressiveness of the disease or a true effect of debulking is not clear, but it does indicate that if debulking can be undertaken, it most likely should.

Recurrent Endometrial Cancer

While most patients with endometrial cancer will be cured, a significant proportion will recur. A large study of recurrent endometrial cancer indicated that half the patients had isolated local recurrences, about one-third had distant metastases, and the remainder had both (53). Vaginal recurrences are frequently curable, most commonly by radiation in women who had not previously had radiotherapy. For women who have a recurrence confined to the central pelvis without lymph node involvement, and who have already undergone radiotherapy, an exenterative procedure may be considered. While most central recurrences in non-irradiated women will respond to radiotherapy, where the lesion is greater than 4 cm in diameter it may not respond completely to radiation, and there is a case for laparotomy and resection of all or most of the tumor to increase the chance of satisfactory control with subsequent radiation.

Endometrial Cancer Found After Routine Hysterectomy

Should this happen, a metastatic work up including a chest X-ray and abdominal and pelvic CT should be performed together with a CA125 assay. Although raised CA125 levels are rare in early stage disease, advanced stage and metastatic endometrial cancer is often associated with a raised CA125 (54).

If extra-abdominal metastases appear to be excluded, any suggestion of pelvic or para-aortic lymphadenopathy, or other intraperitoneal disease is normally an indication for laparotomy.

In the absence of evidence of metastatic disease, it is reasonable to observe patients with stages IA and IB, grade 1 or grade 2 tumors, although oophorectomy is probably wise to exclude synchronous or subsequent ovarian cancer. Where stage IC disease is present in the uterus, and for grade 3 tumors, a laparotomy and staging procedure should be considered.

Who Should Perform Surgery?

The full surgical staging procedure should only be performed by experienced surgeons in appropriately equipped and staffed centers. It is not the procedure for the occasional operator. Similarly, regardless of the surgery planned, obese or unfit women should be operated on in similar centers.

For women with well-differentiated tumors not apparently involving the cervix, with a small mobile uterus and no evidence of adnexal disease on careful examination, an experienced gynecologist can realistically undertake the operation with minimal risk. At the time of surgery, careful palpation of the upper abdomen and nodal groups should be undertaken, peritoneal cytology obtained, and a small omental biopsy obtained. A total abdominal hysterectomy and bilateral salpingo-oophorectomy should be performed, taking care to remove the entire ovary on each side.

Whenever there is doubt about who should perform the surgery, or where the surgery should be performed, consultation with a gynecologic oncologist is prudent.

UTERINE SARCOMAS

The rarity and heterogeneity of this group of uterine tumors containing malignant mesenchymal elements makes it difficult to provide well-documented guidelines for their surgical management. Sarcomas account for approximately 3% of tumors of the uterine body and may be "pure" where they contain only tissue of mesenchymal origin, or "mixed" when malignant mesenchymal tissue and malignant epithelial tissue are both present (55). Pure uterine sarcomas are leiomyosarcomas and endometrial stromal sarcomas, while the malignant mixed Mullerian tumor or carcinosarcoma represents the mixed type of tumor.

The basic surgical procedure that appears to have the best hope of curing uterine sarcomas is a total abdominal hysterectomy and bilateral salpingo-oophorectomy. As will be discussed later, the role of more extensive surgical staging is uncertain, though it may be of value in some situations.

Leiomyosarcoma may occasionally occur in young women. In a GOG study of 59 stage I and stage II leiomyosarcomas, only 3.4% had adnexal metastases (56). In another study of 71 patients with clinical stage I or stage II leiomyosarcomas from Memorial Sloan-Kettering, New York, USA, ovarian metastases were found in only 2.8% (57). Thus, in younger women with no evidence of extrauterine disease, ovarian conservation may be acceptable.

Lissoni et al. reported on eight patients aged between 19 and 32 years who had leiomyosarcoma diagnosed on myomectomy specimens and who were treated conservatively (58). Seven of the patients were alive and well with a median follow-up to 42 months, and three achieved pregnancies. Two pregnancies resulted in normal term deliveries but in one a caesarean section was performed and recurrent leiomyosarcoma demonstrated. This patient died of disseminated disease 26 months after her initial diagnosis.

In leiomyosarcomas, lymph node metastases are uncommon: the GOG study (56) demonstrated a lymph node metastasis rate of 3.5%, while in the Memorial Sloan-Kettering study, no nodal metastases occurred in the absence of gross extrauterine disease and clinically suspicious nodes. These findings indicate that surgical staging is unlikely to be of any benefit in leiomyosarcomas.

Endometrial stromal sarcomas are relatively indolent tumors and tend to recur very late, with at least one-third of the recurrences being found up to 30 years after initial diagnosis (59,60). There is little evidence that surgical staging affects the prognosis, so surgery should be confined to total hysterectomy, bilateral salpingo-oophorectomy and resection of palpably enlarged lymph nodes, together with peritoneal cytology and omental biopsy.

Endometrial sarcomas are extremely aggressive tumors with an extremely poor prognosis and there is no benefit from surgical staging.

Patients with malignant mixed Mullerian tumors, or carcinosarcomas, may benefit from surgical staging. In a pilot study, which started at our institution, patients with disease apparently confined to the corpus and cervix underwent full surgical staging, with subsequent treatment with adjuvant radiation and chemotherapy tailored to the findings (61). A total of 38 patients with clinical stage I and stage II malignant mixed Mullerian tumors were followed for a mean duration of 55 months. The overall survival rate was 74%. Twenty-one patients underwent the proposed multi-modality treatment protocol, comprising a combination of radiation and chemotherapy, and they achieved a 90% disease-free survival. Chemotherapy consisted of two cycles of cisplatin and epirubicin followed by radiotherapy, either to the pelvis or pelvis and para-aortic nodes. Patients who had negative nodes after a complete pelvic lymphadenectomy had been performed were treated with brachytherapy. All other patients received external beam radiation to either the pelvis or pelvis and para-aortic nodes. Two further cycles of chemotherapy were given for patients with surgical stage I disease and four further cycles for those with more advanced disease.

These figures offer hope that surgical staging for malignant mixed Mullerian tumors will allow better tailoring of therapy and improved survival.

SUMMARY

While surgery plays the central role in the treatment of uterine cancer, the exact nature and extent of the surgery is the subject of ongoing debate. Even with advanced or recurrent disease, removal of the uterus, tubes, and ovaries, if feasible, will improve the quality of life for most patients. Particularly with endometrial cancer there is a role for non-oncologists to treat relatively fit women with well-differentiated tumors in the absence of obvious metastatic disease, but it is in the best interests of all concerned to consult with a gynecologic oncology unit in any case where there is doubt as to the most appropriate treatment.

REFERENCES

1. Peel JH. Observations upon the etiology and treatment of carcinoma of the corpus uteri. Am J Obstet Gynecol 1956; 71:718.
2. Stallworthy J, quoted by Gusberg SB. Discussion. Treatment. Gynecol Onocl 1974; 2:429.
3. Jones HW III. Treatment of adenocarcinoma of the endometrium. Obstet Gynecol Survey 1975; 30:147–169.
4. Boronow RC. Endometrial cancer. Not a benign disease. Obstet Gynecol 1976; 47:630.
5. Lewis BV, Stallworthy JA, Cowdell R. Adenocarcinoma of the body of the uterus. J Obstet Gynaecol Br Commonw 1970; 77:343–348.
6. Stallworthy JA. Surgery of endometrial cancer in the Bonney tradition. Ann R Coll Surg Engl 1971; 48:293–305.
7. Boronow RC, Morrow CP, Creasman WT, DiSaia PJ, Silverberg SG, Miller A, Blessing JA. Surgical staging in endometrial cancer: clinical-pathologic findings of prospective study. Obstet Gynecol 1984; 63:825–832.

8. DiSaia PJ, Creasman WT, Boronow RC, Blessing JA. Risk factors and recurrent patterns in stage 1 endometrial cancer. Am J Obstet Gynecol 1985; 151: 1009–1015.
9. Creasman WT, Morrow CP, Bundy BN, Homesley HD, Graham JE, Heller PB. Surgical pathological spread patterns of endometrial cancer. A Gynecologic Oncology Group study. Cancer 1987; 60:2035–2041.
10. Pettersson F (ed). Annual Report on the Results of Treatment in Gynecological Cancer. Vol. 21. Stockholm: International Federation of Gynecology and Obstetrics, 1991.
11. Boronow RC. Surgical staging of endometrial cancer:evolution, evaluation and responsible challenge—a personal perspective. Gynecol Oncol 1997; 66:179–189.
12. Morrow CP, Bundy BN, Kurman RJ, Creasman WT, Heller P, Homesley HD, Graham JE. Relationship between surgical-pathological risk factors and outcome in clinical stage I and II carcinoma of the endometrium: a Gynecologic Oncology Group study. Gynecol Oncol 1991; 40:55–65.
13. Zaino RJ, Kurman RJ, Diana KL, Morrow CP. Prognostic models to predict outcome for women with endometrial adenocarcinoma. Cancer 1996; 77:1115–1121.
14. Wilson TD, Podratz KC, Gaffey TA, Malkasian GD, O'Brien PC, Naessens JM. Evaluation of unfavourable histologic subtypes in endometrial adenocarcinoma. Am J Obstet Gynecol 1990; 162:418–426.
15. Zaino RJ, Kurman RJ, Herbold D, Gliedman J, Bundy BN, Voet R, Advani H. The significance of squamous differentiation in endometrial carcinoma. Cancer 1991; 68:2293–2302.
16. Goff BA, Kato D, Schmidt RA, Ek M, Ferry JA, Muntz HG, Cain JM, Tamimi HK, Figge DC, Greer BE. Uterine papillary serous carcinoma: patterns of metastatic spread. Gynecol Oncol 1994; 54:254–258.
17. Jeffrey JF, Krepart GV, Lotocki RJ. Papillary serous adenocarcinoma of the endometrium. Obstet Gynecol 1986; 67:670–674.
18. Sherman ME, Bitterman P, Rosenshein NB, Dalgado G, Kurman RJ. Uterine serous carcinoma. Am J Surg Pathol 1986; 16:600–610, 1992.
19. Abeler VM, Vergote IB, Kjorstad KE, Trope CG. Clear cell carcinoma of the endometrium. Prognosis and metastatic pattern. Cancer 1996; 78:1740–1747.
20. Schink JC, Lurain JR, Wallemark CB, Chmiel JS. Tumour size in endometrial cancer: a prognostic factor for lymph node metastasis. Obstet Gynecol 1987; 70:216–219.
21. Zaino RJ, Kurman RJ, Diana KL, Morrow CP. Prognostic models to predict outcome for women with endometrial adenocarcinoma. Cancer 1996; 77:1115–1121.
22. Kadar N, Homesley HD, Malfetano JH. Positive peritoneal cytology is an adverse prognostic factor in endometrial cancer only if there is other evidence of extrauterine disease. Gynecol Oncol 1992; 46:145–150.
23. Milosovic MF, Dembo AJ, Thomas GM. The clinical significance of malignant peritoneal cytology in stage I endometrial carcinoma. Int J Gynecol Cancer 1992; 2:225–235.
24. Takeshima N, Nishida H, Tabata T, Hirai Y, Hasumi K. Positive peritoneal cytology in endometrial cancer: enhancement of other prognostic indicators. Gynecolo Oncol 2001; 82:470–473.

25. Koss LG, Schreiber K, Oberlander SG, Moukhtar M, Levine HS, Moussouris HF. Screening of asymptomatic women for endometrial cancer. Obstet Gynecol 1981; 57:681–691.
26. Dijkhuizen FP, Mol BW, Brolman HA, Heintz AP. The accuracy of endometrial sampling in the diagnosis of patients with endometrial carcinoma and hyperplasia. Cancer 2000; 89:1765–1772.
27. Loffer ED. Hysteroscopy with selective endometrial sampling compared with D&C for abnormal uterine bleeding: the value of a negative hysteroscopic view. Obstet Gynecol 1989; 73:16–20.
28. Gucer F, Tamussino K, Reich O, Moser F, Arikan G, Winter R. Two year follow up of patients with endometrial carcinoma after preoperative fluid hysteroscopy. Int J Gynecol Cancer 1998; 8:476–480.
29. Obermair O, Geramou M, Gucer F, Denison U, Graf AH, Kapshammer E. Impact of hysteroscopy on disease free survival in clinically stage I endometrial cancer patients. Int J Gynecol Cancer 2000; 10:275–279.
30. Wallen TE, Malkasian GD, Gaffey TA, O'Brien PC, Fountain KS. Stage II cancer of the endometrium: a pathologic and clinical study. Gynecol Oncol 1984; 18:1–17.
31. Berman ML, Afridi MA, Kambour AI, Ball HG. Risk factors and prognosis in stage II endometrial cancer. Gynecol Oncol 1982; 14:49–61.
32. Kitchener HC. Surgery for endometrial cancer: what type and by whom? Best Practice Res Clin Obstet Gynaecol 2001; 15:407–415.
33. Ryan M, Stainton C, Slaytor EK, Jaconelli C, Watts S, Mackenzie P. Aetiology and prevalence of lower limb oedema following treatment for gynaecological cancer. Aust N Z J Obstet Gynaecol 2003; 143:148–151.
34. Obermair A, Geramou M, Gucer F, Denison U, Grafs AF, Kapshammer E, Medl M, Rosen A, Wierrani F, Neunteufel W, Frech I, Spieser P, Kainz C, Brietenecker G. Endometrial cancer: accuracy of finding a well differentiated tumour at dilatation and curettage compared to findings at subsequent hysterectomy. Int J Gynecol Cancer 1999; 9:383–386.
35. Peterson RW, Quinlivan JA, Casper GR, Nicklin JL. Endometrial adenocarcinoma: presenting pathology is a poor guide to surgical management. Aust N Z J Obstet Gynaecol 2000; 40:191–194.
36. Goff BA, Rice LW. Assessment of depth of myometrial invasion in endometrial adenocarcinoma. Gynecol Oncol 1990; 38:46–48.
37. Franchi M, Ghezzi F, Melpignano M, Cherchi PL, Scarabelli C, Apolloni C, Zanaboni F. Clinical value of intraoperative gross examination in endometrial cancer. Gynecol Oncol 2000; 76:357–361.
38. Schink JC, Lurain JR, Wallemark CB, Chmiel JS. Tumour size in endometrial cancer: a prognostic factor for lymph node metastasis. Obstet Gynecol 1987; 70:216–219.
39. Kilgore LC, Partridge EE, Alvarez RD, Austin JM, Shingleton HM, Noojin F, Conner W. Adenocarcinoma of the endometrium: survival comparisons of patients with and without lymph node sampling. Gynecol Oncol 1995; 56:29–33.
40. Mohan DS, Samuels MA, Selim MA, Shalodi AD, Ellis RJ, Samuels JR, Yun HJ. Long term outcomes of therapeutic lymphadenectomy for stage 1 endometrial adenocarcinoma. Gynecol Oncol 1998; 70:165–171.

41. COSA–NZ–UK Endometrial Cancer Study Groups. Pelvic lymphadenectomy in high risk endometrial cancer. In J Gynecol Cancer 1996; 6:102–107.
42. Orr JW, Holimon JL, Orr PF. Stage 1 corpus cancer: is teletherapy necessary? Am J Obstet Gynecol 1997; 176:777–789.
43. Fanning J. Long term survival of intermediate risk endometrial cancer (stage 1 G3, 1C, II) treated with full lymphadenectomy and brachytherapy without teletherapy. Gynecol Oncol 2001; 82:371–375.
44. Seago DP, Raman A, Lele S. Potential benefit of lymphadenectomy for the treatment of node negative locally advanced uterine cancers. Gynecol Oncol 2001; 83:282–285.
45. Saygili U, Kavaz S, Altunyurt S, Uslu T, Kuyuncuoglu M, Erten O. Omentectomy, peritoneal biopsy and appendectomy in patients with clinical stage 1 endometrial carcinoma. Int J Gynecol Cancer 2001; 11:471–474.
46. Sartori E, Gadducci A, Landoni F, Lissoni A, Maggino T, Zola P, Zanagnolo V. Clinical behaviour 203 stage II endometrial cancer cases: the impact of primary surgical approach and of adjuvant radiation therapy. Int J Gynecol Cancer 2001; 11:430–437.
47. Cornelison TL, Trimble EL, Kosary CL. SEER data, corpus uteri cancer: treatment trends versus survival for FIGO stage II, 1988–1994. Gynecol Oncol 1999; 74:350–355.
48. Mariani A, Webb MJ, Keeney GL, Calori G, Podratz K. Role of wide/radical hysterectomy and pelvic lymph node dissection in endometrial cancer with cervical involvement. Gynecol Oncol 2001; 83:72–80.
49. Aalders J, Abeler V, Kolstad P. Clinical stage II as compared to subclinical intrapelvic extrauterine spread in endometrial carcinoma: a clinical and histopathological study of 175 patients. Gynecol Oncol 1984; 17:64–74.
50. Bruckman JE, Bloomer WD, Marck A, Ehrmann RL, Knapp RC. Stage III adenocarcinoma of the endometrium: two prognostic groups. Gynecol Oncol 1980; 9:12–17.
51. Nicklin JL, Petersen RW. Stage IIIB adenocarcinoma of the endometrium: a clinicopathologic study. Gynecol Oncol 2000; 78:203–207.
52. Bristow RE, Zerbe MJ, Rosenshein NB, Grumbine FC, Montz FJ. Stage IVB endometrial carcinoma: the role of cytoreductive surgery and determinants of survival. Gynecol Oncol 2000; 78:85–91.
53. Aalders J, Abeler V, Kolstad P. Recurrent adenocarcinoma of the endometrium: a clinical and histopathological study of 379 patients. Gynecol Oncol 1984; 17:85–103.
54. Jhang H, Chuang L, Visintainer P, Ramaswamy G. Ca125 levels in the preoperative assessment of advanced stage uterine cancer. Am J Obstet Gynecol 2003; 188:1195–1197.
55. Zaloudek CJ, Norris HJ. Mesenchymal tum s of the uterus. In: Fengolio C, Wolff M, eds. Progress in Surgical Pathology. 3. Vol. 3. New York: New York: Masson, 1981:1–35.
56. Major FJ, Blessing JA, Silverberg SG, Morrow PC, Creasman WT, Currie JL, Yordan E, Brady MF. Prognostic factors in early stage uterine sarcoma. A Gynecologic Oncology Group study. Cancer 1993; 71(4 suppl):1702–1709.

57. Leitao MM, Sonoda Y, Brennan MF, Barakat RR, Chi DS. Incidence of lymph node and ovarian metastases in leiomyosarcomas of the uterus. Gynecol Oncol 2003; 91:209–212.
58. Lissoni A, Cormio G, Bonazzi C, Perego P, Lomonico S, Gabriele A, Bratina G. Fertility sparing surgery in the uterine leiomyosarcoma. Gynecol Oncol 1998; 70:348–350.
59. Chang KL, Crabtree GS, Lim-Tan SK, Kempson RL, Hendrickson MR. Primary uterine endometrial stromal neoplasms. Am J Surg Pathol 1990; 14: 415–438.
60. Chu MC, Mor G, Lim C, Zheng W, Parkash V, Schwartz PE. Low grade endometrial stromal sarcoma; hormonal aspects. Gynecol Oncol 2003; 90:170–176.
61. Manolitsas T, Wain GV, Williams KE, Friedlander M, Hacker NF. Multimodality therapy for patients with clinical stage I and II malignant mixed Mullerian tumours of the uterus. Cancer 2001; 91:1437–1443.

9

Risk Factors and the Role of Radiotherapy in the Treatment of Endometrial Cancer

Ida Ackerman

Department of Radiation Oncology, Toronto Sunnybrook Regional Cancer Centre, University of Toronto, Ontario, Canada

Helen Steed

Department of Gynecology, Cross Cancer Institute, Edmonton, Alberta, Canada

HISTORY OF RADIATION

Pierre Curie announced the discovery of radium in 1898 and the therapeutic application of radium to exposed surfaces of the body began immediately (1). The first suggestion that radium be used interstitially within the center of the cancer was proposed intriguingly by Alexander Graham Bell, inventor of the telephone (1). In 1903 he advocated that a tiny fragment of radium be sealed up in a fine glass tube and inserted into the "heart" of the cancer thus acting directly on the disease.

The first reference in the literature to the employment of radium in the treatment of uterine cancer was in 1905 by Dr. Abbe in New York (2). After this initial innovation for uterine cancer was described, numerous reports were published illustrating the use of radium in the treatment of this common gynecologic cancer (2). Histological examination of the specimens removed after radium treatment described the growths as undergoing progressive regression. They also showed that application of radium before surgery resulted in a "thinning of the neoplastic tissue" (2) thus facilitating the procedure. Dr. Abbe later discussed his earliest case that had been treated with radium after curettage, and stated that she was alive and in perfect health eight years following her radium treatment.

Today, almost 100 years later, both external beam and intracavitary radiation therapy (RT) continue to be widely used in the treatment of uterine cancers. In this chapter we are going to outline the role of this important modality in the current management of uterine malignancies, focusing on the commonest, endometrial carcinoma.

STAGING AND PROGNOSTIC FACTORS

The role of radiotherapy in the treatment of endometrial cancer is intimately related to staging and prognostic factors such as grade, myometrial invasion, and lymph node status. To set the stage for the role and use of RT, we will briefly review the historical clinical and current "surgical staging" of endometrial cancer and the important prognostic factors which guide the use of radiation.

Prior to 1988, endometrial cancer was staged according to a universal clinical staging system International Federation of Gynecology and Obstetrics (FIGO) (Table 1). However, a significant proportion of patients who underwent surgery with pathological assessment of peritoneal and lymph node biopsies were found to have more extensive disease than had been appreciated. Several reports indicated that after surgical evaluation of disease

Table 1 1971 FIGO Clinical Staging for Endometrial Cancer

Stage 0	Carcinoma in situ
Stage I	The carcinoma is confined to the corpus
Stage IA	Length of the uterine cavity is 8 cm or less
Stage IB	Length of the uterine cavity is >8 cm
Sub-grouping of stage I with regard to the histologic grade of the adenocarcinoma:	
Grade 1	Highly differentiated adenomatous carcinoma
Grade 2	Moderately differentiated adenomatous carcinoma with partly solid areas
Grade 3	Predominantly solid or entirely undifferentiated carcinoma
Stage II	The carcinoma has involved the corpus and the cervix but has not extended outside the uterus
Stage III	The carcinoma has extended outside the uterus but not outside the true pelvis
Stage IV	The carcinoma has extended ouside the true pelvis or has obviously involved the mucosa of the bladder or rectum
Stage IVA	Spread of the growth to adjacent organs
Stage IVB	Spread to distant organs

in patients with clinical stage I endometrial cancer, the disease could be upstaged in 12–23% of patients (3–6). The staging system proposed was a comprehensive surgical staging system after several studies showed that the information obtained at the time of surgery is an important indicator of prognosis and overall survival (OS) (Table 2) (6–9). Therefore the current FIGO staging system for endometrial cancer involves surgical staging. This includes an exploratory laparotomy through a midline incision, abdominal and pelvic washings, comprehensive inspection and palpation of the abdomen and pelvis, biopsies of any suspicious peritoneal surfaces, pelvic and para-aortic lymph node dissection in addition to the previously standard total abdominal hysterectomy bilateral salpingo-oophorectomy (TAH BSO).

Following the standard TAH BSO, the important prognostic factors such as the depth of myometrial invasion, tumor grade and histology, the presence of lymph-vascular space invasion (LVS), peritoneal cytology status, cervical involvement, and adnexal spread can be ascertained. The more extensive procedure gives important information regarding the presence or absence of lymph node or peritoneal spread.

There is a strong correlation between histological tumor grade, myometrial invasion, lymph node status, and recurrence. Hendrickson et al. demonstrated that increasing tumor grade and myometrial invasion are associated with an increased risk of pelvic and para-aortic lymph node metastases, adnexal metastases, and recurrences (10). The surgical staging study of the Gynecologic Oncology Group (GOG) reported by Creasman confirmed these findings (6,7). They documented that cancers with high grade (grades 2 and 3) and deeply invasive tumors were more likely to have nodal metastases and recurrences. Endometrial grade 1 carcinomas confined to the inner third of the myometrium have an incidence of positive pelvic nodes of less than 3%, while grade 3 lesions involving the outer third have a 34% incidence of positive

Table 2   1988 FIGO Surgical Staging for Endometrial Cancer

Stage IA	Tumor limited to endometrium
Stage IB	Invasion to less than 1/2 the myometrium
Stage IC	Invasion to more than 1/2 the myometrium
Stage IIA	Endocervical glandular involvement only
Stage IIB	Cervical stromal invasion
Stage IIIA	Tumor invades the serosa and/or adnexa, and /or positive peritoneal cytology
Stage IIIB	Vaginal metastases
Stage IIIC	Metastases to pelvic and/or para-aortic lymph nodes
Stage IVA	Tumor invasion of bladder and/or bowel mucosa
Stage IVB	Distant metastases including intra-abdominal and/or inguinal lymph nodes

pelvic lymph nodes. A similar correlation was seen with para-aortic metastases, as grade 1 carcinomas confined to the inner third of the myometrium did not have positive para-aortic lymph nodes, whereas grade 3 carcinomas in the outer third had a 23% incidence of para-aortic involvement. Lanciano et al. (11) demonstrated that for patients with surgical stage I disease, high grade was an independent predictor of distant metastases, pelvic recurrences, and inferior disease-free survival (DFS).

Morrow et al. (7) demonstrated that any myometrial invasion increased the relative risk of recurrence by four to five times even in patients without documented extrauterine disease extension. This increased risk of recurrence of 20–45% is seen for all grades of tumor involving the outer third of the myometrium (8). Lanciano et al. also illustrated a survival difference in surgically staged patients with different depths of myometrial penetration (11). They described a cause-specific survival (CSS) of 98% for those with surgical stage IA and IB disease versus 87% for those with stage IC disease (10).

Uterine papillary serous carcinoma (UPSC) is an uncommon histological subtype of endometrial cancer with a more aggressive clinical behavior (12–14). It is uniformly high grade and has a tendency for deep myometrial invasion and lymphatic vascular space invasion, lymph node and intraperitoneal metastases, and poor clinical outcomes (13–15).

Overall reported survival rates for all surgical and clinical stages are 35–80% for stages I and II compared to 80–90% for endometrioid adenocarcinoma of the uterus, and 0–25% for stages III and IV (12–15). Clear cell carcinomas are also rare, although often clear cell elements are admixed with papillary serous tumors. A retrospective review of 181 patients with clear cell endometrial carcinoma reported 5- and 10-year actuarial DFS rates of 43% and 39%, respectively (16). The majority of recurrences were outside the pelvis, with two-thirds of the patients relapsing in the abdomen, liver, and lungs.

LVS appears to be an independent risk factor for recurrence and death. Aalders et al. (17) reported recurrences and deaths in 26.7% of patients with clinical stage I disease who had LVS compared with 9.1% for those without LVS ($p < 0.05$). A recent study showed that cancers with LVS were significantly more likely to have nodal disease (35/92 vs. 11/274, $p < 0.001$) (18).

The significance of isolated positive peritoneal cytological finding is less well established. Positive washings are most common in patients with other poor prognostic factors, such as grade 3 histology, deep myometrial invasion, metastatic disease in the adnexa, and positive pelvic or para-aortic lymph nodes (6,19). Milosevic et al. (20) reviewed the literature concerning patients with clinical stage I endometrial cancer and concluded that the poor prognosis associated with positive cytology was more likely a reflection of the other associated poor prognostic factors.

In summary, the prognostic factors outlined are known predictors of relapse and are the hallmark variables used to decide on adjuvant therapy, particularly radiation treatment. While it is recognized that these factors are individually important, the relative importance and which combinations of factors are the most crucial is yet to be determined.

STAGE I DISEASE

RT plays a key role in the treatment of endometrial cancer. It has been used as adjunctive treatment before or after surgery for patients with clinical stages I–III disease. It can also provide a significant chance of cure as definitive therapy in those who are deemed medically unfit for surgery. However, its most frequent application is in the adjuvant setting following surgery for stages I and II. The observation that RT significantly reduces the probability of vaginal and pelvic recurrences following surgical therapy has been recognized for many years and was described by early investigators (21,22). This has now been demonstrated in three prospective randomized trials and is not disputed (17,23,24). Two of these trials involved patients who were not surgically staged (17,23).

Adjuvant Therapy

In 1980, Aalders et al. (17) reported the results of the first prospective randomized trial in 540 clinical stage I patients after TAH BSO. Postoperatively, all patients received a vaginal radium insertion delivering a surface dose of 60 Gy. They were then randomized to either receive 40 Gy with external pelvic irradiation ($n = 263$) or no further treatment ($n = 277$). Patients with proven metastatic disease outside the uterus were excluded. There was a statistically significant decrease in local pelvic relapse in those patients who received pelvic radiotherapy (1.9% vs. 6.9%), but there was no difference in OS. In a post hoc subset analysis, improved OS was seen in those patients with deeply invasive, grade 3 tumors receiving pelvic radiotherapy.

In 2000, Creutzberg et al. (23) reported the Postoperative Radiation Therapy in Endometrial Carcinoma (PORTEC) multi-institutional randomized controlled trial (RCT) of 715 patients treated with TAH BSO randomized to either whole pelvic radiotherapy to 46 Gy ($n = 354$) or to no further treatment ($n = 361$). Inclusion criteria included grade 1 tumors with deep (>50%) myometrial invasion, grade 2 disease with any myometrial invasion, and grade 3 tumors with superficial (<50%) myometrial invasion. Patients with grade 3 disease and outer half myometrial invasion were not eligible for the trial. Adjuvant RT reduced the risk of local regional recurrence from 14% to 4% ($p < 0.001$), but had no impact on five-year OS, which was 81% in the irradiated arm and 85% in the observation arm. Seventy-three percent of the recurrences were in the vagina and the risk of distant metastases was similar in both arms. The authors speculated that the absence of an OS benefit could be attributed to the ability to salvage 79% of patients with isolated local recurrences. The authors concluded that radiotherapy is of marginal benefit in superficial grade 2 tumors and may be avoided, reserving radiotherapy for relapse with an acceptable salvage rate. However, because stage IC and grade 3 patients have a higher risk of local regional failure approaching 20%, adjuvant radiotherapy should be considered.

In 1998 the GOG reported in abstract form the results of a randomized study (24) on 390 surgically staged node-negative patients with stages IB, IC, occult stages IIA and IIB disease and included all grades. One hundred ninety patients were randomized postoperatively to external beam pelvic radiotherapy (EBT) to a dose of 50 Gy in 28 fractions or no further therapy. Eligibility criteria required negative nodes and some degree of myometrial invasion. The majority of patients accrued were stage IB. They found a difference in the two-year progression free survival (PFS) interval of 88% versus 96% ($p = 0.004$), favoring the adjuvant RT arm. Most of the recurrences in the control arm were located in the vagina and vaginal vault.

These three RCTs unequivocally demonstrate that adjuvant pelvic radiotherapy improves pelvic control. Despite this, a corresponding improvement in OS has not as yet been demonstrated. Therefore many have questioned the value of EBT. Should postoperative EBT be offered to patients with grade 3 disease, LVS involvement, or outer half myometrial invasion since pelvic radiotherapy improves local-regional control, whether the patient is surgically staged or not?

Two other approaches have been discussed and debated with regards to adjuvant therapy for endometrial carcinoma. Since the vaginal vault is the most common site of loco-regional recurrence, some authors have advocated the use of vaginal brachytherapy (BT) alone if the patient is fully staged and node-negative. Because surgical staging for endometrial cancer provides a more complete pathologic assessment of the pelvic nodes, there is an opportunity to be more selective in the recommendations for adjuvant RT. Others have suggested that another potential strategy would be to withhold adjuvant treatment initially and limit irradiation only to those who subsequently suffer a pelvic recurrence. This tactic would thus spare many patients treatment-related toxicity with the knowledge that 45–67% can be salvaged with radical radiotherapy at the time of pelvic relapse (25–28).

Adjuvant Brachytherapy Alone

Table 3 outlines the reports using postoperative vaginal vault BT as the sole adjuvant therapy in surgically staged node-negative patients but with unfavorable primary tumor factors, such as deep myometrial invasion, high grade, or microscopic cervical involvement (29–33). Because the vagina has been shown to be the most common site of loco-regional failure among patients who are not irradiated (17,23,33,34), postoperative vaginal BT alone may be substituted for EBT in selected surgically staged patients.

Table 3 Summary of Results of the Use of Vaginal Brachytherapy Alone in Node-Negative Surgically Stage I-Patients

Author	Number of patients	Stage	Therapy	Results	Median follow up (months)
Orr (29)	82 159 69	IA G2,3 IB G1,2,3 IC G1,2,3	6000 cGy to vaginal cuff	100% 5-year OS, 0% RR 97% 5-year OS, 2.5% RR 93% 5-year OS, 4.3% RR	32
Chadha (30)	38	IB G3 IC G1,2,3	21 Gy to depth of 0.5 cm HDR in 3 Fx	93% 5-year OS 87.5% DFS No pelvic or vaginal recurrences	30
Ng (31)	77	IB G3 IC G1,2,3	60 Gy via Cs137 LDR over 3 days, or Ir^{192} 36 Gy over 6 Fx	94% 5-year OS 86% 5-year DFS 14% RR	37
Fanning (32)	66	IA,B G3 IC G1,2,3 II	21 Gy to depth of 0.5 cm via Ir^{192} HDR over 3 Fx	84% 5-year OS 97% 5-year DFS 3% distant recurrences	48 (mean)
Rittenberg (33)	172 53 (subset)	I G1,2,3 IC only	1680 cGy to depth of 0.5 cm Ir^{192} HDR over 3 Fx	97% 2-year OS 95% 5-year OS 2.3% RR 5.7% RR (IC only)	32

Abbreviations: HDR, high-dose rate; Fx, fractions; OS, overall survival; RR, recurrence rate.

The rationale for this approach would be to minimize radiotherapy and its adverse effects without jeopardizing the benefit of local-regional control. Morrow et al. reported a 37% complication rate in those who received postoperative EBT following surgical staging versus only a 4% rate in those who received postoperative vaginal BT alone (7). While these retrospective reports on the use of adjuvant BT alone look promising, the majority of these patients with node-negative disease have an excellent prognosis and the impact of vaginal therapy is unclear (35). There is no RCT comparing external beam therapy to vaginal vault BT in this setting. Given the excellent local control and survival provided with either approach, such a trial would not be feasible especially when one factors in that a significant proportion of these patients die of other causes.

In summary, it is generally agreed by most that it is unlikely that those with stages IA and IB grade-1 tumors, whether surgically staged or not, will benefit from postoperative RT because the risk of recurrence is low and OS is excellent. However, despite the results of clinical trials showing no survival benefit and despite the lower overall relapse rates found in those patients who are surgically staged and node-negative, many gynecologic oncologists continue to refer patients for postoperative RT when the risk of recurrence is deemed to be in excess of 15% (36). Therefore, for many patients with early stage disease and adverse tumor factors as outlined above, RT remains an important adjunctive modality.

Currently, the two most common therapeutic paradigms for the treatment of early stage endometrial cancer are:

- A simple TAH BSO followed by a more liberal use of postoperative EBT based on adverse histopathological risk factors in the uterine specimen, and
- TAH BSO with extended surgical staging, including pelvic and para-aortic node dissection, followed by more limited radiotherapy using vaginal vault therapy alone in those patients who are node-negative but have adverse local disease as outlined previously.

Treatment of Recurrence

Effective treatment with radical pelvic radiation at the time of isolated pelvic relapse has been postulated as a potential explanation for the lack of survival benefit evident in the three randomized trials (17,23,24). This argument on the effectiveness of radiotherapy for "salvage" following recurrence has been previously suggested by Ackerman et al. (27).

The authors used an algorithm to demonstrate the theoretical incremental curative value of postoperative adjuvant pelvic radiotherapy. They concluded that the potential curative value of "routine" adjuvant PRT in clinical stage I high-risk patients is small and not likely to be detected in a clinical trial.

A recent paper from the PORTEC group (37) provides further support for this hypothesis. They updated the results with eight-year local control and survival rates after relapse for patients treated in the PORTEC trial (23). The eight-year actuarial loco-regional recurrence rates were 4% and 15% in the adjuvant RT and control groups, respectively ($p < 0.0001$). There was no difference in the actuarial OS rate between the two groups and the actuarial survival after first relapse was lower in the RT group than in the control group (19% and 51% three-year survival, respectively, $p = 0.004$). The survival after vaginal relapse at five years was significantly better for patients in the control group than for those receiving adjuvant RT (65% and 43%, respectively). This is not surprising as the control group could tolerate and receive higher doses of curative radical RT compared with the patients who have already received radiotherapy. Additionally, these two cohorts (patients who never had radiotherapy and recur, vs. those who recur despite radiotherapy) are unlikely to be comparable, as they may have had biologically different diseases.

Data on the results of radiotherapy for salvage of recurrence are summarized in Table 4 (28,38–42). Pelvic recurrences may present as a vaginal cuff recurrence, pelvic nodal disease, vagina, or a combination. The most common symptom is vaginal bleeding and discharge. Survival results at five years are reported to range from 20% to 60% (38–42). Multiple variables, including histological cell type, grade, initial clinical versus surgical stage, myometrial invasion, and adequate treatment at initial diagnosis have been implicated as valuable prognosticators of recurrences (38). Factors influencing prognosis in vaginal recurrences have been studied and include location, disease-free interval, and relapse after prior RT treatment.

Patients with recurrent endometrial cancer after surgery should be fully evaluated to rule out distant metastatic disease. Isolated pelvic recurrences should be treated with radiation with curative intent. A combination of EBT and BT or interstitial therapy may be used. Tumor doses delivered should be at least 65 Gy, and 75–85 Gy are desirable depending on the tumor volume.

Primary Treatment with Radical Radiation

Approximately 10–20% of endometrial cancer patients have severe medical conditions that render them medically unfit for surgery (43–47). These patients tend to be elderly, obese, and have multiple medical co-morbidities, such that they frequently die from intercurrent disease. Several studies have demonstrated the effectiveness of primary RT in medically unfit patients (43–47). Fishman et al. (43) compared 54 medically unfit clinical stage I and II patients treated with primary radiation alone to matched cases of 108 operable patients. Most patients were treated with intracavitary RT alone to an estimated dose of 40–50 Gy to a lateral myometrial depth of 1.5 cm. The five-year actuarial cancer-specific survivals for patients with

Table 4 Summary of Results of Radiotherapy for Isolated Pelvic Recurrences

Author	Number of patients	Stage	Treatment	Results	Follow-up (median months)
Mandell (38)	20 (13 hx of prior RT)	Clinical stage I	EBT total dose 40–50 Gy BT 21 Gy to a depth of 0.5 cm Ir^{192} in 3 Fx	50% 4-year OS	48
Hoekstra (39)	26 no prior RT	Clinical stage I unknown nodal status	7 EBT total dose 47 Gy 3 BT-HDR 9.8 Gy and LDR 30 Gy to a depth of 0.5 cm 16 EBT + BT	44% 5-year OS	–
Sears (40)	45 no prior RT	IA = 5 IB = 17 IC = 7 II = 3 IIIA = 4 IIIB = 2 IIIC = 1 Unknown = 5	18 EBT total dose 50 Gy 1 BT total dose 40 Gy 26 EBT + BT	44% 5-year OS 51% 5-year DFS 54% 5-year PC	89

Poulsen (28)	93 (91 hx of prior RT)	Clinical stage I, all grades	EBT total dose 40 Gy BT 60 Gy to a depth of 0.5 cm in 3 Fx	10-year actuarial OS 50% lower 1/3 vagina 45% vaginal vault 24% pelvic recurrence	68
Hart (41)	26	I = 14 II = 4 III = 4 IV = 4	EBT total dose 45 Gy BT boost of 30 Gy	50% 2-year OS Median survival = 16 m	15
Wylie (42)	58 no prior RT	I = 58 II = 34 III = 6	EBT total dose 45 Gy BT with Cs137 to dose 40 Gy	63% 5-year OS 10-year actuarial OS: 41% all patients 71% stage I 61% stage II 50% stage III	96

Abbreviations: EBT, external beam therapy; BT, brachytherapy; HDR, high-dose rate; LDR, low-dose rate.

stage I inoperable disease were 80% versus 98% for stage I operable patients. More deaths from intercurrent disease occurred within the unfit group. Nguyen et al. (44) also used intracavitary high-dose rate (HDR) BT alone and demonstrated excellent uterine control rate of 88% at three years. The three-year DFS and OS were 85% and 65%, respectively. Others have used EBT followed by utero-vaginal BT and have demonstrated 5- and 10-year OS and DFS comparable to results obtained using surgery followed by radiation (45–47). Thus a combination of EBT and adequate intracavitary RT in medically unfit patients can be curative in a significant proportion of patients.

STAGE II DISEASE

The management of uterine cancer with involvement of the cervix remains controversial. The initial difficulty is the definitions used to describe stage II cervical cancer. Stage II patients may include those with minimal microscopic involvement of the cervix at the time of surgery or those with obvious clinical cervical involvement, despite the fact that these two groups have very different prognoses. This makes the evaluation of the literature problematic. In addition, the small number of reported cases, retrospective nature of the literature, and lack of randomized prospective studies hinders recommendations for optimal treatment. The treatment options range from extrafascial hysterectomy after RT to radical hysterectomy, with or without radiation (48–53).

Because the routine use of the radical hysterectomy is not feasible in these patients due to the high frequency of medical co-morbidities, the combination of external and intracavitary RT followed by conservative extrafascial hysterectomy found great appeal in the past (51–53). Radical surgery is advantageous when reasonable as it permits accurate staging of disease and offers wide excision of the primary tumor. Most authors were unable to show a survival benefit with radical hysterectomy but advocated its use when the cervix was grossly involved with tumor or preoperative investigations suggested positive cervical stromal involvement.

The surveillance epidemiology and end results (SEER) data (49), however, showed that radical hysterectomy improved survival compared to simple hysterectomy. They reviewed and analyzed 932 patients with FIGO stage II uterine cancer and found a five-year survival of 92.96% in patients treated with radical hysterectomy compared to 84.36% with simple hysterectomy as primary therapy ($p < 0.05$). There was no significant survival difference with the addition of RT in either surgical group. However, this study is limited because it was not randomized and not all patients were known to have FIGO surgical stage II disease with appropriate lymph node assessments. Thus, the inability to detect a significant survival benefit for radiation may possibly be secondary to patient selection and the patients who were treated with radiation may have had more adverse prognostic factors.

When other studies have addressed the survival benefit of radiation, there has been little difference identified between radical surgery alone and combined radiation and surgery, although there is a trend toward a slight survival advantage to combined-modality therapy (50,51,53).

Because clinical stage II endometrial carcinoma is uncommon, individualization of therapy is essential. Patient factors, such as the medical co-morbidities, tumor factors; such as cervical size and the extent of cervical involvement, surgical expertise, and radiotherapy resources need to be considered. If technically feasible, a radical hysterectomy to avoid a "cut-through" procedure and removal of the pelvic lymph nodes initially is reasonable. This approach avoids the increased difficulty of surgery after radiation, and allows an accurate pathologic assessment of the disease including evaluation of nodal involvement. The plan and extent of postoperative radiotherapy can then be made after assessing the pathologic factors and nodal status. However, if the patients are medically unfit or the cervical tumor mass is large with an increased risk of cutting through the tumor, radical radiotherapy followed by a simple hysterectomy, if disease persists, would also be a logical treatment choice. Therefore, a multidisciplinary team review of both clinical presentation and tumor imaging should allow optimal management strategies to be considered.

STAGE III AND IV DISEASE

While the vast majority of patients with endometrial cancer are diagnosed without evidence of extrauterine spread, 10–15% of patients will present with FIGO surgical stage III disease. The five-year survival estimates for women with surgical stage III disease range from 40% to 70% (54,55).

FIGO surgical stage III disease represents a heterogeneous group of patients with both microscopic and macroscopic disease with different prognoses. Most efforts to conduct large prospective clinical trials are hampered by the rarity of these advanced malignancies. Therefore, optimal therapy remains unknown.

Stage IIIA

The majority of patients with extrauterine extension reported in the literature have received adjuvant preoperative or postoperative radiotherapy to either the pelvis or whole abdomen. Adjuvant pelvic radiotherapy has resulted in five-year DFS ranging from 44% to 80% (3,54,56,57). The difficulty in assessing the literature for treatment outcomes for this stage is the various types of patients included in this category ranging from those with microscopic disease only to those with clinical stage III with evidence of gross macroscopic palpable pelvic disease. Some reports indicate a less favorable outcome for patients with clinical stage III endometrial cancer than for those with microscopic pathologic stage III disease. Aalders et al. (58) reported a five-year OS of 40% for patients with surgicopathological stage III disease, compared with 16% for patients with clinical stage III gross disease. Also, Bruckman et al. (59) retrospectively reported on patients managed with adjuvant pelvic RT and low-dose rate vaginal BT. They found a five-year actuarial OS of 80% when only the ovary and fallopian tube were involved, compared with 15% when other extrauterine pelvic structures were involved. Microscopic adnexal metastases alone have a better prognosis and these patients can potentially be observed if there are no other poor prognostic risk factors.

The number of extrauterine disease sites has been shown to directly correlate with probability of disease recurrence. Greven et al. described a decrease in five-year DFS rates of 68%, 56%, and 0% as the number of involved sites increased from one, two, and three or more sites, respectively (60).

The majority of patients with extrauterine disease extension have had adjuvant pelvic radiation treatment (59,61–63). The high rate of abdominal recurrence, however, supports the rationale for the use of abdomino-pelvic RT (APRT) and Table 5 summarizes the favorable results reported by several investigators (64–66). The indications for adjuvant therapy for patients with positive peritoneal cytology as their only adverse risk factor has not been established and it is unclear whether abdominal therapy would improve outcome in these patients (19,20).

Table 5 Outcome for Patients with Surgical-Pathologic Stage-III Endometrial Carcinoma

Author	Number of patients	Treatment type	Clinical outcome	Five-year recurrence sites of failure (%)
Genest (61)	18	Pelvic EBT	70% 5-year DFS	–
Grigsby (62)	30	Pelvic EBT	56% 5-year DFS	23 pelvic 23 distant 10 abdomen
Greven (63)	126	Pelvic EBT	55% 5-year OS	20 pelvis 10 outside pelvis[a]
Greer (64)	27	APRT	80% 5-year CSS	11 distant 15 abdomen
Potish (66)	41	APRT	71% 5-year DFS	5 pelvis 10 distant 20 abdomen
Gibbons (65)	17	APRT	58% 7-year DFS 68% 7-year OS	3 vagina 9 abdomen

[a]Includes both abdomen and distant recurrences.
Abbreviations: EBT, external beam therapy; APRT, abdomino-pelvic radiotherapy; DFS, disease-free survival; CSS, cause-specific survival (reflects death from endometrial cancer); OS, overall survival (reflects death from any cause).

Stage IIIB

Stage IIIB adenocarcinoma of the endometrium is associated with a poor prognosis. Nicklin et al. (67) showed that clinical stage IIIB disease had a statistically worse survival than stage IIIA but not different from patients with stage IIIC or IV disease. Thus, they postulated that these patients require individualized management and should be included with advanced stages IIIC and IV disease in clinical studies.

Stage IIIC

Stage IIIC endometrial carcinoma with pathologically positive pelvic lymph nodes makes up 2–6% of all cases (6,54,60,68). The prognostic significance of nodal involvement limited to pelvic nodes alone has not been well defined. Schorge et al. (54) found that 9 of 13 (69%) patients with positive pelvic nodes and negative para-aortic nodes were disease-free after pelvic RT. Nelson et al. (68) reported a five-year DFS of 81% and actuarial five-year OS of 72% for this group of patients and all patients were treated with postoperative radiotherapy to at least the pelvis. Because distant metastases including upper abdominal recurrences appear to be the predominant pattern of failure in those treated with PRT alone, some patients have been managed with APRT in retrospective studies (64–66). In Nelson's study two of the four recurrences were in the para-aortic region, suggesting a possible role for extended-field RT (EFT) in the presence of positive pelvic nodes.

Patients with histologically proven positive para-aortic lymph nodes are potential candidates for postoperative pelvic and para-aortic irradiation. Table 6 summarizes the series that have reported five-year OS rates between 27% and 53% (69–73). Rose et al. (71) reported a survival advantage for those patients who received postoperative EFT with a five-year OS of 53% versus only 13% for those patients who did not receive radiation. Corn et al. (70) discussed the potential advantage of debulking gross disease in the para-aortic region. Mariani et al. (73) reviewed 51 surgical stage IIIC patients and divided the patients into two groups: (*i*) nodal involvement only, and (*ii*) nodal plus cytological, uterine serosal, adnexal, or vaginal involvement. Their results showed a CSS of 72% and a five-year DFS of 68% for nodal disease only, and CSS of 33% and DFS of 25% for nodal disease plus other extrauterine sites ($p < 0.01$). They suggested that different treatment strategies are needed for these two groups. The same prognostic factors that apply to stage I and II disease, grade and depth of invasion, apply to stage III disease and these need to be assessed and considered when planning treatment (54,62,71–73).

The most promising treatment option for advanced stage III and IV endometrial cancer appears to be combination therapy with radiotherapy and chemotherapy. Various chemotherapy agents including doxirubicin, cisplatin, and paclitaxel have been shown to be effective in endometrial

Table 6 Clinical Outcome for Stage-IIIC Endometrial Carcinoma with Positive Pelvic/Para-aortic Lymph Nodes

Author	Number of patients	Treatment	Clinical outcome	Pattern of failure (% of patients)
Potish (69)	48	EFT[a]	52% 5-year OS	–
Corn (72)	50	EFT[a]	46% 5-year OS	37 pelvis 27 PAN 39 distant
Rose (71)	17	EFT + hormones[b]	53% 5-year OS	17 pelvis 83 distant
McMeekin (72)	47	8 PRT 9 PRT + EFT 17 APRT 8 CT 5 hormones	70% 3-year OS + PAN 87% 3-year OS + isolated PLN	–
Mariani (73)	46	37 PRT 15 PRT + EFT 12 PRT + APRT	53% 5-year CSS 47% 5-year DFS (all patients)	7 pelvic 20 distant 20 both 30 PAN
	Subset anaylsis 22 + LN only	21 PRT 6 PRT + EFT 3 PRT + APRT	72% 5-year CSS 68% 5-year DFS	5 distant 32 PAN 22 [pelvic] + PAN

[a]Includes all patients: EFT alone or EFT with TAH BSO.
[b]Hormones used were megestrol or tamoxifen.
Abbreviations: EFT, extended field radiotherapy; PRT, pelvic radiotherapy; CT, chemotherapy; CSS, cause-specific survival (relates to death from endo-metrial cancer only); OS, overall survival (relates to death from any cause); PAN, para-aortic nodes; PLN, pelvic lymph nodes; LN, lymph nodes.

cancer with response rates between 20% and 42% (74–77). The GOG presented their results recently describing a RCT comparing whole abdominal radiotherapy and chemotherapy for advanced stage III/IV endometrial cancer (78). They found an increased DFS of 58% versus 46% favoring chemotherapy with carboplatin and paclitaxel. Criticisms of this study included the imbalance of the groups with respect to important prognostic factors, such as the number of residual sites of disease, the proportion with substages IIIA–C, and the suboptimal radiotherapy dose delivered.

The rarity of advanced endometrial cancer makes studies difficult, and individualization of therapy in a multidisciplinary clinic optimizing the use of surgery, radiotherapy and chemotherapy is essential.

PALLIATIVE RADIOTHERAPY

Patients with locally advanced or metastatic endometrial cancer who have symptoms of pain and bleeding may receive external irradiation to the pelvis to relieve these symptoms. When palliation is the goal of therapy, it is important to evaluate the patient's performance status. Palliative EBT to control pelvic pain and bleeding is useful. Less commonly intracavitary therapy for bleeding may be used to control bleeding if the local disease extent is appropriately small (79).

Other distant sites that may be treated with palliative irradiation for symptom control include the bony sites for pain, the lung for hemoptysis, the brain for brain metastases and the lymph nodes for painful edema. The doses used are generally 20–30 Gy in 5–10 fractions over 1–2 weeks, although single large doses of 6–8 Gy may be used acutely to stop bleeding.

UTERINE PAPILLARY SEROUS CARCINOMA

UPSC is an uncommon histological type of endometrial cancer comprising 1–10% of all uterine cancers with a poor outcome compared to endometrioid adenocarcinomas (12–15). Based on its similarity to ovarian papillary serous cancer, many investigators recommend that it be treated similarly with surgery followed by chemotherapy (80–82). Others have treated UPSC with surgery followed by pelvic and whole abdomen radiotherapy (14,83–86), or the combination of radiotherapy and chemotherapy (87).

Many studies have addressed the use of both adjuvant pelvic RT and APRT. The use of pelvic radiotherapy alone has been criticized because of the high upper abdominal relapse rate. Kato et al. (14) treated 10 patients with preoperative PRT and 15 patients with postoperative PRT and found that sites of failure included the abdomen, with or without the pelvis, in 45% of patients.

Mallipedi et al. (84) reported on 10 patients with clinical stage I UPSC treated with APRT and 5 of 10 patients survived with no evidence of disease with follow-up of 102–133 months. However, a similar-sized study showed no benefit of APRT when 6/9 relapsed and all relapses were in the radiated field (85). However this study could be criticized since they did include clinical stages I–III. More recently, Lim et al. (86) observed a small survival benefit for APRT. The 58 patients who received 20.5 Gy APRT had a significantly better five-year disease-specific survival than the 20 patients who received less or no radiotherapy. The majority of relapses were still in the pelvis and abdomen despite APRT. One of the limitations of abdomino-pelvic radiotherapy is the limited dose of 20–25 Gy that can be delivered safely.

The optimal management of UPSC remains unknown and many studies are hampered by the lack of accurate surgical assessment of disease extent. Indeed it is unclear if any additional therapy is valuable. We need prospective studies that surgically stage patients and use a combination of modalities to help guide the management of this relatively uncommon endometrial tumor.

UTERINE SARCOMAS

Uterine sarcomas are rare tumors. They are a heterogeneous group of tumors, and thus experience with each individual type of lesion is limited. There are few prospective randomized studies although retrospective studies have evaluated different therapeutic approaches.

Although the value of adjuvant radiation for sarcomas is controversial (88), most authors suggest that it improves local control especially for malignant mixed mesodermal tumors without influencing OS (89,90). The European Organization for Research and Treatment of Cancer (EORTC) recently completed an RCT addressing the value of postoperative adjuvant RT in patients with uterine sarcomas and the results of this trial are eagerly awaited.

IRRADIATION TECHNIQUE AND DOSE

Adjuvant external beam RT is designed to cover potential areas of microscopic disease that include the relevant regional pelvic nodes including the external iliac, internal iliac, and presacral lymph nodes; the upper vagina; and any residual parametrial tissue. Therefore the traditional anterior/posterior pelvic fields generally extend from the L5/S1 interspace superiorly to the inferior aspect of the obturator foramen inferiorly and 1.5–2.0 cm lateral to the widest brim of the bony pelvis laterally. Conventionally a four-field box technique using a high energy 18–20 MV linear accelerator is used and the lateral fields extend from anterior pubic symphysis anteriorly to the S2/S3 interspace posteriorly while the superior and inferior borders remain the same as for the anterior/posterior fields. Some kind of radio-opaque device is used to visualize the upper vagina to ensure that these field borders adequately cover the upper vagina because this is critical. These borders, of course, must be modified according to the individual desired clinical target volume and patient anatomy.

The doses prescribed in the adjuvant setting are between 45 and 50 Gy in 180–200 cGy daily fractions over 4–5 weeks. Depending on the clinical circumstances, additional vaginal vault therapy is given to a dose of 20–40 Gy using low-dose rate therapy or its equivalent using HDR therapy. Vaginal vault BT using applicators such as ovoids, colpostats, or cylinders is employed in addition to external beam therapy in those patients who are not surgically staged and who have microscopic cervical stromal involvement. In addition, it may be used as sole adjuvant therapy in those patients who are surgically staged node-negative but have adverse primary tumor factors. As sole adjuvant therapy, the BT vaginal vault dose is generally the equivalent of 60 Gy.

For whole abdominal and pelvic radiotherapy, the volume of treatment must include the entire peritoneal cavity and the fields are large. The beam arrangements are usually anterior and posterior opposing fields using 6–10 MV linear accelerators. The superior border must clear both diaphragms and inferiorly the field border is just below the obturator foramen. Laterally, the field borders clear the skin. Appropriate shielding is used to shield the heart, and the dose to the kidneys is generally limited to less than 20 Gy. Doses to the abdomen of 20–25 Gy have been reported in 100–125 cGy daily fractions over four weeks and the pelvic volumes as described above are taken to a total dose of 45 Gy. Additional doses to the pelvic and para-aortic nodes may be delivered to a total of 40–45 Gy.

For primary radiation treatment of endometrial cancer, treatment is comparable to the treatment of cervix cancer. External beam pelvic therapy using the volume and technique described above, followed by intracavitary therapy, is utilized bringing the point A dose to approximately 80 Gy.

For treatment of recurrence, therapy is individualized aiming to deliver as high a dose as safely feasible to the gross disease, but a minimum dose of 65 Gy is recommended. For vaginal vault recurrence confined to the mucosa/vaginal vault, intracavitary BT following EBT to deliver a combined vaginal vault dose of 80–85 Gy is desirable and optimizes chances of local control and cure.

RADIOTHERAPY TOXICITY

BT alone or in combination with external beam pelvic or whole abdominal therapy can be associated with both acute and chronic toxicities. The probability of severe complications depends on treatment factors such as the total radiation dose, daily fractionation, the treatment volumes, the use of shielding and treatment techniques, the specific organ involved, and the duration of treatment. Patient factors, especially a previous history of abdominal or pelvic surgery, are also important.

There are minor acute reactions seen during treatment and they affect the rapidly dividing tissues such as skin, gastrointestinal mucosa, bone marrow, and reproductive tissues (91). The most common side effects experienced during pelvic radiotherapy are diarrhea, abdominal cramps, urinary frequency, and urgency. Some minor skin irritation may occur. Many of these minor side effects are underreported if they do not cause an interruption of treatment. Premature menopause is not an issue for the majority of women with endometrial cancer as they are already menopausal.

External beam irradiation may result in severe chronic sequelae. Four to 15% late bowel complication rates requiring surgical intervention have been reported in the past (92,93). The most severe complications were small bowel obstruction, chronic diarrhea, proctitis, rectal and vesico-vaginal fistulas, and vaginal stenosis. These occurred with EBT but the addition of vaginal BT may augment the incidence of fibrosis, stenosis, ulcer, and fistula formation (92,94–97). Other chronic sequelae include the increased risk of insufficiency sacral fractures. More serious bone complications resulting in femoral neck fractures or osteosarcomas are fortunately rare (98).

Complication rates are increased when combination radiotherapy (EBT and BT) is used compared with each individual modality alone (94,99) and if a full lymphadenectomy has been performed (92,93).

More reliable recent prospective toxicity data available from the PORTEC Study concluded that postoperative adjuvant pelvic EBT for clinical stage I endometrial cancer was associated with a 3% risk of severe complications (requiring surgery). There was however a 22% risk of mild, mainly gastrointestinal, side effects, of which the majority were transient (96).

CONCLUSIONS

In summary, there continues to be a significant role for RT in the treatment of endometrial cancer. Since the majority of endometrial cancer patients present with early disease, excellent survival results can be achieved by a variety of regimens, including adjuvant external beam therapy, intracavitary BT alone for node-negative disease, and salvage radiotherapy for isolated pelvic relapse. Primary radical radiotherapy can also offer potential cure for those deemed medically unfit for surgery.

Current studies are focusing on strategies to find the optimal radiotherapy indications in an effort to maximize local control and survival, yet minimize treatment-related morbidity.

Advanced stage III and IV patients are rare, and large prospective studies to optimize treatment strategies are difficult. Individualized treatment using a multidisciplinary team and expertise is desirable.

REFERENCES

1. O'brien FW. The radium treatment of cancer of the cervix. Am J Roent Rad Ther 1947; 57:281–294.

2. Aikins WHB, Harrison FC. Radium in gynaecological conditions. Can Practioner Rev 1912; 37:567–575.

3. Cowles RA, Magarina JF, Masterson BJ, Capen CV. Comparison of clinical and surgical staging in patients with endometrial carcinoma. Obstet Gynecol 1985; 66:413–416.

4. Ayhan A, Yarali H, Urman B, Yuce K, Gunalp S, Havlioglu S. Comparison of clinical and surgical-pathologic staging in patients with endometrial carcinoma. J Surg Oncol 1990; 43:33–35.

5. Wolfson AH, Sightler SE, Markoe AM, Schwade JG, Averette HE, Ganjei P, Hilsenbeck SG. The prognostic significance of surgical staging for carcinoma of the endometrium. Gynecol Oncol 1992; 45:142–146.

6. Creaseman WT, Morrow CP, Bundy BN, Homesley HD, Graham JE, Heller PB. Surgical pathologic spread patterns of endometrial cancer. A Gynecologic Oncology Group study. Cancer 1987; 60:2035–2041.

7. Morrow CP, Bundy BN, Kurman RJ, Creasman WT, Heller P, Homelsey HD, Graham JE. Relationship between surgical-pathological risk factors and outcome in clinical stage I and II carcinoma of the endometrium: a Gynecologic Oncology Group Study. Cancer 1991; 40:55–65.

8. Boronow RC, Morrow CP, Creaseman WT, DiSaia PJ, Silverberg SG, Miller A, Blessing JA. Surgical staging in endometrial cancer: clinical-pathologic findings of a prospective study. Obstet Gynecol 1984; 63:825–832.

9. Announcements. FIGO stages—1988 Revision, Gynecol Oncol 1989; 35: 125–127.

10. Hendrickson M, Ross J, Eifel PJ, Cox RS, Martinez A, Kempson R. Adenocarcinoma of the endometrium: analysis of 256 cases with carcinoma limited to the uterine corpus. Gynecol Oncol 1982; 13:373–392.

11. Lanciano RM, Corn BW, Schultz DJ, Kramer CA, Rosenblum N, Hogan WM. The justification for a surgical staging system in endometrial carcinoma. Radiother Oncol 1993; 28:189–196.

12. Hendrickson M, Ross J, Eifel P, et al. Uterine papillary serous carcinoma: a highly malignant form of endometrial adenocarcinoma. Am J Surg Pathol 1982; 6:93–108.

13. Rosenberg P, Boeryd B, Simonsen E. A new aggressive treatment approach to high grade endometrial cancer of possible benefit to patients with stage I uterine papillary cancer. Gynecol Oncol 1993; 48:32–37.

14. Kato DT, Ferry J, Goodman A, et al. Uterine papillary serous carcinoma: a cliniclpathologic study of 30 cases. Gynecol Oncol 1995; 59:384–389.

15. Jeffrey JF, Krepart GV, Lotocki RJ. Papillary serous adenocarcinoma of the endometrium. Obstet Gynecol 1986; 67:670–674.

16. Abler VM, Vergote IB, Kjorstad KE, Trope CG. Clear cell carcinoma of the endometrium. Cancer 1996; 78:1740–1747.

17. Aalders J, Abeler V, Kolstad P, Onsrud M. Postoperative external irradiation and prognostic parameters in stage I endometrial carcinoma: clinical and histologic study of 540 patients. Obstet Gynecol 1980; 56:419–427.

18. Cohn DE, Horowitz NS, Mutch DG, Kim SM, Manolitsas T, Fowler JM. Should the presence of lymphvascular space involvement be used to assign

patients to adjuvant therapy following hysterectomy for unstaged endometrial cancer? Gynecol Oncol 2002; 87:243–246.

19. Lurain JR. The significance of positive peritoneal cytology in endometrial cancer. Gynecol Oncol 1992; 46:143–147.

20. Milosevic MF, Dembo AJ, Thomas GM. The clinical significance of malignant peritoneal cytology in stage I endometrial carcinoma. Int J Gynecol Cancer 1992; 2:225–235.

21. Price JJ, Hahn GA, Rominger CJ. Vaginal involvement in endometrial carcinoma. Am J Obstet Gynecol 1965; 91:1060–1065.

22. Stander RW. Vaginal metastases following treatment of endometrial carcinoma. Am J Obstet Gyncol 1956; 71:776.

23. Creutzberg CL, van Putten WLJ, Koper PCM, Lybeert MOM, Jobsen JJJ, Warlan Rodenhis CC, et al. Randomized trial of surgery and postoperative radiation therapy versus surgery alone for patients with stage I endometrial carcinoma. Lancet 2000; 355(9213):1404–1411.

24. Roberts JA, Brunetto VL, Keys HM, Zaino R, Spirtos NM, Bloss JD, et al. A phase III randomized study of surgery versus surgery plus adjunctive radiation therapy in intermediate risk endometrial adenocarcinoma. Gynecol Oncol 1998; 68:135 (Abstract #258).

25. Kim YB, Niloff JM. Endometrial carcinoma: analysis of recurrence in patients treated with a strategy minimizing lymph node sampling and radiation therapy. Obstet Gynecol 1993; 82:175–180.

26. Carey MS, O'Connell GI, Kohanson CR. Good outcome associated with a standardized treatment protocol using selective postoperative radiation in patients with clinical stage I adenocarcinoma of the endometrium. Gyneol Oncol 1995; 57:138–144.

27. Ackerman I, Malone S, Thomas G, Franssen E, Balogh J, Dembo A. Endometrial carcinoma-relative effectiveness of adjuvant irradiation vs. therapy reserved for relapse. Gynecol Oncol 1996; 60:177–183.

28. Poulsen M, Roberts SJ. The salvage of recurrent endometrial carcinoma in the vagina and pelvis. Int J Radiat Oncol Biol Phys 1988; 15:809–813.

29. Orr JW, Holimon JL, Orr PF. Stage I corpus cancer: Is teletherapy necessary? Am J Obstet Gynecol 1997; 176:777–789.

30. Chadha M, Nanavati PJ, Liu P, Fanning J, Jacobs A. Patterns of failure in endometrial carcinoma stage Ib grade 3 and IC patients treated with postoperative vaginal vault brachytherapy. Gynecol Oncol 1999; 75:103–107.

31. Ng TY, Perrin LC, Nicklin JL, Cheuk K, Crandon AJ. Local recurrence in high-risk node negative stage I endometrial carcinoma treated with postoperative vaginal vault brachytherapy. Gynecol Oncol 2000; 79:490–494.

32. Fanning J. Long term survival of intermediate risk endometrial cancer (Stage IG3,IC,II) treated with full lymphadenectomy and brachytherapy without teletherapy. Gynecol Oncol 2001; 82:371–374.

33. Rittenberg PV, Lotocki RJ, Heywood MS, Jones KD, Krepart GV. High-risk surgical stage I endometrial cancer: outcomes with vault brachytherapy alone. Gynecol Oncol 2003; 89:288–294.

34. Kucera H, Vavra N, Weghaupt K. Benefit of external irradiation in pathologic stage I endometrial carcinoma: prospective clinical trial of 605 patients who

received postoperative vaginal irradiation and additional pelvic irradiation in the presence of unfavorable prognostic factors. Gynecol Oncol 1990; 38:99–105.
35. Larson DM, Brosie SK, Krawisz BR. Surgery without radiotherapy for primary treatment of endometrial cancer. Obstet Gynecol 1998; 91:355–359.
36. Naumann RW, Higgins RV, Hall JB. The use of adjuvant radiation therapy by members of the Society of Gynecologic Oncologists. Gynecol Oncol 1999; 75:4–9.
37. Creutzberg CL, wan Putten WLC, Koper PC, Lybeert MLM, Jobsen JJ, Warlam-Rodenhuis C, et al. Survival after relapse in patients with endometrial cancer: results from a randomized trial. Gynecol Oncol 2003; 89:201–209.
38. Mandell LR, Dattatreyudu N, Hilaris B. Recurrent stage I endometrial carcinoma: results of treatment and prognostic factors. Int J Radiat Oncol Biol Phys 1985; 11(6):1103–1109.
39. Hoekstra CJM, Koper PCM, van Putten WLJ. Recurrent endometrial adenocarcinoma after surgery alone:prognostic factors and treatment. Radiother Oncol 1993; 27:164–166.
40. Sears JD, Greven KM, Hoen HM, Randal ME. Prognostic factors and treatment outcome for patients with locally recurrent endometrial cancer. Cancer 1994; 74:1303–1308.
41. Hart KB, Han I, Shamsa F, Court WS, Chuba P, Deppe G, Malone J, Christensen C, Porter AT. Radiation therapy for endometrial cancer in patients treated for postoperative recurrence. Int J Radiat Oncol Biol Phys 1998; 41(1):7–11.
42. Wylie J, Irwin C, Pintilie M, Levin W, Manchul L, Milosevic M, Fyles A. Results of radical radiotherapy for recurrent endometrial cancer. Gynecol Oncol 2000; 77(1):66–72.
43. Fishman DA, Roberts KB, Chambers JT, Kohorn EI, Schwartz PE, Chambers SK. Radiation therapy as exclusive treatment for medically inoperable patients with stage I and II endometrioid carcinoma of the endometrium. Gynecol Oncol 1996; 61:181–196.
44. Nguyen TV, Petereit DG. High-dose-rate brachytherapy for medically inoperable stage I endometrial cancer. Gynecol Oncol 1998; 71:196–203.
45. Rouanet P, Dubois JB, Gely S, Pourquier H. Exclusive radiation therapy in endometrial carcinoma. Int J Radiat Oncol Biol Phys 1993; 26:223–228.
46. Kucera H, Knocke TH, Kucera E, Potter R. Treatment of endometrial carcinoma with high-dose-rate brachytherapy alone in medically inoperable stage I patients. Acta Obstet Gynecol Scand 1998; 77:1008–1012.
47. Lehoczky O, Bosze P, Ungar L, Tottossy B. Stage I endometrial carcinoma: treatment of nonoperable patients with intracavitary radiation therapy alone. Gynecol Oncol 1991; 43:211–216.
48. Elia G, Garfinkel DA, Goldberg GL, Davidson S, Runowica CD. Surgical management of patients with endometrial cancer and cervical involvement. Eur J Gynecol Oncol 1995; 16:169–173.
49. Cornelison TL, Trimble EL, Kosary CL. SEER Data, corpus uteri cancer: treatment trends versus survival for FIGO stage II, 1988–1994. Gynecol Oncol 1999; 74:350–355.
50. Rutledge F. The role of radical hysterectomy in adenocarcinoma of the endometrium. Gynecol Oncol 1974; 2:331–335.

51. Kinsella TJ, Bloomer WD, Lavin PT, Knapp RC. Stage II endometrial carcinoma: a 10-year follow-up of combined radiation and surgical treatment. Gynecol Oncol 1980; 10:290–297.
52. Reisinger SA, Staros EB, Feld R, Mohiuddin M, Lewis GC. Preoperative radiation therapy in clinical stage II endometrial carcinoma. Gynecol Oncol 1992; 45:174–178.
53. Leminen A, Forss M, Lehtovirta P. Endometrial adenocarcinoma with clinical evidence of cervical involvement: accuracy of diagnostic procedures, clinical course, and prognostic factors. Act Obstet Gynecol Scand 1995; 74:61–66.
54. Schorge JO, Molpus KL, Goodman A, Nikrui N, Fuller AF Jr. The effect of postsurgical therapy on stage III endometrial carcinoma. Gynecol Oncol 1996; 63:34–39.
55. Lee SW, Russell AH, Kinney WK. Whole abdomen radiotherapy for patients with peritoneal dissemination of endometrial adenocarcinoma. Int J Radiat Oncol Biol Phys 2003; 56(3):788–792.
56. Ayhan A, Taskiran C, Celik C, Aksu T, Yuce K. Surgical stage III Endometrial cacner: anaylsis of treatment outcomes, prognostic factors and failure patterns. Eur J Gynaecol Oncol 2002; 23(6):553–556.
57. Ashman JB, Connell PP, Yamada D, Rotmensch J, Waggoner SE, Mundt AJ. Outcome of endometrial carcinoma patients with involvement of the uterine serosa. Gynecol Oncol 2001; 82:338–343.
58. Aalders J, Abeler V, Kolstad P. Clinical (stage III) as compared to subclinical intrapelvic extrauterine tumor spread in endometrial carcinoma: a clinical and histopathological study of 175 patients. Gynecol Oncol 1984; 17: 64–74.
59. Bruckman JE, Goodman RL, Murthy A, Marck A. Combined irradiation and surgery in the treatment of stage II carcinoma of the endometrium. Cancer 1978; 42:1146–1151.
60. Greven KM, Lanciano RE, Corn B, Case D, Randall ME. Pathologic stage III endometrial carcinoma. Cancer 1993; 71:3697–3702.
61. Genest P, Drouin P, Girard A, et al. Stage III carcinoma of the endometrium: a review of 41 cases. Gynecol Oncol 1987; 26:77–86.
62. Grigsby PW, Perez CA, Kuske RR, et al. Results of therapy, analysis of failures, and prognostic factors for clinical and pathologic stage III adenocarcinoma of the endometrium. Gynecol Oncol 1987; 27:44–57.
63. Greven KM, Curran WJ, Whittington R, et al. Analysis of failure patterns in stage III endometrial carcinoma and therapeutic implications. Int J Radiat Oncol Biol Phys 1989; 17:35–39.
64. Greer BE, Hamberger AD. Treatment of intraperitoneal metastatic adneocarcinoma of the endometrium by the whole-abdomen moving-strip technique and pelvic boost irradiation. Gynecol Oncol 1983; 16:365–373.
65. Gibbons S, Martinez A, Schray M, et al. Adjuvant whole abdominoperlvic irradiaion for high risk endometrial carcinoma. Int J Radiat Oncol Biol Phys 1991; 21:1019–1025.
66. Potish RA. Abdominal radiotherapy for cancer of the uterine cervix and endometrium. Int J Radiat Oncol Biol Phy 1989; 16:1453–1458.

67. Nicklin JL, Petersen RW. Stage 3B adenocarcinoma of the endometrium: a clinicopathologic study. Gynecol Oncol 2000; 78(2):203–207.
68. Nelson G, Randall M, Sutton G, Moore D, Hurteau J, Look K. FIGO Stage IIIC endometrial carcinoma with metastases confince to pelvic lymph nodes: analysis of treatment outcomes, prognostic variables, and failure patterns following adjuvant radiaion therapy. Gynecol Oncol 1999; 75: 211–214.
69. Potish RA, Twiggs LB, Adcock LL, et al. Para-aortic lymph node radiotherapy in cancer of the uterine corpus. Obstet Gynecol 1985; 65:251–256.
70. Corn BW, Lanciano RM, Greven KM. Endometrial cancer with para-aortic adenopathy. Patterns of failure and opportunities for cure. Int J Radiat Oncol Biol Phys 1992; 24:223–227.
71. Rose PG, Cha SD, Tak WK, Fitzgerald T. Radiation thcrapy for surgically proven para-aortic node metastasis in endometrial carcinoma. Int J Radiat Oncol Biol Phys 1992; 24:229–233.
72. McMeekin DS, Lashbrook D, Gold M, Scribner DR, Kamelle S, Tillmanns TD, Mannel R. Nodal distribution and its significance in FIGO stage IIIC endometrial cancer. Gynecol Oncol 2001; 82(2):375–379.
73. Mariani A, Webb MJ, Keeney GL, Haddock MG, Aletti G, Podratz KD. Stage IIIC endometrioid corpus cancer includes distinct subgroups. Gynecol Oncol 2002; 87:112–117.
74. Thigpen JT, Buchsbaum HJ, Mangan C, Blessing JA. Phase II trial of adriamycin in the treatment of advanced or recurrent endometrial carcinoma: a Gynecologic Oncology Group study. Cancer Treat Rep 1979; 63: 21–27.
75. Trope C, Grundsell H, Johnson JE, Cavallin-Stahl FA. A phase II study of cisplatinum for recurrent corpus cancer. Eur J Cancer 1980; 16: 1025–1026.
76. Thigpen JT, Blessing JA, Homesley H, Creasman WT, Sutton G. Phase II trial of cisplatin as first line chemotherapy in patients with advanced or recurrent endometrial carcinoma: a Gynecologic Oncology Group study. Gynecol Oncol 1989; 33:68–70.
77. Ball HG, Blessing JA, Lentz SS, Mutch DG. A phase II trial of taxol in advanced or recurrent adenocarcinoma of the endometrium: a Gynecologic Oncology Group study. Gynecol Oncol 1995; 56:120(abstract).
78. Randall ME, Brunetto G, Muss H, Mannel RS, Spirtos N, Jeffrey F, Thigpen J, Benda J. A RCT of whole abdominal radiotherapy versus combination doxorubicin-cisplatin chemotherapy in advanced endometrial carcinoma: a Gynecology Oncology Group study. ASCO 2003 (abstract #3).
79. Grigsby PW. Update on radiation therapy for endometrial cancer. Oncology 2002; 16(6):777–790.
80. Chambers JT, Merino M, Kohorn EI, et al. Uterine papillary serous carcinoma. Obstet Gynecol 1987; 69(1):109–113.
81. Levenback C, Burke TW, Silva E, et al. Uterine papillary serous carcinoma treated with cisplatin, doxorubicin, and chclophosphamide. Gynecol Oncol 1992; 46:317–321.

82. Price VF, Chambers SK, Carcangiu ML, et al. Intravenous cisplatin, doxorubicin, and cyclophosphamide in the treatment of uterine papillary serous carcinoma (UPSC). Gynecol Oncol 1993; 51:383–389.
83. Craighead PS, Sait K, Stuart GC, Arthur K, Nation J, Duggan M, Guo I. Management of aggressive histologic variants of endometrial carcinoma at the tom Baker Cancer Centre between 1984 and 1994. Gynecol Oncol 2000; 77:248–253.
84. Mallipeddi P, Kapp DS, Teng NN. Long-term survival with adjuvant whole abdominopelvic irradiation for uterine papillary serous carcinoma. Cancer 1993; 71:3076–3081.
85. Frank AH, Tseng PC, Haffty BG, et al. Adjuvant whole-abdominal radiation therapy in uterine papillary serous carcinoma. Cancer 1991; 68:1516–1519.
86. Lim P, Al Kushi A, Gilks B, et al. Early stage uterine papillary serous carcinoma of the endometrium: effect of adjuvant whole abdominal radiotherapy and pathologic parameters on outcome. Cancer 2001; 91(4):752–757.
87. Bancher-Todesca D, Neunteufel W, Williams KE, et al. Influence of postoperative treatment on survival in patients with uterine papillary serous carcinoma. Gynecol Oncol 1998; 71(3):344–347.
88. Kahanpaa KV, Wahlstrom T, Grohn P, Heinonen E, Nieminen U, Widholm O. Sarcoma of the uterus: a clinicopathologic study of 119 patients. Obstet Gynecol 1986; 67:417–424.
89. Spanos WJ, Peters LJ, Oswald MJ. Patterns of recurrence in malignagnt mixed mullerian tumor of the uterus. Cancer 1986; 57:155–159.
90. Echt G, Jepson J, Steel J, Langholz B, Luxton G, Hernandez W. Treatment of uterine sarcomas. Cancer 1990; 66:35–39.
91. Eifel PJ. Radiation therapy. In: Berek JS, Hacker NF eds. Practical Gynecologic Oncology. 3rd ed. Philadelphia: JB Lippincott, 2000:117–158.
92. Greven K, Lanciano R, Herbert S, et al. Analysis of complications in patients with endometrial carcinoma receiving adjuvant irradiation. Int J Radiat Oncol Biol Phys 1991; 21:919–923.
93. Corn BW, Lanciano RM, Greven KM, Noumoff J, Schultz D, Hanks GE, et al. Impact of improved irradiation technique, age and lymph node sampling on the severe complication rate of surgically staged endometrial cancer patients: a multivariate analysis. J Clin Oncol 2003; 12:510–515.
94. Irwin C, Levin W, Fyles A, et al. The role of adjuvant radiotherapy in carinoma of the endometrium: Results in 550 patients with pathologic stage I disease. Gynecol Oncol 1998; 70:247–254.
95. Potish RA, Dusenbery KE. Enteric morbidity of postoperative pelvic external beam and brachytherapy for uterine cancer. Int J Radiat Oncol Biol Phys 1990; 18:1005–1010.
96. Creutzberg CL, van Putten WLJ, Koper PC, Lybeert MLM, Jobsen JJ, Warlam-Rodenhuis CC, De Winter KAJ, Lutgens LC, et al. The morbidity of treatment for patients with stage I endometrial cancer: results from a randomized trial. Int J Radiat Oncol Biol Phys 2001; 51(5):1246–1255.
97. Randall ME, Wilder J, Greven K, et al. Role of intracavitary cuff boost after adjuvant external irradiation in early endometrial carcinoma. Int J Radiat Oncol Biol Phys 1990; 19:49–54.

98. Konski A, Sowers M. Pelvic fractures following irradiation for endometrial carcinoma. Int J Radiat Oncol Biol Phys 1996; 35:361–367.
99. Carey MS, O'Connell GJ, Johanson CR, et al. Good outcome associated with a standardized treatment protocol using selective postoperative radiation in patients with clinical stage I adenocarcinoma of the endometrium. Gynecol Oncol 1995; 57:138–144.

10

Chemotherapy for Uterine Cancer

**Kathryn F. Chrystal, Kerry A. Cheong,
and Peter G. Harper**
*Department of Medical Oncology, Guy's Hospital,
London, U.K.*

INTRODUCTION

Uterine malignancies have a good overall prognosis. The majority of patients present with early stages of the disease and are cured with surgery and radiotherapy. Chemotherapy predominantly has been employed in the management of advanced or recurrent disease where the aim of treatment is usually palliative. The median overall survival in this setting is 7–10 months. Medical oncologists increasingly use chemotherapy for clinical benefit even if this may have little influence on overall survival. Subsequently assessment of quality of life with minimization of toxicity becomes as important as both response rate and survival in evaluating new therapies.

This chapter will review the evidence supporting the role of chemotherapy in uterine malignancies, including the aggressive histological variant, uterine papillary serous carcinoma, and uterine sarcomas. The published literature in this area is limited to mainly phase-II trials and a handful of randomized studies, which have taken years to accrue, given the relative rarity of advanced disease. Previous pelvic radiotherapy inevitably makes second-line chemotherapy difficult with its increased risk of hematological toxicity. These facts make therapeutic decisions based on the current evidence challenging.

ENDOMETRIOID ADENOCARCINOMA

Single Agent Therapy

Many drugs have demonstrated single agent activity, with the most widely investigated being the platinums and anthracyclines. The most active agents are listed in Table 1.

Doxorubicin, the most extensively investigated single agent having been tested in 283 patients, became the standard arm for comparative studies (1–4). Doses of 50–60 mg/m^2 have yielded response rates of 17–37% (4) as did a single study using epirubicin (5). The role of pegylated liposomal doxorubicin with its preferential toxicity profile is being evaluated. An initial study observed a 9.5% response rate in 42 pretreated patients, with two-thirds of the group receiving prior doxorubicin (6).

Historically, cisplatin has been the standard platinum agent investigated as both single agent and in combination. As a single agent it has shown consistent anti-tumor activity with response rates of 20–42% (7–12). As in many tumors, carboplatin with its better side effect profile has also been investigated (13–16). The largest trial using single agent carboplatin demonstrated an overall response rate of 17%, which increased to 24% in chemo-naïve patients (16).

Table 1 Endometrial Carcinoma: Single Agent Activity

Agent	*n*	Prior chemotherapy	Dose	Response rate (%)
Doxorubicin (1–4)	283	2	50–80 mg/m^2	19–37
Epirubicin (5)	27	0	—	26
Cisplatin (7–12)	138	43	50–100 mg/m^2 q21–28	4–42
Carboplatin (13 16)	122	14	300–400 mg/m^2	17–33
Ifosfamide (21,117,118)	117	68	1.2–5 g/m^2	15–25
Paclitaxel (17–20)	98	70	170 mg/m^2 over 3 hours to 250 mg/m^2 over 24 hours q21	27.3–43
5FU (119)	34	—	—	21
Oral etoposide (22)	44	0	50 mg d1-21 q28	14
Topotecan (23,24)	62	22	1 mg/m^2 d1-5 q28	9–20

This is in keeping with the efficacy seen in the three other trials of carboplatin as first-line therapy (13–16).

Paclitaxel as a single agent has comparable efficacy to the "platins" and doxorubicin. Ball et al. reported a response rate of 35.7% in 30 chemo-naïve patients (17). In second-line studies, three trials totaling 70 patients have demonstrated a response rate of 27–43% (18–20). Toxicity was not insignificant and predominantly hematological. Dose reduction was instituted to those with previous pelvic irradiation in an attempt to minimize myelosuppression (17). These promising results have led to paclitaxel being evaluated in combination in phase-III studies.

Ifosfamide demonstrated greater activity than cyclophosphamide in a randomized controlled trial (12.5% compared to 7%) (21). There had been no advantage demonstrated with the addition of cyclophosphamide to doxorubicin in a phase-III trial (3). Oral etoposide in chemo-naïve patients gave a modest response rate of 14% but was well tolerated. Consideration could be given to using this in combination with other active agents (22).

Topotecan, a new topoisomerase I inhibitor, has proven activity in ovarian cancer. Early reports in endometrial carcinoma indicate modest activity (9–20%), however, hematological toxicity has been high with treatment-related deaths in excess of 10% observed, and dose modifications subsequently required, particularly in patients having received prior radiation (23,24).

Combination Regimens

Many active combinations have been identified, some of which are currently being investigated in randomized trials. Table 2 lists the combinations in randomized trials and Table 3 lists active phase-II combinations (25–41). Other combinations evaluated in single studies include carboplatin/vinorelbine, methotrexate, vinblastine, adriamycin, and cisplatin (MVAC), doxorubicin/vincristine/cyclophosphamide/5FU, doxorubicin/etoposide, doxorubicin/cisplatin/vinblastine, and 5FU/cisplatin/etoposide (42–48). The higher response rates of the early combination chemotherapy phase-II studies using doxorubicin and cyclophosphamide (38–40) did raise hopes of benefit; however, in the randomized phase-III studies the doublet did not alter survival or progression-free survival over the anthracycline (3).

The most robust evidence is for the combination of doxorubicin and cisplatin, which remains the standard treatment in all current phase-III trials. Two large randomized trials of the combination against doxorubicin have been completed. Aapro et al. observed a significantly higher response rate for the combination (43% vs. 17%, $p < 0.001$) but failed to demonstrate any overall survival benefit (nine months vs. seven months, $p = 0.0654$). A modest gain in overall survival was revealed when patients were stratified for good performance status ($p = 0.024$ hazard ratio (HR) 1.46, 95% confidence interval (CI) 1.05–2.03) (4). Toxicities as expected were higher for the

Table 2 Endometrial Carcinoma: Randomized Phase-III Trials of Combinations

Agents	*n*	Response rate (%)	PFS (months)	OS (months)
Doxorubicin vs.	177	17	7	7
Doxorubicin/Cisplatin (4)		43	8	9
		$p = < 0.001$		
Doxorubicin vs.	297	27	See text	See text
Doxorubicin/Cisplatin (49)		45		
Doxorubicin vs.	342	46	6.5	11.2
Doxorubicin/Cisplatin (50)		49	5.9	13.2
(circadian scheduling)				
Doxorubicin vs.	356	22	3.2	6.7
Doxorubicin/		30	3.9	7.3
Cyclophosphamide (3)				
Doxorubicin/Cisplatin vs.	314	40	NR	NR
Doxorubicin/Paclitaxel (52)		43		
Doxorubicin/Cisplatin vs.	266	33	NR	NR
Doxorubicin/Cisplatin/		57		
Paclitaxel (53)		$p = < 0.001$		

Abbreviations: PFS, progression free survival; OS, overall survival.

combination with grade 3/4 leucopenia (55.4%) and thrombocytopenia (13.2%) compared to 30.5% and 4.9% for single agent doxorubicin. The second study ($n = 223$), performed by the Gynecologic Oncology Group (GOG) comparing these two regimens, supports these findings. A significantly higher response rate (42% vs. 25% $p = 0.004$) and improved progression-free survival (5.7 months vs. 3.8 months, $p = 0.014$) was demonstrated for the combination. There was no difference in overall survival (9.0 months vs. 9.2 months). Severe toxicity rates were similar to that seen in the EORTC study. Neither of these studies incorporated quality of life analysis.

Attempts to improve the delivery of this combination have been investigated in a phase-III trial of the doxorubicin and cisplatin combination

Table 3 Endometrial Carcinoma: Active Phase-II Combinations

Agents	*n*	Response rate (%)	Complete response (%)
Carboplatin/Paclitaxel (25–27,41)	28	63–78	22–45
Cisplatin/Paclitaxel (28)	24	67	29
Cisplatin/Epirubicin/	30	73	23
Paclitaxel (29)			
Cyclophosphamide/Doxorubicin/	183	45–56	11–20
Cisplatin (30–33)			

administered either standard or in a circadian timed schedule. No difference in response rate or survival was seen (50).

Given its activity as a single agent, paclitaxel has now been tested in combination with both platinums and anthracyclines. Paclitaxel/platinum combinations have been assessed in five phase-II studies with higher response rates than previously reported with single agents (25–29,41). Substantial rates of neurotoxicity were seen with the cisplatin/paclitaxel combination (28) leading to its substitution by carboplatin (27). The results of a randomized phase-II trial comparing paclitaxel/carboplatin and doxorubicin/cisplatin in 70 patients reported, in abstract, a response rate of 35.3% versus 27.6% and progression-free survival at 15 months of 34.7% versus 23.5% in favor of the paclitaxel/carboplatin combination. Longer follow-up is required (51). The combination of paclitaxel/doxorubicin (GOG 163) has in early reports showed no benefit over doxorubicin/cisplatin (52).

Improved responses with doublets prompted the investigation of a three-drug combination with paclitaxel, doxorubicin, and cisplatin (TAP). Paclitaxel was administered on day 2 in an attempt to reduce the high rate of peripheral neuropathy seen with the paclitaxel/cisplatin combination. Growth factor support was required for the triplet due to the high rate of severe hematological toxicity seen in the phase-I study. The TAP combination produced a 57% response rate in contrast to 33% for doxorubicin/cisplatin in the phase-III setting. No survival benefit for TAP has been demonstrated at median follow-up of 18 months although a significant improvement in progression-free interval (PFI) of five months was seen for the triplet. Less grade-4 neutropenia but more grade-3 neurotoxicity was found with TAP (53).

Small studies have been done combining combination chemotherapy with hormonal therapy. The initial high response rates failed to be replicated in larger studies (54–63).

No studies published to date have compared chemotherapy with hormonal therapy or best supportive care. None of these trials described so far have quality of life assessments.

Chemotherapy vs. Whole Abdominal Radiotherapy

Whole abdominal radiotherapy (WART) was compared to chemotherapy with cisplatin and doxorubicin (GOG 122) in a large phase-III trial ($n = 422$). Patients were required to have small volume residual disease (maximum 2 cm) and also included those with a papillary serous histology. Preliminary results demonstrated a significant progression-free and overall survival advantage for combination chemotherapy (HR 0.81 and 0.71, respectively) (64). Quality of life (QoL) analysis revealed no difference in global QoL scores but significantly more frequent and persisting peripheral neuropathy symptoms for the chemotherapy arm (65).

Adjuvant Chemotherapy

Currently there is no evidence to support the use of adjuvant chemotherapy for endometrial carcinoma. Studies which have attempted to answer this question have been underpowered and the definition of "high risk" has been variable, thus confounding attempts at evaluating benefit. The strongest predictor for relapse appears to be the presence of extrauterine disease. Other important prognostic factors include the depth of myometrial invasion, histological grade, cervical or lower uterine segment involvement, lymphovascular invasion, or a papillary serous or clear cell histology (66). The only randomized trial reported involved 181 patients at high risk of recurrence following postoperative radiotherapy. Women were randomized to adjuvant doxorubicin or no further therapy. No progression-free or overall survival advantage was found (67). Four other prospective studies failed to show a benefit with the addition of chemotherapy (68–71). The Radiation Therapy Oncology Group (RTOG) have completed accrual of 436 patients to a randomized trial of adjuvant concurrent cisplatin chemo-radiation followed by cisplatin and paclitaxel versus radiation alone. It is estimated that 2000 women will need to be enrolled in an adjuvant study to show a 5% five-year survival benefit. No advantage has been conferred with the use of adjuvant radiotherapy (72,73) or hormonal therapy (74). The role of adjuvant progestogen therapy has been reviewed by meta-analysis and Cochrane review, with neither finding a significant benefit (75,76).

CONCLUSION

Cytotoxic chemotherapy has a role as palliative treatment in selected patients with advanced endometrial carcinoma. The most active single agents to date are doxorubicin, platinums, and paclitaxel. Combination chemotherapy has demonstrated increased efficacy with improved response rates and progression-free survival but this has not translated into an overall survival benefit. Unfortunately durable responses with chemotherapy, single agent, or combination are few. The absence of robust QoL data makes the relative benefit of any small gain in progression-free survival given the higher toxicities seen with combination therapy difficult to justify.

SEROUS CARCINOMA

Uterine papillary serous carcinoma (UPSC) is an uncommon (2–10% of cases), but clinically aggressive histological subtype of endometrial carcinoma. First reported by Hendrickson et al. as a distinct entity in 1982, he described the histological appearance and pattern of intraperitoneal spread similar to that of epithelial ovarian cancer (77). UPSC often presents as advanced stage disease and has poorer response rates to treatment. Local and distant recurrence after apparent curative surgery is also more common. These factors account for the lower reported five-year survival rates of 35–80% for stages I and II, and 0–25% for stage III/IV disease (78–81).

Both chemotherapy and radiotherapy have been studied in the adjuvant and salvage treatment of UPSC; however, the best agents, multimodality combinations, and timing of treatment are still to be determined. The studies are frequently retrospective and describe small, non-randomized trials.

The majority of the regimens have been platinum-based. Cisplatin, doxorubicin, and cyclophosphamide (CAP) demonstrated modest response rates of 18–27% in two retrospective studies but were associated with significant toxicity (82,83). Paclitaxel has shown promising activity both as a single agent and in combination with carboplatin. In a retrospective review, Zanotti et al. observed an objective response in seven out of 11 patients (64%) with the combination of either carboplatin or cisplatin and paclitaxel as salvage therapy. The median PFI was nine months and toxicity was acceptable (84). A prospective study of a single agent paclitaxel as first-line therapy (200 mg/m^2 over 24 hours) yielded a 77% response rate and median PFI of 7.3 months in 13 evaluable patients. Toxicity was high with 90% grade 3/4 neutropenia and over 50% of patients requiring granulocyte colony-stimulating factor (G-CSF) support (85).

Adjuvant Therapy

Given the high risk of local and distant recurrence in UPSC both chemo-therapy and radiotherapy have been investigated in the adjuvant setting. Evidence from retrospective studies suggests that adjuvant chemotherapy may improve overall survival in high-risk patients and radiotherapy reduces local recurrence.

Price et al. retrospectively evaluated cisplatin, doxorubicin, and cyclo-phosphamide (CAP) in 19 patients without clinical evidence of disease post-surgery [Federation of Gynecology and Obstetrics (FIGO) stages IA–IVB]. This heterogeneous group had a median survival of 31 months and a two years' survival of 58%. FIGO stage was predictive for recurrence and survi-val, with eight of nine stage I and stage II patients remaining disease-free. Local-regional radiation therapy was given to 47% of this group.

A further retrospective study of the postoperative treatment of 23 patients with UPSC (FIGO stages I–IV), examined the role of either chemo-therapy, radiotherapy or both. The combination of platin-based chemother-apy (cisplatin/carboplatin plus cyclophosphamide) and pelvic radiotherapy resulted in significantly improved survival over either treatment alone (80% vs. 30% five-year overall survival; log rank = 0.05) (86).

In a larger review of a subset of 103 patients with aggressive variant histology, Craighead et al. demonstrated a significant reduction in local recurrence in patients with stages IB–III disease treated with adjuvant pelvic radiotherapy but no survival benefit. However, the 17% of patients who received CAP chemotherapy had a longer overall median survival than those who did not undergo chemotherapy (87).

The combination of a platinum and paclitaxel was trialled as adjuvant therapy in nine patients, producing a median PFI of 30 months (84). Radiotherapy was not given to this group.

Steed et al. recently reported their adjuvant series of 108 patients (FIGO stages I–III) treated with either WART (22 Gy whole abdomen +45G pelvic boost) or carboplatin/paclitaxel followed by WART chemotherapy. The five-year survival by stage was 66% (stage I), 40% (stage II), and 15% (stage III). After controlling for stage the WART group had a significantly inferior survival when compared to the combination therapy group (HR 6.1, $p = 0.002$), although follow-up was shorter in the combination group (88). These studies suggest that adjuvant treatment with combination therapy in high-risk patients should be considered.

Prospective evaluation in clinical trials is required to clearly define its role. While no standard chemotherapeutic regimen exists, the combination of a platinum agent and paclitaxel has shown comparable efficacy to other platinum regimens, with more acceptable toxicity. This combination warrants further evaluation and is likely to form the basis of future trials.

UTERINE SARCOMAS

Uterine sarcomas are uncommon tumors, accounting for only 5% of all uterine malignancies (89). Three histological variants make up 95% of this group: carcinosarcoma (otherwise known as mixed Mullerian tumors) comprise 50%, with leiomyosarcoma (LMS) accounting for 30%, and the rarer endometrial stromal sarcoma (EES) 15% (90). Overall these tumors have a poor prognosis with a 50% five-year survival reported for stage I disease, and 0–20% for more advanced disease. This propensity for distant relapse highlights the need for effective systemic therapies.

Retrospective analysis of over 650 patients have identified tumor stage, high mitotic count, and histological type to be independent prognostic variables (91,92). Of the histological subtypes, low-grade EES has been associated with the best prognosis while LMS confers the gravest prognosis, even when adjusting for stage and mitotic count (91).

Chemotherapeutic agents with activity in soft-tissue sarcomas have been the most widely investigated in uterine sarcomas. These include the platinum agents, anthracyclines, epipodophyllotoxins, and more recently the taxanes. Several combinations have undergone investigation, but to date only a handful of randomized phase-III trials have been reported. Initial studies assessing chemotherapeutic responses of uterine sarcoma included all histological subtypes, and therefore the true benefits of chemotherapy in any individual subtype may not have been observed. More recently it has become apparent that these are a heterogeneous group of histologies, which have shown differential responses to chemotherapy and should be studied as separate entities rather than a collective group.

Carcinosarcoma

Single Agents

Ifosfamide® and cisplatin® have demonstrated activity as single agents (Table 4). Ifosfamide ($1.5\,mg/m^2$/day over five days) appears the most active, producing a 34.8% response rate in 28 chemo-naïve patients in the initial phase-II trial (93), later confirmed with a similar response rate in a further study where ifosfamide was the control arm in a randomized trial (94).

Cisplatin ($50\,mg/m^2$ every three weeks) given second-line in 34 patients demonstrated an 18% response rate (95). A subsequent GOG study of 63 chemo-naïve patients produced a similar response of 19% (96). Higher doses of cisplatin ($75–100\,mg/m^2$) in patients yielded a response rate of 42% in 12 patients; however, the small numbers do not allow for any meaningful conclusions about the benefits of cisplatin dose intensification in this population (97).

More recently paclitaxel ($170\,mg/m^2$) has shown encouraging results with four complete and four partial responses [risk ratio (RR) 18.2%] in 44 previously treated patients (98).

No other agents investigated in carcinosarcoma have shown meaningful activity including doxorubicin with response rates of only 0–10% being reported (99,100).

Table 4 Single Agents with Activity in Uterine Sarcoma

Agent	n	Prior chemotherapy	Response rate (%)
Carcinosarcoma: single agent activity			
Ifosfamide (93,94)	222	No	36
Cisplatin (95,96)	63	No	19
	34	Yes	18
Paclitaxel (98)	44	Yes	18
Etoposide (104)	31	Yes	6
Doxorubicin (99,100)	50	No	0–10
Leiomyosarcoma: single agent activity			
Doxorubicin (100)	28	No	25
Ifosfamide (103)	35	No	17
Cisplatin (96)	33	No	3
Paclitaxel (105)	34	No	9.1
Topotecan (107)	36	No	11
Gemcitabine (108)	32	Yes	3
Etoposide (120)	28	Yes	11

Combination Chemotherapy

Three randomized phase-III trials are reported to date comparing single agents to combinations; however, only one of these was performed exclusively in carcinosarcoma (Table 5). Sutton et al. investigated ifosfamide with or without cisplatin in a group of 194 patients with advanced, persistent, or recurrent carcinosarcoma. The combination group had a significantly higher response rate (54% vs. 36%, $p = 0.03$), and a progression-free survival advantage (6.0 m vs. 4.0 m, $p = 0.02$) over the single agent. There was no difference in overall survival between the two groups (MS 9.4 m vs. 7.6 m, $p = 0.07$). The combination resulted in increased toxicity with hematologic, nausea and vomiting, and peripheral neuropathy all reported with greater severity (94).

Other combinations have shown no improvement in efficacy over the single agent; however, these were performed in a heterogeneous patient population before the differential responses of the histological subtypes were evident. Doxorubicin and cyclophosphamide was not superior to doxorubicin alone in a group of mixed sarcoma types (101), and similarly dacarbazine (DTIC) did not show any advantage when added to doxorubicin (100).

Multi-agent combinations such as DEVAC (doxorubicin, DTIC, vindesine, cisplatin, and cyclophosphamide/ifosfamide) have reported response rates of up to 54%, but the toxicity was unacceptable (102).

Combination chemotherapy confers modest improvements in efficacy at the cost of significantly increased toxicity without survival benefit. Where the aim of treatment is palliative, quality of life is paramount. Unfortunately none of the trials we reviewed have included QoL analysis. Thus while the combination of ifosfamide and cisplatin may offer the best efficacy, patients should be carefully selected and counseled as to the ongoing limitations of chemotherapeutic treatment of advanced uterine carcinosarcomas.

Table 5 Uterine Sarcoma—Phase-III Randomized Trials

Agents	n	Response rate %	PFS	OS
All uterine sarcoma subtypes				
Doxorubicin vs.	132	19	No significant	No significant
Dox + Cyclo (101)		19	difference	difference
Doxorubicin vs.	240	16.3	No significant	No significant
Doxorubicin + DTIC (100)		24.2	difference	difference
Carcinosarcoma:				
Ifosfamide vs.	194	36	4.0 m	7.6 m
Ifosfamide + Cisplatin (94)		54	6.0 m, $p = 0.02$	9.4 m, $p = 0.07$

Leiomyosarcoma

Single Agents

The most active agents in LMS are doxorubicin and ifosfamide (Table 4). A 25% response rate was seen among 28 patients treated with doxorubicin 60 mg/m^2 every three weeks (100). Sutton et al. observed response rates of 17% with ifosfamide (103). In contrast to carcinosarcoma, cisplatin has failed to show efficacy in LMS with a response rate of only 3% (96). Negligible activity was seen with oral etoposide, mitozantrone, aziridinylbenzoquinone (AZQ), and aminothiadiazole (ATD) (104).

New agents investigated by GOG include paclitaxel with modest activity in both first- and second-line with three responses in 34 chemo-naïve women (9.1%) (105) and four responses in 48 previously treated (8.4%) (106). Topotecan in 36 chemo-naïve patients achieved one complete and three partial responses (107). Two trials of single agent gemcitabine in soft-tissue sarcomas, which included LMS, indicated poor activity with a 3% response rate (108,109).

Combination Therapy

There have been no randomized trials evaluating combination chemotherapy exclusively for LMS. As discussed earlier two randomized trials including all sarcoma subtypes did not reveal any benefit for the combinations (100,101) (Table 5).

In a phase-II trial, ifosfamide and doxorubicin were evaluated in 34 chemo-naïve women with advanced LMS, resulting in nine partial responses (27.3%) and one complete response (3.0%), for an overall response rate of 30.3%, which is a modest improvement over reported single agent activity. The duration of response was only 4.1 months, and the median overall survival was 9.6 months, increasing to 11.1 months for the responders (110). Toxicity was not insignificant with almost half of the patients experiencing grade 3 or 4 granulocytopenia and two treatment-related deaths.

A further GOG phase-II study investigated the combination of mitomycin, doxorubicin, and cisplatin (MAP). There was significant pulmonary toxicity due to the cumulative mitomycin dose and a response rate of 23% (111).

The gemcitabine and docetaxel combination was both surprisingly "toxic" and surprisingly effective. Despite G-CSF support there was significant hematological toxicity. In 34 patients there were three complete responses and 15 partial responses (53%). The median time to progression was 5.6 months (112). Confirmatory trials are required.

The role of combination therapy in this disease remains contentious. There are increased response rates seen but without direct comparison of efficacy and toxicity and with no quality of life data it is difficult to make firm recommendations.

Adjuvant Chemotherapy

The use of adjuvant chemotherapy following complete surgical resection in uterine sarcoma seems logical given that distant recurrence is common. Studies are limited and made difficult due to the different sensitivity of the histological subtypes and the rarity of the disease.

Currently there is no evidence from prospective studies supporting the use of adjuvant chemotherapy for early uterine sarcoma. Only one randomized controlled trial has been performed to date, in which 156 patients with stages I or II uterine sarcoma (all subtypes) received either doxorubicin $60 \, mg/m^2$, every three weeks for eight cycles, or no further treatment (113). Recurrence rates, PFI and overall survival were equivalent. Given that it is now apparent that doxorubicin only has activity in LMS and not carcinosarcoma, it is possible that a benefit may exist but further studies are required.

Other non-randomized trials have reported a trend towards improved survival for adjuvant chemotherapy (114,115); however, a recent large retrospective review of 208 uterine LMS patients did not demonstrate any association between adjuvant chemotherapy and improved survival (116). At the present time there is no role for the use of adjuvant chemotherapy in uterine sarcoma outside a clinical trial.

CONCLUSIONS

Uterine malignancies are a diverse group of tumors and have been poorly studied due to their relative rarity in the advanced setting. Chemotherapy has largely been employed palliatively where moderate response rates have only been reflected in small gains in progression-free survival. Thus careful evaluation of the patient against potential benefits and toxicities must be employed. The role of adjuvant chemotherapy for endometrial carcinoma and sarcoma remains investigational.

REFERENCES

1. Horton J, Begg CB, Arseneault J, Bruckner H, Creech R, Hahn RG. Comparison of adriamycin with cyclophosphamide in patients with advanced endometrial cancer. Cancer Treat Rep 1978; 62:159–161.
2. Thigpen JT, Buchsbaum HJ, Mangan C, Blessing JA. Phase II trial of adriamycin in the treatment of advanced or recurrent endometrial carcinoma: a Gynecologic Oncology Group study. Cancer Treat Rep 1979; 63:21–27.
3. Thigpen JT, Blessing JA, DiSaia PJ, Yordan E, Carson LF, Evers C. A randomized comparison of doxorubicin alone versus doxorubicin plus cyclophosphamide in the management of advanced or recurrent endometrial carcinoma: a Gynecologic Oncology Group study. J Clin Oncol 1994; 12:1408–1414.
4. Aapro MS, Van Wijk FH, Bolis G, et al. Doxorubicin versus doxorubicin and cisplatin in endometrial carcinoma: definitive results of a randomised study

(55872) by the EORTC Gynaecological Cancer Group. Ann Oncol 2003; 14:441–448.

5. Calero F, Asins-Codoner E, Jimeno J, et al. Epirubicin in advanced endometrial adenocarcinoma: a phase II study of the Grupo Ginecologico Espanol para el Tratamiento Oncologico (GGETO). Eur J Cancer 1991; 27:864–866.

6. Muggia FM, Blessing JA, Sorosky J, Reid GC. Phase II trial of the pegylated liposomal doxorubicin in previously treated metastatic endometrial cancer: a Gynecologic Oncology Group study. J Clin Oncol 2002; 20:2360–2364.

7. Thigpen JT, Blessing JA, Homesley H, Creasman WT, Sutton G. Phase II trial of cisplatin as first-line chemotherapy in patients with advanced or recurrent endometrial carcinoma: a Gynecologic Oncology Group Study. Gynecol'Oncol 1989; 33:68–70.

8. Thigpen JT, Blessing JA, Lagasse LD, DiSaia PJ, Homesley HD. Phase II trial of cisplatin as second-line chemotherapy in patients with advanced or recurrent endometrial carcinoma. A Gynecologic Oncology Group study. Am J Clin Oncol 1984; 7:253–256.

9. Trope C, Grundsell H, Johnsson JE, Cavallin-Stahl E. A phase II study of Cis-platinum for recurrent corpus cancer. Eur J Cancer 1980; 16:1025–1026.

10. Seski JC, Edwards CL, Herson J, Rutledge FN. Cisplatin chemotherapy for disseminated endometrial cancer. Obstet Gynecol 1982; 59:225–228.

11. Deppe G, Cohen CJ, Bruckner HW. Treatment of advanced endometrial adenocarcinoma with cis-dichlorodiammine platinum (II) after intensive prior therapy. Gynecol Oncol 1980; 10:51–54.

12. Edmonson JH, Krook JE, Hilton JF, Malkasian GD, Everson LK, Jefferies JA, Mailliard JA. Randomized phase II studies of cisplatin and a combination of cyclophosphamide-doxorubicin-cisplatin (CAP) in patients with progestin-refractory advanced endometrial carcinoma. Gynecol Oncol 1987; 28:20–24.

13. Long HJ, Pfeifle DM, Wieand HS, Krook JE, Edmonson JH, Buckner JC. Phase II evaluation of carboplatin in advanced endometrial carcinoma. J Natl Cancer Inst 1988; 80:276–278.

14. Green JB, Green S, Alberts DS, O'Toole R, Surwit EA, Noltimier JW. Carboplatin therapy in advanced endometrial cancer. Obstet Gynecol 1990; 75:696–700.

15. Burke TW, Munkarah A, Kavanagh JJ, et al. Treatment of advanced or recurrent endometrial carcinoma with single-agent carboplatin. Gynecol Oncol 1993; 51:397–400.

16. van Wijk FH, Lhomme C, Bolis G, et al. Phase II study of carboplatin in patients with advanced or recurrent endometrial carcinoma. A trial of the EORTC Gynaecological Cancer Group. Eur J Cancer 2003; 39:78–85.

17. Ball HG, Blessing JA, Lentz SS, Mutch DG. A phase II trial of paclitaxel in patients with advanced or recurrent adenocarcinoma of the endometrium: a Gynecologic Oncology Group study. Gynecol Oncol 1996; 62:278–281.

18. Lissoni A, Zanetta G, Losa G, Gabriele A, Parma G, Mangioni C. Phase II study of paclitaxel as salvage treatment in advanced endometrial cancer. Ann Oncol 1996; 7:861–863.

19. Lincoln S, Blessing JA, Lee RB, Rocereto TF. Activity of paclitaxel as second-line chemotherapy in endometrial carcinoma: a Gynecologic Oncology Group study. Gynecol Oncol 2003; 88:277–281.

20. Woo HL, Swenerton KD, Hoskins PJ. Taxol is active in platinum-resistant endometrial adenocarcinoma. Am J Clin Oncol 1996; 19:290–291.
21. Pawinski A, Tumolo S, Hoesel G, et al. Cyclophosphamide or ifosfamide in patients with advanced and/or recurrent endometrial carcinoma: a randomized phase II study of the EORTC Gynecological Cancer Cooperative Group. Eur J Obstet Gynecol Reprod Biol 1999; 86:179–183.
22. Poplin EA, Liu PY, Delmore JE, et al. Phase II trial of oral etoposide in recurrent or refractory endometrial adenocarcinoma: a southwest oncology group study. Gynecol Oncol 1999; 74:432–435.
23. Miller DS, Blessing JA, Lentz SS, Waggoner SE. A phase II trial of topotecan in patients with advanced, persistent, or recurrent endometrial carcinoma: a gynecologic oncology group study. Gynecol Oncol 2002; 87:247–251.
24. Wadler S, Levy DE, Lincoln ST, Soori GS, Schink JC, Goldberg G. Topotecan is an active agent in the first-line treatment of metastatic or recurrent endometrial carcinoma: Eastern Cooperative Oncology Group Study E3E93. J Clin Oncol 2003; 21:2110–2114.
25. Nakamura T, Onishi Y, Yamamoto F, Kouno S, Maeda Y, Hatae M. Evaluation of paclitaxel and carboplatin in patients with endometrial cancer. Gan To Kagaku Ryoho 2000; 27:257–262.
26. Hoskins PJ, Swenerton KD, Pike JA, et al. Paclitaxel and carboplatin, alone or with irradiation, in advanced or recurrent endometrial cancer: a phase II study. J Clin Oncol 2001; 19:4048–4053.
27. Price FV, Edwards RP, Kelley JL, Kunschner AJ, Hart LA. A trial of outpatient paclitaxel and carboplatin for advanced, recurrent, and histologic high-risk endometrial carcinoma: preliminary report. Semin Oncol 1997; 24: S15-78–S15-82.
28. Dimopoulos MA, Papadimitriou CA, Georgoulias V, Moulopoulos LA, Aravantinos G, Gika D, Karpathios S, Stamatelopoulos S. Paclitaxel and cisplatin in advanced or recurrent carcinoma of the endometrium: long-term results of a phase II multicenter study. Gynecol Oncol 2000; 78:52–57.
29. Lissoni A, Gabriele A, Gorga G, et al. Cisplatin-, epirubicin- and paclitaxel-containing chemotherapy in uterine adenocarcinoma. Ann Oncol 1997; 8: 969–972.
30. Turbow MM, Ballon SC, Sikic BI, Koretz MM. Cisplatin, doxorubicin, and cyclophosphamide chemotherapy for advanced endometrial carcinoma. Cancer Treat Rep 1985; 69:465–467.
31. Hancock KC, Freedman RS, Edwards CL, Rutledge FN. Use of cisplatin, doxorubicin, and cyclophosphamide to treat advanced and recurrent adenocarcinoma of the endometrium. Cancer Treat Rep 1986; 70:789–791.
32. De Oliveira CF, van der Burg ME, Osorio ME, et al. Chemotherapy of advanced endometrial cancer with cyclophosphamide, adriamycin and cisplatin (CAP). First Meeting of the International Gynecologic Cancer Society 1987:40.
33. Burke TW, Stringer CA, Morris M, et al. Prospective treatment of advanced or recurrent endometrial carcinoma with cisplatin, doxorubicin, and cyclophosphamide. Gynecol Oncol 1991; 40:264–267.

34. Seltzer V, Vogl SE, Kaplan BH. Adriamycin and cis-diamminedichloroplatinum in the treatment of metastatic endometrial adenocarcinoma. Gynecol Oncol 1984; 19:308–313.
35. Trope C, Johnsson JE, Simonsen E, Christiansen H, Cavallin-Stahl E, Horvath G. Treatment of recurrent endometrial adenocarcinoma with a combination of doxorubicin and cisplatin. Am J Obstet Gynecol 1984; 149: 379–381.
36. Pasmantier MW, Coleman M, Silver RT, Mamaril AP, Quiguyan CC, Galindo A Jr. Treatment of advanced endometrial carcinoma with doxorubicin and cisplatin: effects on both untreated and previously treated patients. Cancer Treat Rep 1985; 69:539–542.
37. Barrett RJ, Blessing JA, Homesley HD, Twiggs L, Webster KD. Circadian-timed combination doxorubicin-cisplatin chemotherapy for advanced endometrial carcinoma. A phase II study of the Gynecologic Oncology Group. Am J Clin Oncol 1993; 16:494–496.
38. Muggia FM, Chia G, Reed LJ, Romney SL. Doxorubicin-cyclophosphamide: effective chemotherapy for advanced endometrial adenocarcinoma. Am J Obstet Gynecol 1977; 128:314–319.
39. Seski JC, Edwards CL, Gershenson DM, Copeland LJ. Doxorubicin and cyclophosphamide chemotherapy for disseminated endometrial cancer. Obstet Gynecol 1981; 58:88–91.
40. Campora E, Vidali A, Mammoliti S, Ragni N, Conte PF. Treatment of advanced or recurrent adenocarcinoma of the endometrium with doxorubicin and cyclophosphamide. Eur J Gynaecol Oncol 1990; 11:181–183.
41. Scudder SA, Liu PY, Smith HO, Wilczynski S, Hannigan EV, Alberts DS. Paclitaxel and carboplatin with amifostine in advanced or recurrent endometrial cancer: a Southwest Oncology Group Trial (S9720). Proc Am Soc Clin Oncol 2001; 20 [abst 819].
42. Pierga JY, Dieras V, Beuzeboc P, et al. Phase II trial of doxorubicin, 5-fluorouracil, etoposide, and cisplatin in advanced or recurrent endometrial carcinoma. Gynecol Oncol 1997; 66:246–249.
43. Pierga JY, Dieras V, Paraiso D, et al. Treatment of advanced or recurrent endometrial carcinoma with combination of etoposide, cisplatin, and 5-fluorouracil: a phase II study. Gynecol Oncol 1996; 60:59–63.
44. Santoro A, Maiorino L, Santoro M, Forestieri V, Forestieri P. Carboplatin and vinorelbine combination for treatment of advanced endometrial carcinoma. Proc Am Soc Clin Oncol 1998; 17 [abst 1444].
45. Sorbe B, Wolmesjo E, Frankendal B. VM-26-vincristine-cisplatin combination chemotherapy in the treatment of primary advanced and recurrent endometrial carcinoma. Obstet Gynecol 1989; 73:343–348.
46. Long HJ III, Langdon RM Jr, Cha SS, et al. Phase II trial of methotrexate, vinblastine, doxorubicin, and cisplatin in advanced/recurrent endometrial carcinoma. Gynecol Oncol 1995; 58:240–243.
47. Kauppila A, Friberg LG. Hormonal and cytotoxic chemotherapy for endometrial carcinoma. Steroid receptors in the selection of appropriate therapy. Acta Obstet Gynecol Scand Suppl 1981; 101:59–64.

48. Alberts DS, Mason NL, O'Toole RV, et al. Doxorubicin-cisplatin-vinblastine combination chemotherapy of advanced endometrial carcinoma: a Southwest Oncology Group Study. Gynecol Oncol 1987; 26:193–201.

49. Thigpen JT, Brady MF, Homesley HD, et al. Phase III trial of doxorubicin with or without cisplatin in advanced endometrial carcinoma: a gynecologic oncology group study. J Clin Oncol 2004; 22:3902–3908.

50. Gallion HH, Brunetto VL, Cibull M, et al. Randomized phase III trial of standard timed doxorubicin plus cisplatin versus circadian timed doxorubicin plus cisplatin in stages III and IV or recurrent endometrial carcinoma: a Gynecologic Oncology Group Study. J Clin Oncol 2003; 21:3808–3813.

51. Weber B, Mayer F, Bougnoux P, et al. What is the best chemotherapy regimen in recurrent or advanced endometrial carcinoma? Preliminary results. Proc Am Soc Clinl Oncol 2003; 22 [abst 1819].

52. Fleming GF, Brunetto VL, Bentley R, et al. Randomized trial of doxorubicin (dox) plus cisplatin (cis) versus dox plus paclitaxel (tax) plus granulocyte colony-stimulating factor (G-CSF) in patients with advanced or recurrent endometrial cancer: a report on Gynecologic Oncology Group (GOG) protocol #163. Proc Am Soc Clin Oncol 2000; 19 [abst 1498].

53. Fleming GF, Brunetto VL, Mundt AJ, Burks RT, Look K, Reid G. Randomized trial of doxorubicin plus cisplatin versus doxorubicin plus cisplatin plus paclitaxel in patients with advanced or recurrent endometrial carcinoma: a Gynaecologic Oncology Group (GOG) study. Proc Am Soc Clin Oncol 2002; 21 [abst 807].

54. Horton J, Elson P, Gordon P, Hahn R, Creech R. Combination chemotherapy for advanced endometrial cancer. An evaluation of three regimens. Cancer 1982; 49:2441–2445.

55. Ayoub J, Audet-Lapointe P, Methot Y, et al. Efficacy of sequential cyclical hormonal therapy in endometrial cancer and its correlation with steroid hormone receptor status. Gynecol Oncol 1988; 31:327–337.

56. Cohen CJ, Bruckner HW, Deppe G, et al. Multidrug treatment of advanced and recurrent endometrial carcinoma: a Gynecologic Oncology Group study. Obstet Gynecol 1984; 63: 719–726.

57. Bruckner HW, Deppe G. Combination chemotherapy of advanced endometrial adenocarcinoma with adriamycin, cyclophosphamide, 5-fluorouracil, and medroxyprogesterone acetate. Obstet Gynecol 1977; 50:10S–12S.

58. Piver MS, Lele SB, Patsner B, Emrich LJ. Melphalan, 5-fluorouracil, and medroxyprogesterone acetate in metastatic endometrial carcinoma. Obstet Gynecol 1986; 67:261–264.

59. Cornelison TL, Baker TR, Piver MS, Driscoll DL. Cisplatin, adriamycin, etoposide, megestrol acetate versus melphalan, 5-fluorouracil, medroxyprogesterone acetate in the treatment of endometrial carcinoma. Gynecol Oncol 1995; 59:243–248.

60. Bafaloukos D, Aravantinos G, Samonis G, et al. Carboplatin, methotrexate and 5-fluorouracil in combination with medroxyprogesterone acetate (JMF-M) in the treatment of advanced or recurrent endometrial carcinoma: a Hellenic cooperative oncology group study. Oncology 1999; 56:198–201.

61. Deppe G, Jacobs AJ, Bruckner H, Cohen CJ. Chemotherapy of advanced and recurrent endometrial carcinoma with cyclophosphamide, doxorubicin, 5-fluorouracil, and megestrol acetate. Am J Obstet Gynecol 1981; 140:313–316.

62. Hoffman MS, Roberts WS, Cavanagh D, Praphat H, Solomon P, Lyman GH. Treatment of recurrent and metastatic endometrial cancer with cisplatin, doxorubicin, cyclophosphamide, and megestrol acetate. Gynecol Oncol 1989; 35:75–77.

63. Lovecchio JL, Averette HE, Lichtinger M, Townsend PA, Girtanner RW, Fenton AN. Treatment of advanced or recurrent endometrial adenocarcinoma with cyclophosphamide, doxorubicin, cis-Platinum, and megestrol acetate. Obstet Gynecol 1984; 63:557–560.

64. Randall ME, Brunetto G, Muss HB, et al. Whole abdominal radiotherapy versus combination doxorubicin-cisplatin chemotherapy in advanced endometrial carcinoma: a randomized phase III trial of the Gynaecologic Oncology Group. Proc Am Soc Clin Oncol 2003; 22 [abst 3].

65. Watkins-Bruner D, Barsevick A, Tian C, et al. Quality of life trade-off to incremental gain in survival on Gynaecologic Oncology Group (GOG) protocol 122: whole abdominal irradiation (WAI) vs. doxorubicin-platinum chemotherapy in advanced endometrial cancer. Proc Am Soc Clin Oncol 2003; 22 [abst 1803].

66. Morrow CP, Bundy BN, Kurman RJ, et al. Relationship between surgical-pathological risk factors and outcome in clinical stages I and II carcinoma of the endometrium: a Gynecologic Oncology Group study. Gynecol Oncol 1991; 40:55–65.

67. Morrow CP, Bundy BN, Homesley HD, et al. Doxorubicin as an adjuvant following surgery and radiation therapy in patients with high-risk endometrial carcinoma, stage I and occult stage II: a Gynecologic Oncology Group Study. Gynecol Oncol 1990; 36:166–171.

68. Smith MR, Peters WA III, Drescher CW. Cisplatin, doxorubicin hydrochloride, and cyclophosphamide followed by radiotherapy in high-risk endometrial carcinoma. Am J Obstet Gynecol 1994; 170:1677–1681; discussion 1681–1682.

69. O'Brien ME, Killackey M. Adjuvant therapy in "high risk" endometrial adenocarcinoma. Proc Am Soc Clin Oncol 1994; 13:249 [abst 781].

70. Jennings S, Dottino P, Johnston C, Cohen C. Adjuvant cisplatin, doxorubicin and etoposide and pelvic radiotherapy for advanced stage or virulent histologic subtypes of endometrial cancer. Proc Am Soc Clin Oncol 1993; 12:268 [abst 858].

71. Burke TW, Gershenson DM, Morris M, et al. Postoperative adjuvant cisplatin, doxorubicin, and cyclophosphamide (PAC) chemotherapy in women with high-risk endometrial carcinoma. Gynecol Oncol 1994; 55:47–50.

72. Aalders J, Abeler V, Kolstad P, Onsrud M. Postoperative external irradiation and prognostic parameters in stage I endometrial carcinoma: clinical and histopathologic study of 540 patients. Obstet Gynecol 1980; 56:419–427.

73. Irwin C, Levin W, Fyles A, Pintilie M, Manchul L, Kirkbride P. The role of adjuvant radiotherapy in carcinoma of the endometrium-results in 550 patients with pathologic stage I disease. Gynecol Oncol 1998; 70:247–254.

74. Vergote I, Kjorstad K, Abeler V, Kolstad P. A randomized trial of adjuvant progestagen in early endometrial cancer. Cancer 1989; 64:1011–1016.
75. Martin-Hirsch PL, Jarvis G, Kitchener H, Lilford R. Progestagens for endometrial cancer. The Cochrane Database of Systematic Reviews 1999; 4, Art No. CD001040.
76. Martin-Hirsch PL, Lilford RJ, Jarvis GJ. Adjuvant progestagen therapy for the treatment of endometrial cancer: review and meta-analyses of published randomised controlled trials. Eur J Obstet Gynecol Reprod Biol 1996; 65: 201–207.
77. Hendrickson M, Ross J, Eifel P, Martinez A, Kempson R. Uterine papillary serous carcinoma: a highly malignant form of endometrial adenocarcinoma. Am J Surg Pathol 1982; 6:93–108.
78. Kato DT, Ferry JA, Goodman A, et al. Uterine papillary serous carcinoma (UPSC): a clinicopathologic study of 30 cases. Gynecol Oncol 1995; 59:384–389.
79. Nicklin JL, Copeland LJ. Endometrial papillary serous carcinoma: patterns of spread and treatment. Clin Obstet Gynecol 1996; 39:686–695.
80. Rosenberg P, Blom R, Hogberg T, Simonsen E. Death rate and recurrence pattern among 841 clinical stage I endometrial cancer patients with special reference to uterine papillary serous carcinoma. Gynecol Oncol 1993; 51: 311–315.
81. Carcangiu ML, Chambers JT. Early pathologic stage clear cell carcinoma and uterine papillary serous carcinoma of the endometrium: comparison of clinico-pathologic features and survival. Int J Gynecol Pathol 1995; 14:30–38.
82. Levenback C, Burke TW, Silva E, et al. Uterine papillary serous carcinoma (UPSC) treated with cisplatin, doxorubicin, and cyclophosphamide (PAC). Gynecol Oncol 1992; 46: 317–321.
83. Price FV, Chambers SK, Carcangiu ML, Kohorn EI, Schwartz PE, Chambers JT. Intravenous cisplatin, doxorubicin, and cyclophosphamide in the treatment of uterine papillary serous carcinoma (UPSC). Gynecol Oncol 1993; 51: 383–389.
84. Zanotti KM, Belinson JL, Kennedy AW, Webster KD, Markman M. The use of paclitaxel and platinum-based chemotherapy in uterine papillary serous carcinoma. Gynecol Oncol 1999; 74:272–277.
85. Ramondetta L, Burke TW, Levenback C, Bevers M, Bodurka-Bevers D, Gershenson DM. Treatment of uterine papillary serous carcinoma with paclitaxel. Gynecol Oncol 2001; 82:156–161.
86. Bancher-Todesca D, Neunteufel W, Williams KE, et al. Influence of post-operative treatment on survival in patients with uterine papillary serous carcinoma. Gynecol Oncol 1998; 71:344–347.
87. Craighead PS, Sait K, Stuart GC, et al. Management of aggressive histologic variants of endometrial carcinoma at the Tom Baker Cancer Centre between 1984 and 1994. Gynecol Oncol 2000; 77:248–253.
88. Steed HL, Manchul L, Fyles A, et al. Treatment of Uterine Papillary Serous Carcinoma with Radiotherapy and Chemotherapy. Proc Am Soc Clin Oncol 2003; 22 [abst 1822].

89. Nordal RR, Thoresen SO. Uterine sarcomas in Norway 1956–1992: incidence, survival and mortality. Eur J Cancer 1997; 33:907–911.
90. Harlow BL, Weiss NS, Lofton S. The epidemiology of sarcomas of the uterus. J Natl Cancer Inst 1986; 76:399–402.
91. Gadducci A, Sartori E, Landoni F, et al. The prognostic relevance of histological type in uterine sarcomas: a Cooperation Task Force (CTF) multivariate analysis of 249 cases. Eur J Gynaecol Oncol 2002; 23:295–299.
92. Olah KS, Dunn JA, Gee H. Leiomyosarcomas have a poorer prognosis than mixed mesodermal tumours when adjusting for known prognostic factors: the result of a retrospective study of 423 cases of uterine sarcoma. Br J Obstet Gynaecol 1992; 99:590–594.
93. Sutton GP, Blessing JA, Rosenshein N, Photopulos G, DiSaia PJ. Phase II trial of ifosfamide and mesna in mixed mesodermal tumors of the uterus (a Gynecologic Oncology Group study). Am J Obstet Gynecol 1989; 161: 309–312.
94. Sutton G, Brunetto VL, Kilgore L, et al. A phase III trial of ifosfamide with or without cisplatin in carcinosarcoma of the uterus: a Gynecologic Oncology Group Study. Gynecol Oncol 2000; 79:147–153.
95. Thigpen JT, Blessing JA, Orr JW Jr, DiSaia PJ. Phase II trial of cisplatin in the treatment of patients with advanced or recurrent mixed mesodermal sarcomas of the uterus: a Gynecologic Oncology Group Study. Cancer Treat Rep 1986; 70:271–274.
96. Thigpen JT, Blessing JA, Beecham J, Homesley H, Yordan E. Phase II trial of cisplatin as first-line chemotherapy in patients with advanced or recurrent uterine sarcomas: a Gynecologic Oncology Group study. J Clin Oncol 1991; 9:1962–1966.
97. Gershenson DM, Kavanagh JJ, Copeland LJ, Edwards CL, Stringer CA, Wharton JT. Cisplatin therapy for disseminated mixed mesodermal sarcoma of the uterus. J Clin Oncol 1987; 5:618–621.
98. Curtin JP, Blessing JA, Soper JT, DeGeest K. Paclitaxel in the treatment of carcinosarcoma of the uterus: a gynecologic oncology group study. Gynecol Oncol 2001; 83:268–270.
99. Gershenson DM, Kavanagh JJ, Copeland LJ, Edwards CL, Freedman RS, Wharton JT. High-dose doxorubicin infusion therapy for disseminated mixed mesodermal sarcoma of the uterus. Cancer 1987; 59:1264–1267.
100. Omura GA, Major FJ, Blessing JA, et al. A randomized study of adriamycin with and without dimethyl triazenoimidazole carboxamide in advanced uterine sarcomas. Cancer 1983; 52:626–632.
101. Muss HB, Bundy B, DiSaia PJ, et al. Treatment of recurrent or advanced uterine sarcoma. A randomized trial of doxorubicin versus doxorubicin and cyclophosphamide (a phase III trial of the Gynecologic Oncology Group). Cancer 1985; 55:1648–1653.
102. Pautier P, Genestie C, Fizazi K, et al. Cisplatin-based chemotherapy regimen (DECAV) for uterine sarcomas. Int J Gynecol Cancer 2002; 12:749–754.
103. Sutton GP, Blessing JA, Barrett RJ, McGehee R. Phase II trial of ifosfamide and mesna in leiomyosarcoma of the uterus: a Gynecologic Oncology Group study. Am J Obstet Gynecol 1992; 166:556–559.

104. Curtin JP, Silverberg SJ, Thigpen JT, Spanos WJ. Corpus: mesenchymal tumors. In: In: Hoskins WJ, Perez CA, Young RC, eds. Principles and Practice of Gynecologic Oncology. Philadelphia: Lippincott-Raven, 1997: 897–918.
105. Sutton G, Blessing JA, Ball H. Phase II trial of paclitaxel in leiomyosarcoma of the uterus: a gynecologic oncology group study. Gynecol Oncol 1999; 74:346–349.
106. Gallup DG, Blessing JA, Andersen W, Morgan MA. Evaluation of paclitaxel in previously treated leiomyosarcoma of the uterus: a gynecologic oncology group study. Gynecol Oncol 2003; 89:48–51.
107. Miller DS, Blessing JA, Kilgore LC, Mannel R, Van Le L. Phase II trial of topotecan in patients with advanced, persistent, or recurrent uterine leiomyosarcomas: a Gynecologic Oncology Group Study. Am J Clin Oncol 2000; 23:355–357.
108. Svancarova L, Blay JY, Judson IR, et al. Gemcitabine in advanced adult soft-tissue sarcomas. A phase II study of the EORTC Soft Tissue and Bone Sarcoma Group. Eur J Cancer 2002; 38:556–559.
109. Okuno S, Edmonson J, Mahoney M, Buckner JC, Frytak S, Galanis E. Phase II trial of gemcitabine in advanced sarcomas. Cancer 2002; 94:3225–3229.
110. Sutton G, Blessing JA, Malfetano JH. Ifosfamide and doxorubicin in the treatment of advanced leiomyosarcomas of the uterus: a Gynecologic Oncology Group study. Gynecol Oncol 1996; 62:226–229.
111. Edmonson JH, Blessing JA, Cosin JA, Miller DS, Cohn DE, Rotmensch J. Phase II study of mitomycin, doxorubicin, and cisplatin in the treatment of advanced uterine leiomyosarcoma: a Gynecologic Oncology Group study. Gynecol Oncol 2002; 85:507–510.
112. Hensley ML, Maki R, Venkatraman E, et al. Gemcitabine and docetaxel in patients with unresectable leiomyosarcoma: results of a phase II trial. J Clin Oncol 2002; 20:2824–2831.
113. Omura GA, Blessing JA, Major F, et al. A randomized clinical trial of adjuvant adriamycin in uterine sarcomas: a Gynecologic Oncology Group Study. J Clin Oncol 1985; 3:1240–1245.
114. Peters WA III, Rivkin SE, Smith MR, Tesh DE. Cisplatin and adriamycin combination chemotherapy for uterine stromal sarcomas and mixed mesodermal tumors. Gynecol Oncol 1989; 34:323–327.
115. Piver MS, Lele SB, Marchetti DL, Emrich LJ. Effect of adjuvant chemotherapy on time to recurrence and survival of stage I uterine sarcomas. J Surg Oncol 1988; 38:233–239.
116. Giuntoli RL II, Metzinger DS, DiMarco CS, et al. Retrospective review of 208 patients with leiomyosarcoma of the uterus: prognostic indicators, surgical management, and adjuvant therapy. Gynecol Oncol 2003; 89:460–469.
117. Sutton GP, Blessing JA, Homesley HD, McGuire WP, Adcock L. Phase II study of ifosfamide and mesna in refractory adenocarcinoma of the endometrium. A Gynecologic Oncology Group study. Cancer 1994; 73:1453–1455.
118. Sutton GP, Blessing JA, DeMars LR, Moore D, Burke TW, Grendys EC. A phase II Gynecologic Oncology Group trial of ifosfamide and mesna in advanced or recurrent adenocarcinoma of the endometrium. Gynecol Oncol 1996; 63:25–27.

119. Carbone PP, Carter SK. Endometrial cancer: approach to development of effective chemotherapy. Gynecol Oncol 1974; 2:348–353.
120. Thigpen T, Blessing JA, Yordan E, Valea F, Vaccarello L. Phase II trial of etoposide in leiomyosarcoma of the uterus: a Gynecologic Oncology Group study. Gynecol Oncol 1996; 63:120–122.

11

Minimal Access Surgery in Endometrial Cancer

Robbert Soeters and Lynette Denny
*Department of Obstetrics and Gynaecology, Groote Schuur Hospital,
Cape Town, South Africa*

INTRODUCTION

Minimal access surgery has in the last 20 years developed into a subspecialty with applications in all aspects of gynecological surgery. The main applications of minimal access surgery in gynecology are hysteroscopy and laparoscopy. The application of hysteroscopy has been dealt with elsewhere. In this chapter the laparoscopic approach in patients with early endometrial cancer will be discussed.

Laparoscopy has come a long way from the days that it was only considered a diagnostic tool. Operative laparoscopy, which took off in the 1980s had, apart from laparoscopic sterilization, its main application in organ sparing surgery such as the treatment of ovarian cysts and the dissection of adhesions and became the accepted form of surgical treatment for endometriosis.

The publication of the first laparoscopic hysterectomy by Reich in 1989 signaled a new era of gynecological operative laparoscopy. In this publication the authors described a rather complicated technique where the hysterectomy is performed completely laparoscopically (1). The introduction and development of laparoscopic assisted vaginal hysterectomy (LAVH) and bilateral salpingo-oophorectomy brought this form of surgery, after adequate training, well within the reach of general gynecologists.

THE ROLE OF VAGINAL HYSTERECTOMY IN THE MANAGEMENT OF ENDOMETRIAL CANCER

Prior to the development of a laparoscopic approach to the management of endometrial carcinoma, a number of studies showed that there is a place for vaginal hysterectomy in the treatment of endometrial carcinoma (2–4). Lelle et al. published their results of vaginal hysterectomy in 60 patients with early endometrial cancer who were not considered candidates for the conventional abdominal approach (4). The operative mortality was 0% and the complication rate was 14%. The crude 5- and 10-year survival rates were 91.1% and 87.1%, respectively. Although the authors stated that an abdominal approach remained the standard of care in patients with early stage endometrial cancer, they also concluded that there is a definite place for vaginal hysterectomy in patients with good prognostic criteria who are at high-operative risk. There are, however, problems associated with the vaginal approach as a treatment modality for patients with endometrial cancer. For example, in this study, only 12% of patients had a bilateral salpingo-oophorectomy and in 7% of the cases morcellation was necessary to remove the uterus. Morcellation, however, did not seem to have a detrimental effect on prognosis as all four patients who had this operative complication survived (4).

A major disadvantage of a vaginal approach is the inability to carry out a thorough inspection of the abdominal cavity for unsuspected metastases. A laparoscopic approach would facilitate adequate surgical staging without compromising the prognosis. Moreover, using this technique, a bilateral salpingo-oophorectomy can be safely carried out and the risk of morcellation can be avoided.

LAPAROSCOPIC-ASSISTED VAGINAL HYSTERECTOMY (LAVH)

A number of early reports have described series of patients with benign disease who underwent LAVH (5–7). These and later publications demonstrated all the advantages of the abdominal approach for hysterectomy such as full inspection of the abdominal cavity and dissection of adhesions in combination with the advantages of a vaginal approach to hysterectomy. These latter advantages include decreased morbidity, blood loss, postoperative discomfort, pain, length of hospitalization, and speedier recovery from surgery. The extent of the laparoscopic part and the subsequent vaginal part during the LAVH may, however, differ from surgeon to surgeon. The laparoscopic part may vary from a diagnostic laparoscopy to a laparoscopic freeing of the entire uterus. Johns and Diamond addressed this aspect of a laparoscopic approach during hysterectomy and felt that reports should include the extent of the laparoscopic portion of the operation (8).

LAPAROSCOPIC LYMPHADENECTOMY

The development of laparoscopic pelvic and para-aortic lymphadenectomy has been a further logical step in the application of laparoscopy for patients with early endometrial cancer. Publications by Querleu in 1991 and by Childers in 1992 and 1993 (9–11) described the technique of laparoscopic pelvic and para-aortic lymphadenectomy.

APPLICATION OF LAVH AND LYMPHADENECTOMY FOR ENDOMETRIAL CANCER

The description by Childers and Surwitt of two cases of combined laparoscopic and vaginal surgery for the management of two cases of stage I endometrial cancer was the first of many in the treatment by minimal access surgery for such patients (12). The same group subsequently published the first substantial series of 53 patients with stage I endometrial cancer who underwent laparoscopic assisted surgical staging (13). Initially, 59 patients with stage I endometrial cancer were considered candidates for this procedure. Significantly, six patients were found to have intraperitoneal disease and were taken out of the study. The remaining 53 patients all had an LAVH. Twenty-nine patients had pelvic and para-aortic lymphadenectomy according to protocol guidelines, i.e., >50% myometrial invasion and/or tumor grade 2 or 3. In two patients lymphadenectomy could not be carried out due to obesity. One significant complication (ureteric injury) in this series was encountered. Another complication was a cystotomy, which resulted in a laparotomy and total abdominal hysterectomy, bilateral salpingo-oophorectomy (BSO), and repair of the bladder defect (13).

Since this publication, many more patients with early stage endometrial cancer have been reported to have undergone a laparoscopic approach. Clearly, as with all novel surgical procedures, the laparoscopic approach is subject to a learning curve. Eltabbakh reported on 75 consecutive patients with clinical stage I endometrial cancer ($n = 72$) and uterine sarcoma ($n = 3$) (14). All patients underwent LAVH, BSO, and pelvic lymph node sampling. These patients were divided into three equal groups ($n = 25$) based on date of surgery. Patient characteristics such as age, body mass index (BMI), number of previous laparotomies, and extent of adhesions were similar among the three study groups. Para-aortic lymph node sampling ($n = 16$; five in group 1, five in group 2, and six in group 3) was also evenly distributed among the three groups. The author operated on all patients. The study demonstrated that, with experience, the operative time decreased significantly (231.8 minutes for group 1 vs. 167.7 minutes for group 3; $p < 0.001$). Furthermore, the number of pelvic lymph nodes which were harvested increased as a function of the learning curve (7.8 for group 1 vs. 11.9 for group 3; $p < 0.05$) (14).

COMPLICATIONS OF LAPAROSCOPY

Although the complication rate of laparoscopy has been reported to be lower than that of an open procedure, a few complications can be directly attributed to laparoscopy. These include injuries to small and large bowel and the ureter. These injuries may go unnoticed during the procedure, thereby further aggravating the seriousness of the complication. Postoperative pain is a significant indication of possible intra-abdominal trauma and bowel injury should be excluded.

Injury to the great vessels during insertion of either the Verres needle or the trochar is a potentially life threatening complication and requires an emergency laparotomy. Scribner et al. described a patient who required laparotomy after she developed bowel herniation through a 12 mm trochar incision. This patient subsequently developed a pulmonary embolism and died. Another patient in the same series died after vascular injury due to trochar insertion (15).

Not all laparoscopic procedures as treatment for patients with endometrial cancer are completed, as some require conversion from laparoscopy to laparotomy. The published conversion rate varies from 6% to 7%, but has been reported to be as high as 12.5% and is mainly due to gross obesity, uncontrollable bleeding, and unexpected intraperitoneal cancer (15–17).

A worrying aspect of laparoscopic surgery in patients with endometrial carcinoma is that the procedure may increase tumor spread. Sonada et al. found a high incidence of positive peritoneal cytology in patients with early stage endometrial cancer who underwent laparoscopy (18). Vergote et al. suggested that this might be attributed to the use of an intrauterine manipulator during the procedure (19). These authors have used Pozzi forceps on the cervix to manipulate the uterus and found no increase of positive peritoneal cytology compared to patients who underwent total abdominal hysterectomy (TAH) (19). Chu et al. described three cases with early endometrial cancer who developed vaginal cuff recurrence within nine months after LAVH. The authors suggested that the use of an intrauterine manipulator might cause this phenomenon (20). Other authors, however, found similar rates of vaginal recurrences for patients treated with LAVH and TAH (17–22).

Finally, in a recent publication, Muntz et al. reported a large port-site recurrence in a patient who had LAVH–BSO and lymphadenectomy for a stage IA grade 2 endometrial cancer (23). It has been suggested that implantation of tumor cells takes place in the port site during the procedure where CO_2 is used to insufflate the abdomen (23,24). Another possible source for port-site metastases may be tumor contamination of laparoscopic instruments.

CLINICAL OUTCOME OF LAPAROSCOPIC VERSUS OPEN ABDOMINAL SURGICAL APPROACH TO MANAGEMENT OF ENDOMETRIAL CANCER

Few retrospective studies have compared the clinical outcome of patients who had laparoscopy with those who underwent laparotomy. Gemignani et al. described 69 patients who had an LAVH and compared these with 251 historical patients who were treated using the abdominal approach. Progression-free survival for both groups was similar. Underlining the disadvantages of a retrospective review, it appeared that the mean weight in the LAVH group (71.3 kg) was significantly lower than that of the laparotomy group (81.9 kg). Furthermore, only 16% in the laparoscopy group had lymph node sampling as opposed to 45% in the TAH group. There was, however, no significant difference in the mean lymph node yield obtained by both methods ($p = 0.29$) (22).

Malur et al. published the only prospective study comparing survival data of LAVH and the abdominal approach (25). Seventy patients with stages I–III endometrial cancer were prospectively randomized to either a laparoscopic-vaginal or an abdominal approach. Pelvic and para-aortic lymph node sampling was evenly distributed between the two groups. Although the number of patients entered into the study was relatively small, it appeared that progression-free survival and overall survival of the two groups were very similar, suggesting the validity of the laparoscopic approach for patients with endometrial cancer (25).

The Gynecologic Oncology Group is currently performing a randomized prospective trial comparing laparoscopy to laparotomy in staging of patients with early endometrial cancer (LAP2). Such a trial, with enough patient numbers, should give valid answers without the limitations of a retrospective study.

COST BENEFIT OF LAPAROSCOPIC SURGERY

Costing of a relative new procedure, like laparoscopic surgery, is of utmost importance. Published data are, however, conflicting. Eltabbakh et al. found that the total costs of laparoscopy (LAVH) were significantly higher than that of laparotomy (TAH–BSO), but it should be noted that the laparoscopy patients were compared to historical controls (TAH–BSO) (16). Conversely, Scribner et al. found that the overall costs of laparoscopy were similar to that of laparotomy, while Gemignani et al. found that the overall mean total charges to be significantly less compared to that of laparotomy (22,26). In all publications discussing cost benefits it appears that the theater cost for laparoscopy is higher compared to those of patients undergoing laparotomy. These differences are, however, offset by less hospital in-patient costs for patients who underwent laparoscopy. Furthermore, it appears that economic related costs like return to full activity and return to work are significantly less for the patients who undergo laparoscopy compared to those who undergo laparotomy (16,22,26).

CONTRAINDICATIONS TO LAPAROSCOPIC SURGERY FOR TREATMENT OF ENDOMETRIAL CANCER

A number of absolute and relative contraindications should be taken into consideration before one embarks on an LAVH in a patient with endometrial carcinoma. Absolute contraindications include:

- advanced endometrial carcinoma or suspected concomitant adnexal pathology,
- previous pelvic or abdominal radiation,
- an enlarged uterus (>12 weeks),
- severe cardiopulmonary symptoms precluding Trendelenberg position, and
- severe hip disease precluding lithotomy position.

Relative contraindications include:

- endometriosis resulting in severe adhesions,
- minimal uterine mobility and/or limited vaginal access,
- severe adhesions as a result of previous abdominal surgery or pelvic inflammatory disease, and
- gross obesity.

A number of relative contraindications may be dealt with during the laparoscopy in such a manner that the LAVH is made possible.

With the use of laparoscopic techniques in gynecological oncology it is important to bear in mind that the same principles of an open approach apply.

These principles include indications and an intimate knowledge of surgical anatomy.

SETTING UP FOR LAPAROSCOPIC SURGERY

Before the procedure, the patient should be counseled as to the extent and possible complications of the operation. The patient should be made aware that there might be anesthetic complications. General surgical complications such as bleeding, infections, and trauma to adjacent organs should be discussed. Above all, the possibility of a conversion from a laparoscopic to an open procedure in case of unexpected complication should be emphasized. Omission of preoperative counseling may have far reaching legal consequences, if a complication for which the patient has not been counseled is encountered. In general, patients undergoing operative laparoscopy should have a bowel preparation one day prior to surgery. The risk of bowel injury and having to perform a colostomy may be thus reduced. Patients with endometrial carcinoma are considered to be at high risk for intraoperative thrombo-embolic events. Doppler studies of the common femoral vein in patients undergoing laparoscopic cholecystectomy have shown greatly reduced flow caused by high intraperitoneal pressure and reduced venous return from the legs (27). It is thus imperative that optimum precautions are taken to decrease the occurrence of thrombo-embolic events. This means that elasticized support stockings and intermittent pneumatic compression should be utilized during the procedure. Pharmacological prophylaxis is also mandatory and may be either low-dose unfractionated heparin or low-molecular weight heparin. These measures should be continued until the patient leaves the hospital after the procedure. Preoperative antibiotics are recommended to minimize the chance of postoperative infection.

Surgery for high-risk stage I (grades 1–2 and >50% myometrial invasion, grade 3 and any invasion), and stage II endometrial carcinoma presently includes extra-fascial hysterectomy and bilateral salpingo-oophorectomy. Several studies have demonstrated the merits (diagnostic and therapeutic) of a pelvic lymphadenectomy (28,29). The survival benefits of para-aortic lymphadenectomy, however, remain unproven in patients with high-risk stages I and II endometrial cancer. Faught et al. demonstrated that in selected high-risk patients, 80 para-aortic lymphadenectomies had to be performed to benefit four patients (30). For these reasons para-aortic lymphadenectomy is not part of the surgical treatment of patients with high-risk endometrial cancer at Groote Schuur Hospital, Cape Town, South Africa.

If a patient is found to have low-risk endometrial cancer after diagnostic endometrial sampling, frozen section is performed during definitive surgery after LAVH to identify unsuspected high-risk factors. If no such factors are detected on frozen section, the operation is considered to be complete. Otherwise a pelvic lymphadenctomy is carried out.

LAPAROSCOPIC SURGERY

Laparoscopic surgery, more so than open surgery, is a team approach. This means that the surgeon, surgical assistant, scrub nurse, and anesthetist must have an intimate knowledge of the possibilities and limitations of laparoscopic surgery.

During an open approach the position of the patient should be relatively stationary throughout the procedure. During a laparoscopic approach, however, the position of the patient will change from modified lithotomy/Lloyd Davis position to a lithotomy position and from Trendelenburg to a supine position. An operating table which is electronically controlled should be utilized for these reasons.

An equipment tower including video monitor, CO_2 insufflator, light source, and camera box should be available in the theater. The tower should be positioned so that the surgeon and other members of the team at all times have an uninterrupted view of the monitor and the other equipment which is part of the tower.

The authors, throughout the procedure, use a 0° 10 mm telescope. A camera is attached to the telescope and is white balanced prior to the procedure. The camera should have focus and zoom adjustments. Easy access to still picture facilities should be available on the camera as well.

The authors use electro-surgical equipment, which includes Liga-Sure® and bipolar current. This combination enables a safe coagulation technique for the surgeon. The operating laparoscopy tray should only comprise instruments which are used during the procedure. Too many instruments on the traytable may only hinder the surgical team rather than being of assistance. Spare instruments should, however, be readily available in the theater. The basic instruments should include two grasping forceps, one pair of disposable scissors, and one pair of forceps for electrocautery. Suction and irrigation should be combined in one instrument, but should under ideal circumstances only be used at the end of the procedure.

Prior to the laparoscopic procedure, the bladder is emptied followed by an examination under anesthetic, and a single tooth vulsellum forceps is put on the cervix for manipulation of the uterus. For a sub-umbilical insertion of the trochar, the authors use the disposable so-called Step trochar® (Tyco). This trochar enables the surgeon to insert a Verres needle and 10 mm introducer through the same sleeve to reduce the risk of accidental trauma. In patients who have undergone previous abdominal surgery an open approach is advisable. Two smaller disposable 5 mm Pediport trochars® (Tyco) are used for suprapubic insertion.

After a pneumoperitoneum is created by insufflation of CO_2, the main sub-umbilical trochar is inserted. The two smaller trochars are subsequently introduced in the left and right iliac fossa, respectively, just lateral to the deep epigastric vessels, under direct vision. The direction of the trochars should be towards the anterior pelvis. If a pelvic lymphadenectomy is intended, an additional non-disposable 10 mm trochar is introduced in the midline just above the pubic hairline.

A careful inspection of uterus, adnexae, Pouch of Douglas, and peritoneal surfaces is carried out. Normal saline is introduced in the Pouch of Douglas and subsequently aspirated for cytological analysis. The upper abdomen is then carefully examined. Possible adhesions are dissected and biopsied. After identification of the ureter at the pelvic brim, the infundibulo-pelvic ligament is grasped and cauterized followed by dissection. The round ligament on the ipsilateral side is then grasped, cauterized, and dissected. The contralateral infundibulo-pelvic ligament and round ligament are then cauterized and dissected. The bladder peritoneum is dissected and pulled down with a grasper.

Setting up the vaginal part of the procedure follows careful laparo-scopic hemostasis. The patient is put in a lithotomy position and the cervix is exposed. The cervix is radially injected with Por-8 and a local anesthetic. The cervix is circumcised and the Pouch of Douglas is entered followed by opening of the vesico-uterine space. After clamping, dissection and suturing of the uterosacral and cardinal ligaments, the uterine artery pedicles are dealt with in the same fashion. As the infundibulo-pelvic ligaments are already dissected during the laparoscopic part, the uterus and adnexae can now safely be removed. After careful hemostasis and inspection of the main pedicles the vagina is closed. Care should be taken that the pelvic peritoneum is closed together with the vaginal epithelium.

For the pelvic lymphadenectomy, the patient is taken out of lithotomy position and the legs of the patient are taken out of the leg supports and stretched without any flexion of the hips. The patient is kept in Trendelenburg position. The remainder of the round ligament is grasped and pulled anteriorly so that the retroperitoneal space is made visible and the peritoneum is further dissected parallel to the round ligament. The internal and external iliac arteries and veins and ureter are identified. The paravesical space is now entered and the obturator nerve identified (Fig. 1). The tissue between the posterior aspect of the external iliac vein and obturator nerve is gently removed by traction and dissection. The tissue may then be pulled through the suprapubic 10 mm port. The external iliac artery and vein are now separated and the tissue between these structures and between the external iliac artery and psoas muscle is removed (Fig. 2) and also extracted

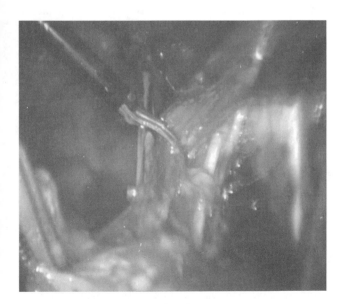

Figure 1 Exposure of obturator nerve.

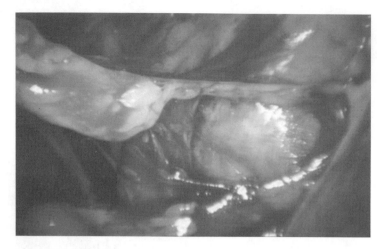

Figure 2 Removal of lymph nodes over the psoas muscle.

through the suprapubic 10 mm port. The bifurcation of the common iliac artery into internal and external iliac artery is identified by grasping with gentle anterior traction of the pedicle of the infundibulo-pelvic ligament. Care must be taken that bleeding which may occur during this step is dealt with as this may obstruct the view of the common iliac artery. The nodes alongside the common iliac artery are removed by traction after the position of the ureter has again been identified. Next, the nodes at the bifurcation are removed followed by removal in a caudal direction of the nodal tissue lateral to and alongside the internal iliac by traction and gentle blunt dissection by the closed tip of an atraumatic grasper. Careful hemostasis is completed followed by a similar procedure on the contralateral side. After the bilateral laparoscopic pelvic lymphadenectomy has been completed, an inspection of the pedicles is carried out. If necessary a soft silicone drain is left in the pelvis to monitor pelvic blood/lymph loss.

The abdomen is desufflated. The trochars are removed. To decrease the risk of herniation, it is recommended that the underlying fascia and peritoneum should be closed at the port-sites of large, i.e., 10 mm, trochars. Closure of the fascia defect caused by the 5 mm trochar ports has been suggested when extensive manipulation has taken place (31).

REFERENCES

1. Reich H, DeCaprio J, McGlynn F. Laparoscopic hysterectomy. J Gynecol Surg 1989; 5:213–215.
2. Peters WA III, Andersen WA, Thornton WN Jnr, Morley GW. The selective use of vaginal hysterectomy in the management of adenocarcinoma of the endometrium. Am J Obstet Gynecol 1983; 146:285–289.

3. Bloss JD, Berman ML, Bloss LP, Buller RE. Use of vaginal hysterectomy for the management of stage I endometrial cancer in the medically compromised patient. Gynecol Oncol 1991; 40(1):74–77.
4. Lelle RJ, Morley GW, Peters WA. The role of vaginal hysterectomy in the treatment of endometrial carcinoma. Int J Gynecol Cancer 1994(4):342–347.
5. Minelli L, Angiolillo M, Caione C, Palmara V. Laparoscopically-assisted vaginal hysterectomy. Endoscopy 1991; 23(2):64–66.
6. Liu CY. Laparoscopic hysterectomy. A review of 72 cases. J Reprod Med. 1992; 37(4):351–354.
7. Mage G, Canis M, Wittiez A, Pouly MA, Bruhat MA. Hysterectomie et coelioscopie. J Gynecol Obstet Biol Reprod 1990; 19:569–573.
8. Johns DA, Diamond MP. Laparoscopic assisted vaginal hysterectomy. J Reprod Med 1994; 39(6):424–428.
9. Querleu D, Leblanc E, Castelain B. Laparoscopic pelvic lymphadenectomy in the staging of early carcinoma of the cervix. Am J Obstet Gynecol 1991; 164:579–581.
10. Childers J, Hatch K, Surwit EA. The role of laparscopic lymphadenectomy in the management of cervical carcinoma. Gynecol Oncol 1992; 47:38–43.
11. Childers J, Surwit EA. Laparoscopic para-aortic lymph node biopsy for diagnosis of a non-Hodgkin's lymphoma. Surg Laparoscop Endoscop 1992; 2: 139–142.
12. Childers JM, Surwit EA. Combined laparoscopic and vaginal surgery for the management of two cases of stage I endometrial cancer. Gynecol Oncol 1992; 45(1):46–51.
13. Childers JM, Brzechffa PR, Hatch KD, Surwit EA. Laparocopically assisted surgical staging (LASS) of endometrial cancer. Gynecol Oncol 1993; 51(1): 33–38.
14. Eltabbakh GH. Effect of Surgeon's experience on the surgical out come of laparoscopic surgery for women with endometrial cancer. Gynecol Oncol 2000; 78:58–61.
15. Scribner DR, Walker JL, Johnson GA, McMeekin SD, Gold MA, Mannel RS. Surgical management of early-stage Endometrial cancer in the elderly: Is laparoscopy feasible? Gynecol Oncol 2001; 83:563–568.
16. Eltabbakh GH, Shamonki MJ, Moody JM, Garafano LL. Laparoscopy as the primary modality for the treatment of women with endometrial carcinoma. Cancer 2001; 91(2):378–387.
17. Magrina JF, Mutone NF, Weaver AL, Magtibay PM, Fowler RS, Cornella JL. Laparoscopic lymphadenectomy and vaginal or laparoscopic hysterectomy with bilateral salpingo-oophorectomy for endometrial cancer: morbidity and survival. Am J Obstet Gynecol 1999; 181(2):376–381.
18. Sonada Y, Zerbe M, Smith A, Lin O, Barakat RR, Hoskins WJ. High incidence of positive peritoneal cytology in low risk endometrial cancer treated by laparoscopically assisted vaginal hysterectomy. Gynecol Oncol 2001; 80:378–382.
19. Vergote I, De Smet I, Amant F. Letter to the editor. Gynecol Oncol 84; 537.
20. Chu CS, Randall TC, Banders CA, Rubin SC. Vaginal cuff recurrence of endometrial cancer treated by laparoscopic-assisted vaginal hysterectomy. 2003, 88; 62–65.

21. Lim BK, Lavie O, Bolger B, Lopes T, Monaghan JM. The role of laparoscdopic surgery in the management of endometrial cancer. BJOG 2000; 107(1):24–27.
22. Gemignani ML, Curtin JP, Zelmanovich J, Patel DA, Venkatraman Laparoscopic-assisted vaginal hysterectomy for endometrial cancer: clinical outcomes and hospital charges. Gynecol Oncol 1999; 73(1):5–11.
23. Muntz HG, Goff BA, Madsen BL, Yon JL. Port-site recurrence after laparoscopic surgery for endometrial carcinoma. Obstet Gynecol 1999; 93:807–809.
24. Kadar N. Port-site recurrences following laparoscopic operations for gynaecological malignancies. Br J Obstet Gynaecol 1997; 104(11):1308–1313.
25. Malur S, Possover M, Michels W, Schneider A. Laparocopic assisted vaginal versus abdominal surgery In patients with endometrial cancer—a prospective randomized trial. Gynecol Oncol 2001; 80:239–244.
26. Scribner DR Jr, Mannel RS, Walker JL, Johnson GA. Cost analysis of laparoscopic versus laparotomy for early endometrial cancer. Gynecol Oncol 1999; 75(3):460–463.
27. International Consensus Statement Cardiovascular Disease Educational & Research Trust; International Union of Angiology Chest 1998; 114:531s–549s.
28. Kilgore LC, Partridge EE, Alvarez RD, et al. Adenocarcinoma of the endometrium: survival comparisons of patients with and without pelvic node sampling. Gynecol Oncol 1995; 56(1):29–33.
29. Mohan DS, Samuels MA, Selim MA, Abdelwahab DS, Ellis RJ, Samuels JR, Yun HJ. Long-term outcomes of therapeutic pelvic lymphadenectomy for stage I endometrial adenocarcinoma. Gynecol Oncol 1998; 70(2):165–171.
30. Faught W, Krepart GV, Lotocki R, Heywood M. Should selective par-aortic lymphadenectomy be part of surgical staging for endometrial cancer? Gynecol Oncol 1994; 55(1):51–55.
31. Nezhat FR, Nezhat CH, Seidman DS. Incisional Hernias after Advanced Laparoscopic Surgery. J Am Assoc Gynecol Laparosc 1996; 3(4 suppl):S34–S35.

12

Follow-Up and Detection of Relapsed Disease in Uterine Cancer

Fabio Landoni, Angelo Maggioni, and Guilherme Cidade Crippa
European Institute of Oncology, Milan, Italy

BACKGROUND

By definition, surveillance following primary cancer therapy is the observation and follow-up of asymptomatic patients who are clinically free of disease (FOD) with the aim of identifying relapses while they are still localized and theoretically amenable to secondary treatment.

Approximately 80% of uterine cancers are confined to the uterus at initial diagnosis (70.2% are International Federation of Gynecology and Obstetrics (FIGO) stage I and 12.4% are FIGO stage II) (1). Of the 17.4% with extrauterine disease, 13.3% are FIGO stage III, and 4.1% are FIGO stage IV. Stage of disease is one factor that significantly influences the risk of recurrence. Overall survival (OS) for all stages, from the time of diagnosis, is 92.1%, 82.6%, 81.9%, 78.8%, and 76.5% at one, two, three, four, and five-years, respectively, and 73% at 10 years (2). The variation in disease-free survival (DFS) and OS with stage is illustrated in Table 1.

Risk of relapse is also related to histological subtype. Uterine papillary serous carcinoma (UPSC) and clear cell carcinomas have a significantly worse outcome when compared with endometrioid carcinomas. Approximately 40% of clinical stage I UPSC die of their disease within three years of diagnosis and, although the incidence of clinical stage I UPSC is 4–10% of all endometrial carcinomas, it accounts for about one-quarter of the entire endometrial cancer mortality. Fifty-two percent (22/42) of the

Table 1 OS (%) and DFS (%) by FIGO Surgical Stage

Stage	2 years		3 years		5 years	
	DFS	OS	DFS	OS	DFS	OS
Ia	93.5	95.3	91.1	92.4	87.1	88.9
Ib		96.0		93.5		90.0
Ic		91.0		88.0		80.7
IIa	84.4	89.0	79.8	83.1	75.9	79.9
IIb		87.5		81.1		72.3
IIIa	74.9	77.0	69.3	71.0	63.1	63.4
IIIb		61.7		48.0		38.8
IIIc		70.4		63.4		51.1
IVa	67.3	39.5	49.1	27.9	36.9	19.9
IVb		32.0		21.8		17.2

Source: From Ref. 1.

UPSC patients reported by Rosenberg et al. (3) died of their cancer during the observation period (median of 70 months), compared to only 7.5% (59/789) of patients with endometrioid adenocarcinomas.

Comparing life table survival for all stage I patients with a population life table (*Vital Statistics of the United States, 1980*) for women of equal age, Burke et al. (4) found no differences between the two groups. This suggests that early-stage endometrial cancer has no significant impact on overall life expectancy. Despite the fact that these patients have a relatively low recurrence rate, they generally undergo intensive surveillance for three to five years. This can partly be explained by the fact that the prognosis of those who develop recurrent disease is poor.

A further indication for follow-up, particularly in those high-risk groups who have been treated with adjuvant radiation, is to detect evidence of treatment morbidity.

Limited data are available regarding the morbidities associated with adjuvant radiotherapy for endometrial cancer. Reports of complication rates are often confusing given the heterogeneity of treatment techniques applied over a protracted period. Corn et al. (5) evaluating 235 patients found severe complications in 13 patients, giving rise to a five-year actuarial risk of 5.5%. The median time to their development was 45 months (range 2–161 months). On reviewing the literature, they reported complications ranging from 12.7% to 7.7% (over a sample of 378 patients). A further review by Shumsky et al. (6) suggested an incidence of 9.5% of acute complications (radiation enteritis/proctitis), which usually resolved within three months and a severe late complication rate of 5.5–6.5%, most becoming apparent within three years of treatment.

The frequency and duration of post-treatment surveillance differs widely among institutions and even among clinicians practicing in the same hospital. This is almost certainly a reflection of the lack of robust data by which to guide practice. While it is possible to question the whole ethos of post-treatment surveillance, the purpose of this chapter is to examine what current practice hopes to achieve and how it might achieve it. Given the time and resources that are targeted for post-treatment surveillance, it seems reasonable to examine the validity of follow-up and its associated investigations.

PATTERNS OF RECURRENCE

Recurrence Rate

Of 6260 patients of all stages reported in the FIGO Annual Report (1), 1640 relapsed after primary therapy (26.2%). The recurrence rate by stage (among relapsed patients with an available surgical stage for analysis) is shown in Table 2.

Considering all stages, the recurrence rate as reported in the literature varies from 7.3% to 18% (2–4,7–16).

Time to Recurrence

Shumsky et al. (14) describe a recurrence rate for all stages of 6.2/100 for the first year, 4.3/100 for the second, and 2/100 per year thereafter. This observation was based on a series of 317 patients of whom 53 (16%) relapsed. The majority of relapsed cases are recognized within three years of primary therapy, the median time to recurrence ranging from 12.8 to 22 months (Table 3).

Table 2 Recurrence Rate by FIGO Stage

Stage	n	Relapses (%)
Ia	975	128 (13.1)
Ib	2035	273 (13.4)
Ic	986	209 (21.2)
IIa	342	82 (24)
IIb	367	109 (29.7)
IIIa	457	188 (41.1)
IIIb	101	66 (65.3)
IIIc	200	103 (51.5)
IVa	57	42 (73.7)
IVb	174	142 (81.6)

Source: From Ref. 1.

Table 3   Recurrence Time Characteristics

Reference	Median (months)	Range	% at 1 year	% at 2 years	% at 3 years
Agboola et al. (2)	18.5	3–194	—	—	80
Burke et al. (4)	15	—	—	—	—
Berchuck et al. (7)	—	—	—	—	82
Gadducci et al. (8)	17.5	6–64	—	—	—
Podczaski et al. (11)	12.8	2–125	47	70	—
Reddoch et al. (12)[a]	14.8	—	51	82	95
Shumsky et al. (14)	—	—	—	58	70
Morice et al. (15)	22	5–67	—	—	85

[a] All 39 relapsed patients reported by Reddoch et al. developed recurrent disease by 39 months.

Variations in time to recurrence have been noted with histological subtype. Rosenberg et al. (3) noted that all recurrences among the UPSC patients occurred within 38 months and the median time to recurrence was 18 months. In other adenocarcinomas, all recurrences had occurred by 105 months with a median time of 26 months. However, these figures do not represent significant differences in median recurrence-free interval between patients with UPSC and those with other adenocarcinomas of different grades.

Site of Recurrence

An overview of the available literature is shown in Table 4. Summarizing the data suggest the following sites' frequencies of recurrence:

Local	35.2% (from 25% to 53.8%)
Distant	53.1% (from 41% to 70.8%)
Local plus distant recurrence	11.7% (from 3.7% to 27%)

The heterogeneity of the groups reported by different authors renders a meaningful analysis of sites of recurrence difficult. It does appear, however, that a higher proportion of patients fail at a distant site following postoperative adjuvant pelvic radiotherapy (PRT) (16,17). If one accepts that the use of postoperative adjuvant radiotherapy influences the site of first relapse, the prevalence of distant relapses almost certainly reflects the fact that this treatment is preferentially prescribed to high-risk patients. Sartori et al. (16) in an Italian study of the Co-operation Task Force (CTF) reported on 1606 endometrial cancer patients evaluating the factors

Table 4 Sites of Recurrence

Reference	n	Local (%)	Distant (%)	Local + distant (%)
			Site of Recurrence	
Agboola et al. (2)	50	19 (38)	31 (62)	—
Burke et al. (4)	38	11 (29)	18 (47.3)	9 (23.7)
Berchuck et al. (7)	44	12 (27)	20 (46)	12 (27)
Gadducci et al. (8)	24	6 (25)	17 (70.8)	1 (4.2)
Pastner et al. (10)	13	7 (53.8)	6 (46.2)	—
Podczaski et al. (11)	47	16 (34)	29 (61.7)	2 (4.3)
Reddoch et al. (12)	39	15 (38.6)	16 (41)	8 (20.5)
Shumsky et al. (14)	53	25 (47.1)	22 (41.5)	6 (11.4)
Morice et al. (15)	27	7 (26)	19 (70.3)	1 (3.7)
Total	335	118 (35.2)	178 (53.1)	39 (11.7)

influencing survival in relapsed cases. They reported the site of recurrence in patients treated with surgery alone and those that received adjuvant PRT. Vaginal/pelvic relapses occurred in 61.2% of the patients treated with surgery alone and in 34.3% of those treated with adjuvant PRT. Distant relapses were found in 38.8% of the patients treated with surgery alone and in 65.7% of those treated with adjuvant PRT.

Of the 1640 relapsed patients reported in the FIGO Annual Report (1), 652 had a site of recurrence recorded in addition to stage. The sites of recurrence according to stage are presented in Table 5. For those who presented with disease confined to the uterus the recurrence sites are presented in Table 6.

The site of recurrence differs significantly between patients with UPSC and other adenocarcinomas. Forty-six percent of the recurrences in the UPSC group reported by Rosenberg et al. (3) occurred in the abdomen

Table 5 Sites of Recurrences According to the Stage

Site	I (%)	II (%)	III (%)	IV (%)
		Stage		
Local	138 (47)	58 (51.8)	46 (23.4)	13 (26.5)
Distant	129 (43.9)	40 (35.7)	117 (59.4)	30 (61.2)
Local + Distant	27 (9.1)	14 (12.5)	34 (17.2)	6 (12.3)
Total	294	112	197	49

Source: From Ref. 1.

Table 6 Sites of Recurrences According to the Stage for Stages I and II

	Stage				
Site	Ia (%)	Ib (%)	Ic (%)	IIa (%)	IIb (%)
Local	26 (59.1)	73 (57.5)	39 (31.8)	25 (61)	33 (46.5)
Distant	17 (39.6)	46 (36.2)	66 (53.6)	13 (31.7)	27 (38)
Local + Distant	1 (2.3)	8 (6.3)	18 (14.6)	3 (7.3)	11 (15.5)
Total	44	127	123	41	71

Source: From Ref. 1.

outside the pelvis whereas the most dominant site of recurrence in the adenocarcinoma group was the vagina.

RECURRENCE RISK GROUPS

The risk factors for relapse in patients with endometrial cancer can be defined in relation to the characteristics of the intrauterine tumor and the presence or absence of extrauterine disease. In one large series, Morrow et al. (9) analyzed the surgical-pathological findings in relation to postoperative treatment and recurrence in 895 endometrial cancer patients.

The uterine risk factors considered were:

- histological grade,
- depth of myometrial invasion,
- vascular space invasion (VSI), and
- cervical extension.

The extrauterine risk factors were:

- pelvic node metastases,
- aortic node metastases,
- adnexal metastases,
- positive pelvic peritoneal cytology, and
- gross tumor breakthrough of the uterine serosa with or without peritoneal implants.

Only 1 of the 99 patients without myometrial invasion experienced a recurrence. The frequency of recurrence observed for patients with tumor grades 1–3 was 4.4%, 8.6%, and 16.1%, respectively. Analyzing the recurrence rate for cases having a single risk factor, the frequency of recurrence for the different categories of risk ranged from 14.3% to 40% with an average of 20.1%. The subjects with two positive risk factors had a median recurrence frequency of 43.1%, with 63.3% for those with three or more risk factors (Table 7).

Table 7 Rates of Recurrences According to Tumor Risk Factors

Risk factor	Recurrence rate (%)
Specific Factor	
Pelvic nodes	5/18 (27.7)
Aortic nodes	2/5 (40)
Adnexal tumor	1/7 (14.3)
Gross disease	1/4 (25)
Cytology	6/32 (18.8)
VSI	9/34 (26.5)
Isthmus/Cervix	15/94 (16)
Overall	
One factor	39/194 (20.1)
Two factors	31/72 (43.1)
Three or more factors	38/60 (63.3)

Abbreviation: VSI, vascular space invasion.
Source: From Ref. 9.

Forty-eight cases (5.4%) presented with aortic node metastases, of which 28 (58.3%) progressed. In the study population, patients with aortic node metastases account for nearly a quarter of all recurrences. Considering separately positive pelvic nodes, gross adnexal metastases, or outer myometrial invasion, patients with one or more of these features constituted only 25% of the study population but accounted for 98% (47/48) of the cases with aortic node metastases. Of the positive aortic node group, 36% were tumor-free for more than five years (median 21.2 months); the corresponding rate for the aortic node-negative group was 85%. In the authors' opinion (9), the 390 patients who, after surgical staging, were found to have no evidence of extrauterine disease, no cervical invasion, and no capillary space involvement could be considered at low risk for recurrence.

In a similar fashion, Shumsky et al. (6) divided endometrial cancer patients into low or high risk of recurrence. Evaluating 369 patients with endometrial carcinoma, the authors defined those at low risk as FIGO stage IA, grade 1 or 2 adenocarcinoma, or stage IB, grade 1 adenocarcinoma. In these groups the five-year recurrence rate was 2.7–4.1%. High-risk cases were defined as those with FIGO stage IA, grade 3 adenocarcinoma, stage IB, grade 2 or 3 adenocarcinoma, stage equal to or greater than IC adenocarcinoma any grade, and aggressive histologies (Table 8). This high-risk group of women had a five-year recurrence rate of 21.4–23.4%. Using the same criteria on a different population, Gadducci et al. (8) reported similar outcomes with a five-year DFS of 94.2 % in low-risk compared with 76.0% in high-risk patients ($p = 0.0472$). Of the 24 relapsed patients, three were in the low-risk group and 21 in the high-risk.

Table 8 Recurrence Risk Groups

Low-risk	• Stage IA grade 1 or 2 adenocarcinoma
	• Stage IB grade 1 adenocarcinoma
High-risk	• Stage IA grade 3 adenocarcinoma
	• Stage IB grade 2 or 3 adenocarcinoma
	• Stage equal to or greater than IC adenocarcinoma any grade
	• Aggressive histologies

Source: From Ref. 6.

Focusing on UPSC patients, Rosenberg et al. (3) reported 841 patients with clinical stage I endometrial carcinoma. The median follow-up time for the whole group was 70 months. A total of 62 patients recurred, giving an overall recurrence rate of 7.4%. The UPSC patients had a recurrence rate of 31%, whereas 6% of patients with other adenocarcinomas recurred. In a series published by Reddoch et al. (12), all recurrences except one were seen in patients with high-risk histology. High-risk histology was defined as grades 2 and 3 endometrioid adenocarcinoma, or variant cell types such as clear cell and papillary serous carcinoma. Only one of 148 patients (0.7%) with grade I endometrioid adenocarcinoma recurred.

In an attempt to evaluate the effect of loco-regional control on subsequent metastatic dissemination, Corn et al. (18) defined local recurrence as that occurring within the radiation field and distant recurrence as that occurring outwidth the radiation field (e.g., a recurrence in the para-aortic nodes could be considered as a local recurrence if this patient had received para-aortic radiotherapy). Over a sample of 394 patients (all treated with surgery followed by adjuvant radiotherapy), followed from 2 to 151 months (median 62 months), the authors evaluated what they defined as freedom from distant failure (FFDR) as a function of local disease status. Within the context of their model, the earlier a local failure developed, the more likely it was associated with distant metastasis ($p < 0.05$). Also evaluating the OS, they observed that those women who failed locally had a nearly fourfold risk of failing distantly compared to those who remained locally controlled (FFDR, $p = 0.02$; OS, $p = 0.0002$). Only local control, grade of differentiation (1/2 vs. 3 FFDR $p = 0.004$; OS $p = 0.0001$), and pathological stage (I vs. II/III FFDR and OS, $p = 0.0001$) were independently related to the likelihood of achieving freedom from distant relapse at five years.

PROGNOSIS AFTER RECURRENCE

The management of advanced or recurrent endometrial carcinoma is varied, but the overall consensus in the literature is that regardless of management strategies, the outcomes are universally poor. Both the site of recurrence and the nature of the initial treatment influence the prognosis after recurrence. Patients with vaginal/pelvic relapses and those not previously exposed to adjuvant radiation appear to have a more favorable outcome after treatment of relapse. Those who have received PRT and/or present with a pelvic or distant recurrence are likely to have a poor outcome. This may reflect a biologically aggressive radio-resistant tumor. Sartori et al. (16) reported a global 5- and 10-year survival rate after recurrence of 26% and 22%, respectively. When survival was considered by relapse site, the survival at 5 and 10 years was 68% for vaginal relapses; 29% and 18%, respectively, for pelvic relapses; and 8% for distant relapses ($p < 0.00001$).

Burke et al. (4) reported that among the 11 patients with isolated pelvic relapses (29% of all recurrences), two with isolated vaginal cuff recurrence were salvaged by additional irradiation, but despite additional therapy, the other nine patients died of disease with a median survival of 21 months. Of the 27 patients (71%) with distant failure, all died of disease with a median survival of 22 months, resulting in a salvage rate of 18% for pelvic-recurrence patients and 0% for distant failures.

Following documented recurrence, Podczaski et al. (11) reported actuarial OS at 12, 24, and 36 months as 42%, 24%, and 17%, respectively. Only 5 of the 47 patients (11%) continued to be clinically disease free from 28 to 111 months after the treatment of recurrent cancer. Patients with recurrent disease limited to the vagina had a one-year actuarial survival of 76%, whereas patients with involvement of other sites had a survival of 31%. The site of recurrence ($p = 0.002$), and the interval from primary therapy to relapse ($<$ or ≥ 1 year, $p = 0.002$) were also covariates related to patient survival after relapse. Patients with recurrent tumor who did not receive postoperative radiation had a 12- and 24-month actuarial survival of 54% and 34%, respectively. In contrast, patients who had received post-operative radiotherapy had 12- and 24-month survivals of 37% and 20%, respectively ($p = 0.05$). Analyzing subgroups with the intent of determining the effect of radiotherapy on OS and DFS is difficult, if not impossible, as there is an inherent bias. Patients with risk factors for relapse are more likely to receive postoperative radiation.

According to Gadducci et al. (8), the median survival time after recurrence is 10 months, being longer in patients who relapsed after 17.5 months compared with those who relapsed earlier ($p = 0.02$). Second-line therapy was able to salvage 8 of 44 recurrent cases as reported by Berchuck et al. (7) (18%). These included 6 out of 12 (50%) with isolated vaginal disease, and 2 out of 34 (6%) with other patterns of recurrent disease ($p = 0.01$). In a small series of 39 recurrences (12) no patient with systemic disease was salvaged by chemotherapy. In fact, only three of 39 patients (8%) were salvaged by additional therapy, including two with a vaginal vault recurrence (one microscopic diagnosed by Pap smear and one with a palpable vaginal vault lesion), and one with an isolated skin lesion, all cured by surgical excision and radiotherapy. Agboola et al. (2) reported an OS rate for relapsed patients of 44% at five years and 22% at 10 years, with a median survival after a recurrence of 9.5 months (range 1–103).

Among the 27 relapsing patients described by Morice et al. (15), 19 (70.4%) died at a median time of 12.2 months (range 2–70), six patients were alive with progressive disease, and only one patient was alive free of disease five years after treatment (one with a vaginal recurrence treated by colpectomy).

All of the UPSC patients with recurrence reported by Rosenberg et al. (3) died of their disease within 21 months of diagnosis of recurrence (median survival time after recurrence, seven months). In the remaining adenocarcinoma patients who had recurred, 39% (19/49) were alive without disease after a median observation time after recurrence of 10.5 months.

When grade of tumor is used to determine the outcome following relapse, the proportion of recurring patients dead of cancer at the end of follow-up are 54% for grade 1, 47% for grade 2, and 82% for grade 3, with an overall mortality for all grades of 61%. In fact, Agboola et al. (2) reported that, after recurrence, survival was influenced by the grade of disease ($p = 0.05$); higher grade was associated with increased risk of dying from cancer after recurrence by a risk ratio of 1.56 [95% confidence interval (CI) 0.69–2.44].

DETECTION AND SURVEILLANCE

Surveillance Programs

There is no general agreement with regard to standard follow-up programs for patients treated for uterine cancer (Table 9), as confirmed by the reported survey of Barnhill et al. (19). A questionnaire was mailed to members of the Society of Gynecologic Oncologists (SGO) to obtain information regarding the follow-up practices for asymptomatic, disease-free patients who had previously been treated for endometrial cancer. The majority of respondents stated that they followed up every three months during the first year after completion of therapy, three to four months in the second year, six months to the end of the fifth year and annually thereafter. Eighty-four percent of respondents performed a Pap smear at each visit, and all performed a pelvic examination. The majority also recommended a yearly chest X-ray for the first three years after completion of therapy. There was also support for performing serum CA125 surveillance. The average response suggesting serum CA125 level was four times each year during the first two years, then twice each year for the next three years. Between 11% and 18% of respondents did not recommend routine CA125 testing during the five years after completion of therapy. Perhaps, the most interesting result from this survey was the very haphazard and non-uniform approach to

Table 9 Surveillance Protocols

Reference	Clinical visit	Pap smear	Chest X-ray	Others
Agboola et al. (2)	Every three months on first year Every four months on second year Every six months from the third to the fifth years Annually thereafter	At every clinical visit	Annually	When clinically indicated
Berchuck et al. (7)	Every three months on first year Every four months on second and third years Every six months for the next two years	At every clinical visit	Annually	When clinically indicated
Gadducci et al. (8)	Every 3–4 months for the first two years Every six months for the next three years Annually thereafter	At every clinical visit	Every six months for the first two years Annually for the next three years Individually increasing intervals thereafter	Pelvic ultrasound at every clinical visit Abdominal-pelvic CT scan annually for 5 years Others when clinically indicated
Podcazki et al. (11)	Every three months on first and second years Every six months on the next three years Annually thereafter	Every six months for the first five years	Annually	Intravenous pyelogram annually Others when clinically indicated
Reddoch et al. (12)	Every three months for the first two years Every four months on third year Every six months on fourth and fifth years	At every clinical visit	Annually	CA125 for selected patients Others when clinically indicated
Morice et al. (15)	Every three months on first year Every four months on second year Every six months on third year Annually thereafter	At every clinical visit	Annually	Abdominal-pelvic ultrasound annually

follow-up with very little if any of the interventions based on an impact on outcome.

Shumsky et al. (14) described routine follow-up at their institution apparently based upon using different protocols in relation to known risk. These included clinical visits every three months for the first year, every four months for the second year, and every six months thereafter for a minimum of five years. At each visit a vaginal vault Pap smear and physical examination was performed. Chest X-rays were performed biannually. After evaluation of the results, the same authors conducted another study (6) dividing the patients by risk group. They concluded that for low risk, patients should not be routinely followed up but rather offered a consultation for the purposes of educating and informing them of the signs and symptoms suggestive of recurrent disease. Thereafter, they were discharged to their family practitioners for annual health examinations. Suspected or confirmed recurrences should be promptly referred back to the cancer center. In contrast, the high-risk patients should be examined every six months for three years, and discharged after three years of uneventful follow-up. Routine vaginal cytology was only recommended in the third year prior to discharge. Other investigations (CT scans, CA125, and chest X-rays) were only recommended when signs or symptoms suspicious for recurrence were present (Table 10).

Table 10 Suggested Follow-Up Protocol by Risk Groups

Reference	Risk group	Clinical visit	Pap smear	Chest X-ray
Shumsky et al. (14)	Not considered	Every three months on first year Every four months on second year Every six months until fifth year	At every clinical visit	Biannually
Shumsky et al. (6)	Low	No follow-up Education for signs and symptoms heralding recurrences Discharge to family physicians for annual health examinations		
	High	Every six months for three years Discharged after three years	On third year (prior to discharge)	Targeted for signs or symptoms suspicious for recurrences

Source: From Ref. 6, 14.

Detection and Outcome

There has recently been an increasing amount of interest in linking post-treatment surveillance to eventual outcome. Shumsky et al. (14) reported that 75% (40/53) of their patients who relapsed presented with symptoms at or shortly after the time of recurrence and initiated their own visits. The vast majority of these attended their family physician instead of the regional cancer center. Only 11 of 53 patients (21%) were detected by routine protocol at the cancer center, five by physical exam and six by chest X-ray. Of the six symptomatic patients assessed at the cancer center, all waited between two and four months for their scheduled visit. It was reported that on the routine follow-up visits in the institution, only one recurrence was detected for every 206 routine follow-up visits (17/3503). A total of 3503 vaginal smears were performed with no improvement in diagnosing recurrences earlier. In the report, Pap smear alone detected none of the 11 cases of isolated vaginal recurrence. Radiographic evidence of lung metastases was the only evidence of recurrence in seven patients (six asymptomatic ones) and none of these survived. Detecting and treating recurrences earlier should have led to improved survival, but did not. There was no difference in long term survival after recurrence between patients whose recurrence was identified at routine follow-up and those identified at patient-initiated visits ($p = 0.55$). These results prompted us to suggest different surveillance protocols that took into account the risk factors for relapsed disease (Table 10).

Berchuck et al. (7) reported that at diagnosis of recurrence, 61% of patients had symptoms related to their cancer, 68% had physical findings suggestive of recurrence, and 84% had either symptoms and/or physical findings. Pap smears were performed at each clinic visit and findings consistent with recurrent cancer were seen in 25% of the relapsing patients at the time of diagnosis of recurrence. But, among the 12 patients with isolated vaginal recurrences, only three had Pap smears suggestive of recurrent disease in the absence of symptoms or visible signs of disease. One of these three patients (33%) was salvaged with second-line therapy compared to 5 out of 9 patients (56%) who presented with symptoms or physical findings. Chest radiographs were performed annually and demonstrated recurrent disease in nine (20%) cases. Three of them presented with an abnormal chest radiograph, which was the only evidence of recurrent disease, and all of these died of disease within two years of diagnosis, as did the sole patient who was found to have isolated lung metastases after evaluation of symptoms. The authors calculated that as a group, the 354 patients would have to undergo approximately 5000 physical examinations and Pap smears and 1700 chest radiographs to salvage 8 of 44 relapsing patients. Seven of these eight patients presented with signs and/or symptoms of their recurrent disease and could have been diagnosed based on these clinical findings.

Overall, 14% (1/7) of the patients with recurrence diagnosed exclusively by laboratory and/or radiological investigations were salvaged by second-line therapy versus 19% (7/37) of the patients with signs and/or symptoms of recurrent disease. Furthermore, there was no obvious difference in eventual survival when those diagnosed by investigation were compared with those who presented as a result of symptoms.

Twenty-three of 47 relapses reported by Podczaski et al. (11) (49%) were symptomatic. Of the 24 patients without symptoms at the time of recurrence, 13 had an abnormal physical examination, nine had an abnormal chest X-ray, one patient had an abnormal vaginal smear, and one patient (with local and distant recurrence) had both an abnormal physical examination and an abnormal chest X-ray. The combination of history and physical examination would have detected 79% of the recurrences. In terms of diagnostic procedures, the routine chest X-ray was the most useful, detecting 42% of the recurrences in the asymptomatic group (10 of 24). Only eight (17%) patients were salvaged with second-line therapy. The salvage rate for patients whose vaginal recurrences were detected only by Pap smear in the absence of clinical signs was no better than that of patients with visible recurrences. Radiographic evidence of lung metastases was the only evidence of recurrence in three patients and none of these survived. Therefore, there would appear to be no advantage in terms of salvage or OS if one compares symptomatic patients initiating their own visits with asymptomatic patients diagnosed as a result of routine investigation at follow-up.

Similar outcomes were noted by Agboola et al. (2). This study examined 50 cases of recurrent endometrial cancer, 25 of which (50%) were identified during a routine follow-up visit. Twenty-three recurrences (46%) were diagnosed during a patient-initiated interval visit as a result of symptoms. In two cases it was not possible to determine which mode of presentation prompted diagnosis. Twenty-one recurrences (42%) were detected by physical examination (seven at patient-initiated visits, 13 at routine visits and one unknown); chest X-ray detected nine recurrences (18%) (two at patient-initiated visits and seven at routine visits), and a Pap smear taken during a routine visit detected two recurrences. Of the 50 recurrences, 20 (40%) were detected in asymptomatic patients (10 local recurrence and 10 distant) and 30 (60%) were detected when the patients had symptoms (9 local and 21 distant). Most of the symptomatic recurrences were detected at patient-initiated visits [23/30 (76.7%)]. There was no significant difference in OS between symptomatic patients (median 42 months, range 11–147) versus asymptomatic patients [median 47 months, range 12–134 ($p = 0.33$)] (Fig. 1). Similarly, no survival differences were noted between patients in whom a recurrence was diagnosed at a routine visit (median 44 months, range 12–134) versus a patient-initiated visit [median 45 months, range 11–134 ($p = 0.97$)] (Fig. 2). In addition, there was no significant difference

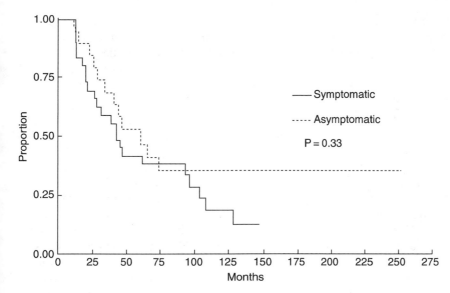

Figure 1 Overall survival rates (from time of initial diagnosis) of patients who were symptomatic and asymptomatic at time of diagnosis of recurrent endometrial cancer.

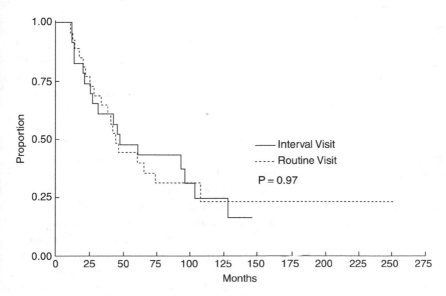

Figure 2 Overall survival rates of patients in whom recurrence of cancer was diagnosed at interval visits or at routine visits.

in survival after detection of recurrence in symptomatic patients (median seven months, range 1–103) versus asymptomatic patients [median 31 months, range 1–96) ($p = 0.135$)] and between patients diagnosed with a recurrence at a routine visit (median 24 months, range 1–103) versus interval visits [median seven months, range 1–89 months ($p = 0.25$)]. There were seven routine chest radiographic examinations with positive results from a total of 2057 (0.34%). There were seven Pap smears with positive results from a total of 4830 (0.14%): four patients had clinically evident disease when the Pap smear was taken, one continued to be free of disease three years later, and two patients had clinically evident disease within three months of the smear being taken. Irrespective of whether the patient has symptoms or not, or if the recurrence was diagnosed at a routine or a patient-initiated visit, survival rates after recurrence are not significantly different.

With regard to cost, we conclude that despite the lack of evidence that early detection of pulmonary metastases leads to improvements in survival, the continuation of routine X-ray examinations might be supportable on economic grounds, as the incremental cost per case detected was small in their institution. There would, however, be no economic or clinical justification for routine Pap smears in the follow-up of endometrial cancer.

Reddoch et al. (12) reported on 39 cases of relapsed endometrial cancer. Sixteen (41%) presented with symptoms that resulted in the diagnosis. (In the four patients who required radiological investigation to make the diagnosis, the investigation had been prompted by their physical findings.) Twenty-three (59%) were asymptomatic when the diagnosis of relapse was made. Of those asymptomatic patients, recurrence was diagnosed by physical examination in 13 (57%), serum CA125 level in 6 (26%), computed tomography (CT) scan in two, and chest X-ray and Pap smear accounted for one diagnosis each. Overall, 29 (74%) patients had their recurrent disease diagnosed and/or confirmed as a direct result of suspicious symptoms or clinical findings. The authors concluded that there seemed to be no benefit in obtaining Pap smears every three or four months for the first two years after therapy. Furthermore there seemed to be little point in including routine chest X-rays in routine follow-up protocols. Finally, the use of a routine measurement of serum CA125 should be reserved for patients at high risk for systemic recurrence. Having evaluated the results obtained from their initial surveillance protocol (Table 9) they suggested a novel protocol. This included a pelvic examination and Pap smear annually performed in the primary-care sector but no chest radiography. A Pap smear and a pelvic exam six months following primary therapy and a serum CA125 measurement should be reserved for high-risk cases (Table 11). Within the context of their sample, they concluded that this follow-up scheme would have detected 95% of the relapses while eliminating 46% of clinic visits, 67% of Pap smears, and 100% of chest radiographs.

Table 11 Suggested Follow-Up Protocol by Risk Groups According to Reddoch et al.

Risk group	Clinical visit	Pap smear	Chest X-ray	Others
Low	Annually until fifth year	Annually until fifth year	No	No
High	Every six months on first year Annually thereafter	Every six months on first year Annually thereafter	No	CA125[a]

[a]Every six months on first year; annually thereafter.
Source: From Ref. 12.

Two further small studies came to similar conclusions. Gadducci et al. (8) reported 11 (45.8%) patients who were symptomatic and 13 (54.2%) who were asymptomatic at the time relapse was diagnosed. Survival was similar in both groups, suggesting that intensive follow-up protocols confer no survival advantage. Morice et al. (15) noted that 81% (22/27) of relapsing patients presented with symptoms at the time of diagnosis. Pap smear was unable to demonstrate the presence of cancer cells in any of the three patients who had abnormal vaginal appearances during the gynecological examination. All of them had positive biopsies confirming vaginal cuff recurrence. All seven patients who presented with pulmonary relapses were symptomatic and the radiological confirmation of recurrence was prompted by their symptoms. In none of them did the chest X-ray obtained at a routine visit detect the disease prior to the development of symptoms.

There has been recent interest in the use of serum CA125 in the management of endometrial cancer. The role of the serum CA125 levels in post-treatment surveillance, however, is not clearly defined. Pastner et al. (10) reported on the measurement of the serum CA125 preoperatively and before each follow-up visit on 125 patients with surgically staged endometrial cancer. Of 13 recurrent patients, six had isolated vaginal recurrence and none of these had an elevated serum CA125 level at the time of recurrence. The remaining seven patients had pelvic (1), abdominal (4), or pulmonary (2) recurrences, and all had elevated serum CA125 levels at the time recurrence was noted. Four patients who received postoperative pelvic radiation had severe, chronic radiation enteritis. These four patients presented with elevated serum CA125 levels coincident with the development of significant partial small bowel obstruction that persisted until surgical exploration. No evidence of recurrent disease was found in any of these patients and their levels subsequently returned to normal. Rose et al. (13) reported 266 women who underwent post-treatment surveillance with 1101 CA125 measurements. Serial CA125 levels were elevated in 19 of 33 relapsing patients (58%). A comparison between the CA125 level at recurrence and a pre-treatment value was possible in 22 of the 33 patients. In every case in which CA125 was elevated at recurrence, a pre-treatment level was also elevated. One recurrence was detected based on an elevated CA125 level. Although the patient was asymptomatic, an abdominal CT scan demonstrated recurrent disease in the liver. CA125 levels were falsely elevated in 11 patients, following pelvic (4) and pelvic and para-aortic radiation therapy (5). Patients receiving para-aortic radiation therapy often maintained persistently elevated CA125 levels, whereas most patients with pelvic radiation and elevated CA125 levels had normalizing values within three months. One patient with intestinal obstruction secondary to radiation injury had a CA125 level of 914 U/mL, with no evidence of disease at her laparotomy for intestinal bypass.

CONCLUSIONS

The primary objective of follow-up is to identify relapses at a stage when, theoretically, they are amenable to secondary treatment. However, there is no evidence that intensive surveillance appreciably improves survival. In fact, follow-up protocols are inefficient in detecting recurrences earlier and do not improve survival outcome. Outcome following recurrences of endometrial cancer may be more dependent on the disease process, the initial therapy, and success of salvage treatment rather than the timing of diagnosis.

Several studies have demonstrated wide variations in surveillance practices and an associated large variation in costs. One consistent feature of the literature is that despite close follow-up, most recurrences are detected in the interval between routine follow-up visits. The most frequent reason for detection of recurrence is the patient herself presenting with symptoms or signs that indicate recurrence. Furthermore, when patients present because of signs or symptoms of disease, there does not appear to be any difference in survival when they are compared to those detected at a routine scheduled follow-up. Finally, no improvement in survival can be demonstrated between symptomatic and asymptomatic patients.

The present lack of efficient methods for treating recurrence does not justify the service costs and the increase in the patient's anxiety that is associated with more active outpatient surveillance.

Given the time and resource allocation diverted toward follow-up it seems reasonable to assume that this practice can no longer be justified. The case for follow-up is largely based upon the desire to salvage the few and perhaps provide some reassurance to those who require it. There is also the consideration of testing new strategies in relapsed patients. It would seem reasonable at this point to reach a compromise and attempt to individualize follow-up. Part of this approach should include patient education in order that significant symptoms prompt early investigation.

There may be some justification in adopting a risk assessment strategy as suggested by Shumsky et al. (6). In addition there is also some justification for including patients with lymph-vascular space invasion (LVSI) as high risk (9,20).

It is likely that not all will agree in considering FIGO stage IAG3 as high risk. We feel that it should. As the FIGO Annual Report (1) has indicated, the OS for this group of patients at one, two, three, four, and five years is 97.2%, 85.7%, 78.3%, 70.5%, and 68.6%, respectively. The survival rate for the FIGO stage IAG3 at five years (68.6%) is the worst of all stage I and stage II patients with the exception of ICG3 (62.9%), IIAG3 (57.3%), and IIBG3 (58.5%). Even stages IIIAG1 (78.6%), IIIBG1 (76.7%), and IIIAG2 (69.3%) do better at five years than IAG3.

We do not agree, however, with the general concept that this division is sufficient to allocate patients to different follow-up protocols, and more importantly, we do not agree with more intensive follow-up for patients considered to be at high risk.

Allocation of risk groups is important from a prognostic point of view. However, in defining a realistic follow-up protocol it is essential to consider whether or not postoperative adjuvant radiotherapy has been used. Most high-risk patients will have been treated with adjuvant radiation and most of the low-risk patients will not.

In the high-risk patients, one might intuitively select more intensive follow-up. The literature suggests that the majority of such patients belong to a group with more aggressive tumors that, consequently, receive adjuvant radiotherapy, have a greater frequency of distant relapses, less options for therapy at relapse, and, despite therapy, a worse prognosis after recurrence. There seems little point in offering intensive surveillance given these adverse factors. In our opinion, the patients most likely to benefit from intense surveillance are the high- or low-risk patients who have not been previously irradiated, as conceivably these represent the group with the greatest chance of responding to further therapy. Thus one strategy does not suit all and the challenge is to define protocols that will reduce clinical visits, patient's anxiety, and costs without compromising the diagnosis of relapses, the therapeutic chances, or the prognosis after treatment of relapse.

We believe that four groups can be defined with associated different follow-up protocols. These are low- and high-risk patients with and without previous PRT (i.e., the standard adjuvant therapy). The suggested follow-up protocol for each is shown in Table 12.

One exception to this grouping perhaps is the group of women who initially present with either intraperitoneal disease or para-aortic disease. Most of these will have been treated primarily with aortic radiotherapy

Table 12 Follow-Up Protocol for Endometrial Cancer Patients

Group	Clinical visit	Pap smear	Chest X-ray	Others
Low-risk No PRT[b]	Every six months until third year Annually thereafter	No	No	CA125[a]
Low-risk PRT[b]	Every six months until third year Annually thereafter	No	No	CA125[a]
High-risk No PRT[b]	Every four months on first year Every six months on second and third year Annually thereafter	No	No	Pelvic CT scan annually until third year CA125[a]
High-risk PRT[b]	Every six months until third year Annually thereafter	No	No	CA125[a]

[a]If elevated preoperative levels. There are insufficient data to justify any particular interval.
[b]PRT, pelvic radiotherapy.

and/or chemotherapy. We feel that such women should be offered a more individualized approach rather than allocated a standard protocol. It is important to emphasize that when patients are followed up, a meticulous pelvic and physical examination should be performed, as another consistent feature of the available literature is that most recurrences are heralded by symptoms and signs that can be assessed by an alert physician.

Routine vaginal cytology for endometrial carcinoma surveillance is not warranted given the lack of a preinvasive stage. A relapse on the vaginal vault tends to infiltrate the whole thickness of the wall before neoplastic cells can be collected by surface cytology. At that point, a recurrent endometrial cancer in the vaginal mucosa or pelvis is either a visible or palpable lesion that can usually be detected by gynecologic examination. This requires a diagnostic biopsy, not screening cytology (8,15).

Routine chest X-rays and measurement of serum CA125 levels are also unnecessary, as the prognosis is not improved by early diagnosis before the onset of symptoms. One justification for their use might be within clinical trials whose objectives are to test new strategies for the treatment of recurrent disease.

Some of these conclusions might be difficult to accept and interpreted as "abandoning" the cancer patient. This is not the case. All patients deserve the most appropriate evidence-based management and the literature does not support our current empiric practices. It is time that cancer physicians become more realistic and accept that current practice appears to be largely focused upon their own fears and on the necessity for reassurance of success rather than on the patient's real needs and expectations.

REFERENCES

1. Pecorelli S (ed). FIGO annual report 24th volume (1993–1995). J Epidemiol Biostat 2001; 6(1):45–86.
2. Agboola OO, Grunfeld E, Coyle D, Perry GA. Costs and benefits of routine follow-up after curative treatment for endometrial cancer. CMAJ 1997; 157:879–886.
3. Rosenberg P, Blom R, Hogberg T, Simonsen E. Death rate and recurrence pattern among 841 clinical stage I endometrial cancer patients with special reference to uterine papillary serous carcinoma. Gynecol Oncol 1993; 51: 311–315.
4. Burke TW, Heller PB, Woodward JE, Davidson SA, Hoskins WJ, Park RC. Treatment failure in endometrial carcinoma. Obstet Gynecol 1990; 75:96–101.
5. Corn BW, Lanciano RM, Greven KM, Noumoff J, Schultz D, Hanks GE, Fowble BL. Impact of improved irradiation technique, age, and lymph node sampling on the severe complication rate of surgically staged endometrial cancer patients: a multivariate analysis. J Clin Oncol 1994; 12:510–515.
6. Shumsky AG, Brasher PMA, Stuart GCE, Nation JG. Risk specific follow-up for endometrial carcinoma patients. Gynecol Oncol 1997; 65:379–382.
7. Berchuck A, Anspach C, Evans AC, Soper JT, Rodriguez GC, Dodge R, Robboy S, Clarke-Pearson DL. Post-surgical surveillance of patients with FIGO stage I/II endometrial adenocarcinoma. Gynecol Oncol 1995; 59:20–24.
8. Gadducci A, Cosio S, Fanucchi A, Cristofani R, Genazzani AR. An intensive follow-up does not change survival of patients with clinical stage I endometrial cancer. Anticancer Res 2000; 20:1977–1984.
9. Morrow CP, Bundy BN, Kurman RJ, Creasman WT, Heller P, Homesley HD, Graham JE. Relationship between surgical-pathological risk factors and outcome in clinical stages I and II carcinoma of the endometrium: a Gynecologic Oncology Group Study. Gynecol Oncol 1991; 40:55–65.
10. Pastner B, Orr JW, Mann WJ Jr. Use of serum CA125 measurement in posttreatment surveillance of early-stage endometrial carcinoma. Am J Obstet Gynecol 1990; 162:427–429.
11. Podczaski E, Kaminski P, Gurski K, MacNeill C, Stryker JA, Singapuri K, Hackett TE, Sorosky J, Sorosky J, Zaino R. Detection and patterns of treatment failure in 300 consecutive cases of "early" endometrial cancer after primary surgery. Gynecol Oncol 1992; 47:323–327.
12. Reddoch JM, Burke TW, Morris M, Tornos C, Levenbach C, Gershenson DM. Surveillance for recurrent endometrial carcinoma: development of a follow-up scheme. Gynecol Oncol 1995; 59:221–225.
13. Rose PG, Sommers RM, Reale FR, Hunter RE, Fournier L, Nelson BE. Serial serum CA125 measurements for evaluation of recurrence in patients with endometrial carcinoma. Obstet Gynecol 1994; 84:12–16.
14. Shumsky AG, Stuart GCE, Brasher PM, Nation JG, Robertson DI, Sangkarat S. An evaluation of routine follow-up of patients treated for endometrial carcinoma. Gynecol Oncol 1994; 55:229–233.

15. Morice P, Levy-Piedbois C, Ajaj S, Pautier P, Haie-Meder C, Lhomme C, Duvillard P, Castaigne D. Value and cost evaluation of routine follow-up for patients with clinical stage I/II endometrial cancer. Eur J Cancer 2001; 37(8):985–990.
16. Sartori E, Laface B, Gadducci A, Maggino T, Zola P, Landoni F, Zanagnolo V. Factors influencing survival in endometrial cancer relapsing patients: a Cooperation Task Force (CTF) study. Int J Gynecol Cancer 2003; 13:458–465.
17. Ackerman I, Malone S, Thomas G, Franssen E, Balogh J, Dembo A. Endometrial carcinoma—relative effectiveness of adjuvant irradiation vs. therapy reserved for relapse. Gynecol Oncol 1996; 60:177–183.
18. Corn BW, Lanciano RM, D'Agostino R Jr, Kiggundu E, Dunton CJ, Purser P, Greven KM. The relationship of local and distant failure from endometrial cancer: defining a clinical paradigm. Gynecol Oncol 1997; 66:411–416.
19. Barnhill D, O'Connor D, Farley J, Teneriello M, Armstrong D, Park R. Clinical surveillance of gynecologic cancer patients. Gynecol Oncol 1992; 46: 275–280.
20. Cohn DE, Horowitz NS, Mutch DG, Kim SM, Manolitsas T, Fowler JM. Should the presence of lymphvascular space involvement be used to assign patients to adjuvant therapy following hysterectomy for unstaged endometrial cancer? Gynecol Oncol 2002; 87:243–246.

13

The Role of Surgery in Advanced and Relapsed Disease

J. Michael Straughn and Ronald D. Alvarez
Division of Gynecologic Oncology, University of Alabama, Birmingham, Alabama, U.S.A.

IMPORTANCE OF SURGICAL STAGING

The cornerstone of therapy for patients with epithelial endometrial cancer has been surgery, specifically extra-fascial hysterectomy (EH) and bilateral salpingo-oophorectomy. Historically, patients with endometrial cancer were clinically staged and the use of preoperative or postoperative radiation therapy was extremely common. During the 1980s, it became evident that clinical staging understaged a large number of patients with endometrial cancer. In 1988, data from several trials led the International Federation of Gynecology and Obstetrics (FIGO) to recommend a change from clinical staging to surgical staging. Since that time, surgical staging has been more routinely incorporated into the management of women with endometrial cancer. Surgical staging includes EH, bilateral salpingo-oophorectomy, peritoneal cytology, and pelvic and para-aortic lymphadenectomy. This strategy allows one to accurately determine the extent of disease, thus allowing for better assessment of prognosis and for individualization of postoperative therapy. Fortunately, the majority of patients with endometrial cancer have stage I disease (i.e., disease confined to the uterus); however, a subset of these early stage patients, even those who received adjuvant therapy for high-risk factors, will relapse either locally in the pelvis, distantly, or a combination of both. Approximately 25% of all patients with endometrial cancer will have extrauterine disease at the time of diagnosis including metastases to the cervix, adnexa, upper abdomen, and lymph nodes. Distant metastases to the lung, brain, liver, and bone occur more commonly in patients with recurrent disease. The purpose of this chapter is to evaluate the surgical options for patients with advanced and relapsed epithelial cancer of the uterus.

ROLE OF RADICAL HYSTERECTOMY

Some patients with endometrial cancer will present with clinical evidence of disease in the cervix (stage II). Historically, radical hysterectomy (RH) was utilized for patients with clinical stage II disease, but this procedure became less commonly used in this setting because of the high rate of nodal involvement and complications from radical surgery (1). Therefore, preoperative radiation therapy (external radiation and intracavitary radiation) followed by an EH six weeks later became the standard of care for patients with stage II endometrial cancer. This combination therapy was found to have acceptable five-year survival rates (70%) and low morbidity (2,3). Nahhas et al. compared the outcomes of patients who underwent external radiation and intracavitary radiation therapy followed by EH to patients who underwent external radiation therapy only followed by RH. Patients who underwent RH after external radiation therapy had slightly more complications (blood loss and voiding dysfunction) with no improvement in survival (4).

The role of RH for clinical stage II endometrial cancer has been revisited in several recent articles. In contrast to previous reports, several authors have found that RH with bilateral salpingo-oophorectomy and pelvic/para-aortic lymphadenectomy is safe and effective in patients with clinical stage II disease (5–7). An Italian study retrospectively evaluated 203 patients with stage II endometrial cancer (5). One hundred thirty-five patients underwent an EH and bilateral salpingo-oophorectomy and 68 patients underwent a type II modified RH with bilateral salpingo-oophorectomy. Adjuvant radiation therapy was administered to 77% of patients who underwent EH versus 41% of the patients who underwent RH. About 59% of the stage IIA patients and 73% of the stage IIB patients received adjuvant radiation therapy. Five-year overall survival was statistically improved in the patients who underwent RH versus EH (94% vs. 79%; $p < 0.05$). Complication rates were similar between the patients who underwent EH followed by radiation therapy versus RH followed by radiation therapy (12% vs. 25%). Of note, the use of adjuvant radiation therapy (compared to observation) did decrease local recurrence rates (11% vs. 19%) but did not improve five-year overall survival (80% vs. 76%).

In a report of 48 patients with surgical stage II endometrial cancer, there were no recurrences in patients who underwent EH followed by a combination of teletherapy and brachytherapy ($n = 20$) (6). Three of seventeen patients (18%) who underwent EH followed by either teletherapy or brachy-therapy recurred. All patients ($n = 11$) who underwent RH in this same series did not recur, and significant surgical morbidity was not encountered. There-fore, the authors concluded that RH was a reasonable strategy for patients who had clinical evidence of stage II disease at the time of diagnosis.

Mariani et al. reported their experience with stage II patients under-going RH (7). They found that patients who underwent an RH and negative lymphadenectomy did not recur with or without adjuvant radiation therapy. In spite of these encouraging reports of radical surgery for patients with stage II disease, one must realize that many patients may not be good candi-dates for radical surgery due to obesity or other medical comorbidities. Clinically, it can be difficult to distinguish a patient with stage II endome-trial cancer from a patient with stage IB adenocarcinoma of the cervix. A histopathologic evaluation and consultation with a gynecologic pathologist should be performed to determine the origin of the primary; however, even with expert consultation, this may be difficult to determine. Ultimately, the clinical scenario may provide more insight regarding the primary than the histopathologic information. For example, older, more obese patients are more likely to have a primary of the endometrium than of the endocervix. Radical surgery is an excellent option particularly when there is doubt about whether a cervical primary exists.

ROLE OF PRIMARY CYTOREDUCTION IN PATIENTS WITH ADVANCED DISEASE

During the past 25 years, the role of cytoreductive surgery has been incorpo-rated into the management of patients with advanced ovarian cancer. How-ever, the role of debulking in patients with advanced endometrial cancer has been less clear. Vaginal involvement in patients with endometrial cancer is uncommon but some patients will present with vaginal metastases at the time of diagnosis (8). Treatment options for patients with vaginal involvement include either preoperative radiation therapy followed by EH or primary surgery followed by radiation therapy. Patients presenting with significant uterine bleeding and vaginal metastases usually require surgery followed by postoperative radiation therapy in order to control the uterine bleeding in a timely fashion. Several studies have shown that vaginal involvement is an independent predictor of poor prognosis (9). There are no data to suggest that patients with vaginal involvement benefit from radical vaginectomy or pelvic exenteration.

Isolated involvement of the adnexa may be discovered preoperatively or intraoperatively in patients with endometrial cancer. A pathologic evalua-tion is necessary to determine whether disease in the adnexa is primary or metastatic; usually disease in the ovary is metastatic from the endometrium (10). However, patients occasionally will have synchronous primaries of the uterus and the ovary. The most common presentation is a stage I endometrioid adenocarcinoma of the endometrium and ovary. Generally, patients with synchronous isolated primaries of the ovary and endometrium have a favorable prognosis and can be managed without adjuvant therapy particularly when the tumor is well-differentiated (11).

The primary goal of pelvic and para-aortic lymphadenectomy is to determine the presence of metastatic disease in the lymph nodes. At the time of surgical staging, one may discover grossly enlarged lymph nodes. When this situation is encountered, the surgeon may choose to perform a complete pelvic and para-aortic lymphadenectomy to debulk these lymph nodes or may perform a lymph node sampling to simply confirm metastatic disease. Two reports from the University of Minnesota have reported that debulking of macroscopically enlarged lymph nodes improves survival in patients with advanced cervical cancer (12,13). Kilgore et al. reported that with patients with endometrial cancer who underwent lymphadenectomy, both low-risk (stage I) and high-risk patients (stages II and III) had an improvement in survival compared to patients who did not undergo lymphadenectomy (14). Several authors have suggested that patients with grossly enlarged lymph nodes benefit from lymphadenectomy followed by postoperative extended-field radiation therapy (15–17).

Mariani et al. reported a survival benefit in patients with metastatic nodal disease who underwent a complete pelvic and para-aortic lymphadenectomy (18). Fifty-one patients underwent complete surgical staging and were found to have positive pelvic or para-aortic lymph nodes. All patients underwent a pelvic lymphadenectomy; however, 38 patients did not undergo a para-aortic lymphadenectomy while 13 patients did have a formal dissection of the para-aortic lymph nodes (five or more nodes). About 40 (78%) patients received postoperative radiation therapy, four received chemotherapy, and five received hormonal therapy. Five-year overall survival was significantly improved in these patients with nodal metastases who underwent both a pelvic and para-aortic lymphadenectomy compared to patients who underwent a pelvic lymphadenectomy alone (77% vs. 42%; $p = 0.05$). Additionally, five-year recurrence-free survival was also significantly improved in the para-aortic lymphadenectomy group (76% vs. 36%; $p = 0.02$). The authors found that surgical morbidity and long-term complications were not increased in the para-aortic lymphadenectomy group.

On occasion, patients with endometrial cancer will present with gross intraperitoneal disease much like that encountered in patients with ovarian cancer. Investigators from M.D. Anderson Cancer Center have reported their experience with advanced stage adenocarcinoma of the endometrium (19). Thirty-one patients were treated with surgical debulking followed by whole abdominal and pelvic boost radiation therapy. About 27 patients (17 stage III and 10 stage IV) were cytoreduced to a residual disease measuring ≤ 2 cm; the five-year survival for this cohort of patients was 80%. All patients with residual disease >2 cm died from their disease.

In a review of 47 patients with stage IV endometrial cancer, 29 patients underwent a surgical approach with debulking of all gross bulky disease while 18 patients did not undergo surgical resection (20). Using cytotoxic chemotherapy and/or hormonal therapy, the overall survival was 18 months for the patients who underwent surgical cytoreduction versus eight months for those patients who did not undergo surgery ($p = 0.0001$). Of note, the authors did not report the size of the residual disease.

Chi et al. reported their experience at Memorial Sloan-Kettering Cancer Center with 55 stage IV endometrial cancer patients (6 stage IVA and 49 stage IVB) (21). Twenty-four patients (group 1) were optimally cytoreduced to ≤ 2 cm of residual disease, 21 patients (group 2) underwent suboptimal cytoreduction (>2 cm), and 10 patients (group 3) had no cytoreduction performed. There were no statistically significant clinicopathologic differences between the three groups. Ninety-eight percent of patients received some form of postoperative therapy (radiation, chemotherapy, or hormonal therapy). Median survival rates were statistically different for the three groups (31 months—group 1, 12 months—group 2, and 3 months—group 3; $p < 0.01$). The authors concluded that aggressive cytoreduction improved survival in patients with stage IV endometrial cancer.

Bristow et al. reported their experience with 65 patients with stage IVB endometrial carcinoma (22). Optimal cytoreduction, defined as residual tumor ≤ 1 cm in maximal diameter, was accomplished in 36 patients while 29 patients had suboptimal cytoreduction. The median survival rates were 34 and 11 months, respectively ($p = 0.0001$).

Uterine papillary serous carcinoma (UPSC) is an aggressive form of endometrial carcinoma that accounts for approximately 10% of cases. UPSC often behaves clinically like papillary serous adenocarcinoma of the ovary and has a propensity for intraperitoneal spread even with minimal myometrial invasion. Patients with a preoperative endometrial biopsy suggesting UPSC should be considered at high risk for extrauterine disease and should undergo a complete pelvic/para-aortic lymphadenectomy, omentectomy, peritoneal biopsies, and debulking of any intra-abdominal disease. Several authors have reported a survival benefit in patients with advanced UPSC who were able to undergo optimal debulking (23–25). In one series of 43 patients with stage III or stage IV UPSC, patients with microscopic residual disease after surgical debulking had a median survival of 40 months versus 20 months for patients with macroscopic residual disease ($p < 0.001$) (25).

Although these retrospective studies indicate a survival benefit with aggressive cytoreduction, the question remains: Is the benefit the result of tumor biology or surgical effort or some combination therein? It will be difficult to answer this question without randomized, prospective studies; however, the available retrospective data does suggest that the amount of residual disease after surgical debulking impacts survival (Table 1).

Table 1   Results of Cytoreductive Surgery in Patients with Advanced Endometrial
Cancer

Author	Patients	Cytoreductive Status	Survival	p value
Greer et al. (19)	31 Stage III/IV	27—Optimal	5YS—80%	N/A
		4—Suboptimal	5YS—0%	
Goff et al. (20)	47 Stage IV	29—Optimal	18 months	0.0001
		18—Suboptimal	8 months	
Chi et al. (21)	55 Stage IV	24—Optimal	31 months	<0.01
		21—Suboptimal	12 months	
		10—None	3 months	
Bristow et al. (22)	65 Stage IV	36—Optimal	34 months	0.0001
		29—Suboptimal	11 months	

ROLE OF SECONDARY CYTOREDUCTION IN PATIENTS WITH RELAPSED DISEASE

The majority of patients with surgical stage I endometrial cancer will remain disease-free at five years; however, a subset of patients will recur. In a large retrospective study of 513 stage I patients, 239 patients were classified as intermediate risk and 88% of these patients were observed without adjuvant radiation (26). There were 16 recurrences (8%) in this cohort of observed patients; 50% of these patients had an isolated recurrence in the vagina and 88% were salvaged with radiation therapy. Patients with an isolated pelvic recurrence who have not previously been irradiated should be treated with combination radiation therapy (teletherapy and brachytherapy). Salvage rates for patients with recurrent endometrial cancer vary depending on the location of relapse, but survival is excellent for patients with an isolated vaginal recurrence (27–30).

Occasionally, patients will present with isolated, recurrent disease in the pelvis or abdomen. In this setting, a surgical approach can be considered much like that done in patients with isolated recurrent ovarian cancer. An Italian study reported on 20 patients with recurrent endometrial cancer isolated in the pelvis or abdomen (31). Included in this study were patients with large vaginal recurrences (>4 cm) who were not considered candidates for radiation therapy. All patients underwent extensive surgical cytoreduction including bowel resection, omentectomy, vaginectomy, and peritoneal stripping. Thirteen of 20 patients (65%) had all gross disease removed at the time of cytoreduction; local control was achieved in 85% of these patients. The five-year overall survival was 32% in the cohort of patients who underwent cytoreduction versus 0% in the cohort of patients that could not be cytoreduced ($p < 0.05$). Of note, 10% of patients died in the immediate postoperative period. The decision to perform a secondary cytoreduction and subsequent adjuvant therapy has to be highly individualized for the patient with isolated pelvic or abdominal recurrence; however, these data suggest that survival may be prolonged when all disease is removed. Authors have reported surgical resections of metastatic lesions to the lung, liver, and brain; however, patients with distant metastases have poor outcomes in spite of aggressive therapy.

ROLE OF PELVIC EXENTERATION IN PATIENTS WITH RELAPSED DISEASE

In the 1940s, Alexander Brunschwig developed the procedure known as a pelvic exenteration. It was originally developed as a palliative procedure for large pelvic malignancies; however, the indications for this procedure have been modified and limited primarily to patients with a central recurrence of cervical cancer. Patients with endometrial cancer who recur centrally after failing primary surgery and definitive radiation therapy have limited options. Most patients are not able to receive further radiation therapy since the surrounding tissues have already reached their maximum tolerated dose. A small subset of patients with a central recurrence and no evidence of distant metastases may benefit from pelvic exenteration. A multi-institutional study reported on 20 patients with recurrent endometrial cancer who underwent pelvic exenteration with curative intent (32). They reported a five-year disease-free survival of 45% and a major complication rate of 60%. Barakat et al. reported their experience with 44 patients who underwent pelvic exenteration for recurrent endometrial cancer (33). The majority of these patients (77%) had a hysterectomy with bilateral salpingo-oophorectomy as their primary therapy with preoperative or postoperative radiation therapy. Fifty-two percent of patients underwent a total exenteration while 46% of patients had an anterior exenteration performed. Postoperative complications occurred in 80% of patients including urinary/intestinal fistulas, pelvic abscess, sepsis, pulmonary embolus, and cerebrovascular accident. There was one intraoperative death and six postoperative deaths. Median survival was 10 months for the entire group, but there were nine (20%) long-term survivors (>5 years). Although overall long-term survival is poor for patients after exenterative surgery, a small subset of patients may benefit from this procedure.

CONCLUSION

The majority of patients diagnosed with endometrial cancer have an excellent prognosis, but some patients will be faced with the difficulties resulting from advanced or relapsed disease. Surgical staging is critically important to identify patients with advanced disease and some therapeutic benefit from lymphadenectomy may occur, although the outcome of the ongoing A

Study of Endometrial Cancer (ASTEC) trial in the United Kingdom may shed further light on this. RH for selected patients with clinical stage II endometrial cancer should be carefully considered. In patients with metastatic intraperitoneal disease, every effort should be made to render a patient optimally debulked. A small subset of patients with isolated relapsed endometrial cancer may benefit from cytoreduction or pelvic exenteration. Improvements in adjuvant therapies may further clarify the role of surgery in patients with advanced or recurrent endometrial cancer.

REFERENCES

1. Rutledge F. The role of radical hysterectomy in adenocarcinoma of the endometrium. Gynecol Oncol 1974; 2:333–347.
2. Larson DM, Copeland LJ, Gallager HS, Kong JP, Wharton JT, Stringer CA. Stage II endometrial carcinoma: results and complications of a combined radiotherapeutic-surgical approach. Cancer 1988; 61:1528–1534.
3. Kinsella TJ, Bloomer WD, Lavin PT, Knapp RC. Stage II endometrial carcinoma: 10-year follow-up of combined radiation and surgical treatment. Gynecol Oncol 1980; 10:290–297.
4. Nahhas WA, Whitney CW, Stryker JA, Curry SL, Chung CK, Mortel R. Stage II endometrial carcinoma. Gynecol Oncol 1980; 10:303–311.
5. Sartori S, Gadducci A, Landoni F, Lissoni A, Maggino T, Zola P, Zanagnolo V. Clinical behavior of 203 stage II endometrial cancer cases: the impact of primary surgical approach and of adjuvant radiation therapy. Int J Gynecol Cancer 2001; 11:430–437.
6. Eltabbakh GH, Moore AD. Survival of women with surgical stage II endometrial cancer. Gynecol Oncol 1999; 74:80–85.
7. Mariani A, Webb MJ, Keeney GL, Calori G, Podratz KC. Role of wide/radical hysterectomy and pelvic lymph node dissection in endometrial cancer with cervical involvement. Gynecol Oncol 2001; 83:72–80.
8. Mackillop WJ, Pringle JF. Stage III endometrial carcinoma: a review of 90 cases. Cancer 1985; 56:2519–2523.
9. Behbakht K, Yordan EL, Casey C, DeGeest K, Massad LS, Kirschner CV, Wilbanks GD. Prognostic indicators of survival in advanced endometrial cancer. Gynecol Oncol 1994; 55:363–367.
10. Aalders J, Abeler V, Kolstad P. Clinical (stage III) as compared to subclinical intrapelvic extrauterine tumor spread in endometrial carcinoma: a clinical and histpathological study of 175 patients. Gynecol Oncol 1984; 17:64–74.
11. Eifel P, Hendrickson M, Ross J, Ballon S, Martinez A, Kempson R. Simultaneous presentation of carcinoma involving the ovary and uterine corpus. Cancer 1982; 50:163–170.
12. Cosin JA, Fowler JM, Chen MD, Paley PJ, Carson LF, Twiggs LB. Pretreatment surgical staging of patients with cervical carcinoma. Cancer 1998; 82:2241–2248.
13. Downey GO, Potish RA, Adcock LL, Prem KA, Twiggs LB. Pretreatment surgical staging in cervical carcinoma: therapeutic efficacy of pelvic lymph node dissection. Am J Gynecol Oncol 1989; 160:1055–1061.

14. Kilgore LC, Partridge EE, Alvarez RD, Austin JM, Shingleton HM, Noojin F, Conner W. Adenocarcinoma of the endometrium: survival comparisons of patients with and without pelvic node sampling. Gynecol Oncol 1995; 56:29–33.
15. Corn BW, Lanciano RM, Greven KM, Schultz DJ, Reisinger SA, Stafford PM, Hanks GM. Endometrial cancer with para-aortic adenopathy: patterns of failure and opportunities for cure. Int J Radiat Oncol Biol Phys 1992; 24:223–227.
16. Rose PG, Cha SD, Tak WK, Fitzgerald T, Reale F, Hunter RE. Radiation therapy for surgically proven para-aortic node metastasis in endometrial carcinoma. Int J Radiat Oncol Biol Phys 1992; 24:229–233.
17. Feuer GA, Calanog A. Endometrial carcinoma: treatment of positive para-aortic nodes. Gynecol Oncol 1987; 27:104–109.
18. Mariani A, Webb MJ, Galli L, Podratz KC. Potential therapeutic role of para-aortic lymphadenectomy in node-positive endometrial cancer. Gynecol Oncol 2000; 76:348–356.
19. Greer BE, Hamberger AD. Treatment of intraperitoneal metastatic adenocarcinoma of the endometrium by the whole-abdomen moving-strip technique and pelvic boost irradiation. Gynceol Oncol 1983; 16:165–173.
20. Goff BA, Goodman AK, Muntz HG, Fuller AF, Nikrui N, Rice LW. Surgical stage IV endometrial carcinoma: a study of 47 patients. Gynecol Oncol 1994; 52:237–240.
21. Chi DS, Welshinger M, Venkatraman ES, Barakat RR. The role of surgical cytoreduction in stage IV endometrial carcinoma. Gynecol Oncol 1997; 67:56–60.
22. Bristow RE, Zerbe MJ, Rosenshein NB, Grumbine FC, Montz FJ. Stage IVB endometrial carcinoma: the role of cytoreductive surgery and determinants of survival. Gynecol Oncol 2000; 78:85–91.
23. Bristow RE, Asrari F, Trimble EL, Montz FJ. Extended surgical staging for uterine papillary serous carcinoma: survival outcome of locoregional (stages I–III) disease. Gynecol Oncol 2001; 81:279–286.
24. Bristow RE, Duska LR, Montz FJ. The role of cytoreductive surgery in the management of stage IV uterine papillary serous carcinoma. Gynecol Oncol 2001; 81:92–99.
25. Memarzadeh S, Holschneider CH, Bristow RE, Jones NL, FU YS, Karlan BY, Berek JS, Farias-Eisner R. FIGO stages II and IV uterine papillary serous carcinoma: impact of residual disease on survival. Int J Gynecol Cancer 2002; 12:454–458.
26. Straughn JM, Huh WK, Kelly FJ, Leath CA, Kleinberg MJ, Hyde J, Numnum TM, Zhang Y, Soong SJ, Austin JM, Partridge EE, Kilgore LC, Alvarez RD. Conservative management of Stage I endometrial carcinoma after surgical staging. Gynecol Oncol 2002; 84:194–200.
27. Ackerman I, Malone S, Thomas G, Franssen E, Balogh J, Dembo A. Endometrial carcinoma—relative effectiveness of adjuvant irradiation versus therapy reserved for relapse. Gynecol Oncol 1996; 60:177–183.
28. Pirtoli L, Ciatto S, Cionini L, Taddei G, Colafranceschi M. Salvage with radiotherapy of postsurgical relapses of endometrial cancer. Tumori 1980; 66:475–480.

29. Mandell L, Nori D, Hilaris B. Recurrent stage I endometrial carcinoma: results of treatment and prognostic factors. Int J Radiat Oncol Biol Phys 1985; 11:1103–1109.
30. Poulsen M, Roberts S. The salvage of recurrent endometrial carcinoma in the vagina and pelvis. Int J Radiat Oncol Biol Phys 1988; 15:809–813.
31. Scarabelli S, Campagnutta E, Giorda G, DePiero G, Sopracordevole F, Quaranta M, DeMarco L. Maximal cytoreductive surgery as a reasonable therapeutic alternative for recurrent endometrial carcinoma. Gynecol Oncol 1998; 70:90–93.
32. Morris M, Alvarez RD, Kinney WK, Wilson TO. Treatment of recurrent adenocarcinoma of the endometrium with pelvic exenteration. Gynecol Oncol 1996; 60:288–291.
33. Barakat RR, Goldman NA, Patel DA, Venkatraman ES, Curtin JP. Pelvic exenteration for recurrent endometrial cancer. Gynecol Oncol 1999; 75:99–102.

14

Endometrial Carcinoma and Hormone Replacement Therapy

Michael S. Marsh

Guy's, Kings, and St. Thomas' Medical School, London, U.K.

ENDOMETRIAL CANCER AND UNOPPOSED ESTROGEN USE

The relationship between unopposed estrogen use and endometrial cancer has been firmly established over the last 30 years by numerous experimental and epidemiological studies (1–6). The relative risks from different studies vary widely: the overall estimated increase in relative risk for users compared with nonusers from a recent meta-analysis was reported as 2.3 [95% confidence interval (CI) 2.1–2.5], with a much higher risk ratio (RR) associated with prolonged duration of use (RR 9.5 for 10 or more years) (7). Unsurprisingly, the incidence of endometrial hyperplasia is increased in postmenopausal women on unopposed estrogen therapy, with an incidence of approximately 15–20% per year (3,8,9).

The risk of developing the disease appears to be proportional to the duration of estrogen therapy. After 10 years of estrogen replacement therapy (ERT), the risk is elevated about 10-fold compared to that in a lifetime nonuser (10). However, unopposed oral estrogens may have a rapid effect on the endometrium and have been reported to produce precancerous endometrial lesions such as endometrial hyperplasia in only a few months. The progression of such lesions to cancer may take place in only a few years (11).

The risk of endometrial cancer with oral unopposed estrogens may not be avoided by using low-dose preparations or less potent estrogens.

Long-term administration of oral unopposed low-dose estrogens (0.3 mg conjugated equine estrogens) has been reported to cause a five-fold increase in the risk of endometrial cancer (12).

The use of unopposed biologically weak estrogens such as estriol given orally also appears to increase the risk of endometrial cancer although in contrast to stronger estrogens, the effect may subside soon after ceasing the treatment. In a Swedish nationwide population-based case–control study, detailed information on hormone replacement was obtained from 789, cases of endometrial cancer and 3368 controls (13). After multivariate adjustment, oral use of estriol 1–2 mg daily was reported to increase the relative risk of both endometrial cancer and endometrial atypical hyperplasia: the odds ratios for at least five years of use compared with never-use were 3.0 (95% CI 2.0–4.4) and 8.3 (4.0–17.4), respectively. The excess relative risk was lost rapidly after cessation of treatment. Women who stopped exposure more than one year before the index date (six months before diagnosis) had no discernible increase in relative risk compared with those who had never used estriol. This study may have been weakened by recall and detection bias. In contrast, another cohort study did not find endometrial proliferation with an oral dose of 2 mg estriol given daily (14).

Modifying the regimen of estrogen administration does not appear to reduce the added risk. Both interrupted and continuous estrogen administration are associated with endometrial abnormalities (15). For example, interrupting estrogen treatment for 5–7 days/mo is not associated with lower risk than daily use (7).

Although the risk of developing endometrial cancer decreases in a time-dependent manner after cessation of ERT, the residual excess risk even after short term unopposed use of potent estrogens may remain for many years. In a case–control study of the risk of adenocarcinoma of the endometrium and conjugated estrogen use, it was reported that in women who had used estrogen for at least one year and then discontinued treatment, the risk of endometrial cancer remained significantly elevated even after estrogen-free intervals of over 10 years (10). Pooled data suggest that women who have taken conjugated estrogen for one or more years may remain at increased risk for at least 15 years after they discontinue use, and that such women should be considered for long-term gynecologic surveillance (4,6,10,16–19).

VAGINAL ESTROGEN TREATMENT

The association of unopposed vaginal estrogen with increased endometrial cancer risk has been known for more than 20 years. In an early hospital-based case–control study of the epidemiology of endometrial cancer in women aged 45–74 years, Kelsey et al. (20) reported an increase in endometrial cancer risk with vaginal estrogen use, but did not have information about type or duration.

It is clear that for more potent estrogens such as estradiol and conjugated equine estrogen (CEE), the risk is dependent on the dose and type of estrogen used. Conjugated equine estrogen cream given at 1.25 mg/day will produce levels of estradiol and estrone similar to the same dose given orally, and are likely to have the same effects on the endometrium as oral treatment. However, when given at a lower dose (0.1 mg/day), it will not cause a detectable rise in plasma estrogen levels (21).

However, the effect on risk of dosage and type of estrogen with less potent estrogens such as estriol is less clear. Only weak associations were observed between vaginal application of low-potency estrogen formulations and relative risk of endometrial neoplasia in the Swedish nationwide population-based case–control study mentioned above (13). Use of vaginally administered low-potency estrogen formulations was reported by 14.7% of cases and 11.3% of controls. About 49% of vaginal treatment episodes consisted of estriol (0.5 mg), 44% dienoestrol (0.5 mg), and 7% estradiol (25 g). After multivariate adjustment, the odds ratio associated with ever-use was 1.2 (95% CI 1.0–1.6). In the multivariate analysis, use of vaginal oestriol (used by 49 cases and 195 controls) gave an odds ratio of 1.1 (0.8–1.6), and vaginal dienoestrol (used by 46 cases and 188 controls) an odds ratio of 1.0 (0.7–1.5) compared with never-use of these formulations, suggesting no difference in effect between these two preparations. This is in contrast to data that suggest dienoestrol is a more potent estrogen.

An analysis of the use of vaginal estriol in 12 published studies (214 subjects) that provided acceptable biopsy data suggested that single daily treatment with unopposed intravaginal estriol in the recommended doses in postmenopausal women is safe and does not cause an increased risk of endometrial proliferation or hyperplasia (22).

It is clear that potent estrogens such as conjugated equine estrogens and estradiol at sufficient dose are likely to produce effects on the endometrium that are similar to oral administration. What is less clear is whether weaker unopposed intravaginal estrogens such as estriol may have the same effect. Current information suggests that if weaker intravaginal estrogens do have an effect to increase endometrial cancer risk, it is likely to be numerically very small.

THE ADDITION OF PROGESTOGENS

Progesterone has a well-established anti-estrogenic effect on the endometrium. In an estrogen-primed endometrium, progestogens down-regulate nuclear estrogen receptors by inhibiting receptor synthesis and accelerating their turnover, and down-regulate the genes required for epithelial growth, leading to reduced epidermal growth factor production. They promote differentiation of glands and stroma, decidualization, and secretory activity of the endometrium; increase blood vessel volume; and stimulate secretion of insulin growth factor binding protein 1. Progestogens also stimulate 17-hydroxysteroid dehydrogenase production, which converts 17-beta estradiol (17-E2) to the weaker estrogen, estrone sulphate, and induce endometrial sloughing and uterine bleeding. Adding a progestogen to ERT is mandatory to avoid endometrial hyperstimulation in women with an intact uterus. Except in some cases of women with endometriosis, progestogens should not be used in hormone replacement therapy (HRT) after hysterectomy. In the rare cases when progestogen use is contemplated in hysterectomized women, the likely unfavorable effects on breast cancer and cardiovascular disease risk should be considered.

The histological changes produced by progestogens are dose and duration dependent. In a 28-day estrogen regimen, progestogen supplementation for less than 10 days/mo has been shown to be associated with an elevated risk of endometrial abnormalities compared to that in a nonuser, while the use of a progestin for 10–12 days or more per month, depending on its potency and half life, decreases the excess risk (23). The currently recommended duration of progestogens to protect the endometrium is 12–14 days each month (24). The minimum dosages of various progestogens, which provide endometrial protection when added for at least 12 days each month have been established and are incorporated into commercially available sequential HRT preparations, e.g., norethindrone acetate (NETA) 0.7–1.0 mg, levonogestrel (LNG) 0.150 mg, medroxyprogesterone acetate (MPA) 5–10 mg, dydrogesterone 10–20 mg, and micronized progesterone 200 mg. LNG and NETA are also delivered via a skin patch (Table 1).

Long-cycle HRT regimens, in which progestogens are added to continuous estrogens every two or three months have been shown to be associated

Table 1 Examples of Commercially Available Sequential HRT Estrogen/Progestogen Combinations

Estrogen	Progestogen	Formulation
Estradiol, 2 mg	Norethisterone, 1 mg	Tabs
Estradiol, 1/2 mg	Levonorgestrel, 0.25/0.5 mg	Tabs
Estradiol, 1/2 mg	Dydrogesterone, 10 mg	Tabs
Estradiol, 2 mg	Dydrogesterone, 20 mg	Tabs
Estradiol, 50 µg	Norethisterone, 1 mg	Patches + Tabs
Estradiol, 50 µg	Norethisterone, 170 µg	Patches
Estradiol, 40/80 µg	Dydrogesterone, 10 mg	Patches + Tabs
Estradiol, 2 mg	Medroxyprogesterone acetate, 20 mg	Tabs
Conj. equine estrogens 0.625 mg	Medroxyprogesterone acetate, 10 mg	Tabs
Conj. equine estrogens 0.625/1.25 mg	Norgestrel, 150 µg	Tabs

with an increased risk of endometrial hyperplasia (25). Such regimens should be used with caution and the endometrium should be carefully monitored during treatment. It is not known whether long-cycle therapy elevates the risk of endometrial carcinoma after treatment is stopped, as occurs with unopposed estrogen.

It is likely that the majority of commercially available sequential HRT preparations do not cause any clinically significant increase in the risk of endometrial carcinoma. However, many studies concerning uterine safety of different available preparations are not placebo-controlled and are of short duration. The randomized placebo-controlled postmenopausal estrogen/progestin interventions (PEPI) trial studied sequential E-P treatment and demonstrated an endometrial protective effect of 10 mg daily of MPA or 200 mg daily of micronized progesterone for 12 days/mo added to CEE 0.625 mg over a three-year period (26). Other studies have demonstrated endometrial safety of sequential 5 mg MPA monthly over one year and cyclic addition of 10 mg dydrogesterone to 2 mg oral 17-E2 daily over two years (27–29).

Longer-term studies of sequential HRT using endometrial cancer as the endpoint have produced conflicting results. The case–control study of Pike et al. (23) found a nearly twofold increased risk for endometrial cancer associated with cyclic HRT regimens if progestogens were used for fewer than 10 days/mo, but no increased risk among women who took progestogens for longer duration. In contrast, Beresford et al. demonstrated a trend towards an increase in endometrial cancer risk with time, even among those women who took 10 mg of MPA daily for 10 or more days per month. Women who used any sequential therapy in any form had a relative risk of endometrial cancer of 1.4 (1.0–1.9). Among women using less than 10 days of added progestogen per month, the relative risk was 3.1 (1.7–5.7), whereas that for women with 10–21 days of added progestogen was 1.3 (0.8–2.2). However, use of these regimens for five or more years was associated with risks of 3.7 (1.7–8.2) and 2.5 (1.1–5.5), respectively, relative to nonusers of hormones (30).

Weiderpass et al. demonstrated an increased endometrial cancer risk with sequential HRT, a risk which was confined to women with fewer than 16 days of progestogens per cycle (RR for >5 years of use = 1.6; 95% CI = 1.1–2.4) (31). In this study 81% of subjects received progestogen treatment for 10 days, which does not reflect the currently commonly used regimens, which incorporate 12–14 days of progestin therapy.

Studies of the effects of continuous combined HRT, in which estrogens and progestogens are both given daily (Table 2), show very low or zero rates of endometrial hyperplasia (26,32,33). In contrast to the studies of sequential therapy, where current data suggest no effect on endometrial cancer risk, or a very slight increase, continuous combined HRT appears to reduce the risk (31,34). In the case–control study of Weiderpass et al.

Table 2 Examples of Commercially Available Continuous Combined HRT Estrogen/
Progestogen Combinations

Estrogen	Progestogen	Formulation
Estradiol, 2 mg	Norethisterone, 1 mg	Tabs
Estradiol, 2 mg	Norethisterone, 0.7 mg	Tabs
Estradiol, 1 mg	Dydrogesterone, 5 mg	Tabs
Estradiol, 50 µg	Norethisterone, 170 µg	Patches
Estradiol, 1/2 mg	Medroxyprogesterone acetate, 2.5/5 mg	Tabs
Conj. equine estrogens 0.625 mg	Medroxyprogesterone acetate, 5 mg	Tabs

(31), 46.6% of women had used continuous estrogen–progestin. Five or more years of treatment gave an odds ratio $= 0.2$ (95% CI $= 0.1$–0.8).

Data from Women's Health Initiative (WHI), a randomized controlled HRT primary prevention trial of 16,608 postmenopausal women aged 50–79 years taking placebo or 0.625 mg CEE+2.5 mg medroxyprogesterone acetate per day, demonstrated that endometrial cancer rates were not increased by five years of this continuous combined hormone therapy (34). The estimated hazards ratio for endometrial cancer was 0.83 (95% CI $= 0.47$–1.47).

Both the WHI and Heart and Estrogen Progest in Replacement Study (HERS) II studies used the same continuous combined therapy (0.625 mg CEE+2.5 mg medroxyprogesterone acetate per day). Combined data from both studies shows 24 endometrial cancer cases in the HRT groups versus 30 in the placebo groups, corresponding to a pooled relative risk of 0.76 (95% CI $= 0.45$–1.31) (34–36).

TIBOLONE AND ENDOMETRIAL CANCER RISK

Tibolone is a synthetic steroid with estrogenic, androgenic, and progestogenic properties which is used as an alternative to estrogen receptor protein (ERP).

Tibolone becomes biologically active after its breakdown into three metabolites: 3-OH-tibolone, 3-OH-tibolone, and delta 4-ketoisomer. The first two metabolites bind only to estrogen receptors, whereas the last has an affinity for progesterone and androgen receptors. In the endometrium, tibolone is transformed into the metabolite delta-4-isomer by 3–hydroxysteroid dehydrogenase isomerase. This metabolite has intrinsic progestogenic activity and causes minimal stimulation of the endometrial tissue (37).

Satisfactory long-term data on the effects of tibolone on the risk of endometrial cancer are unavailable, but short-term endometrial studies suggest that the likely effect is neutral or protective (38,39).

Volker (37) studied 150 healthy postmenopausal women treated with 2.5 mg/day of tibolone and found no biopsy evidence of stimulation of the endometrium in 98.2% and 91.9% of subjects at 12 and 24 months, respectively. A change from an atrophic to a weak proliferative pattern was observed in 1.8% at 12 months, increasing to 6.5% after two years of continuous use. One case of endometrial hyperplasia was detected and no cancer was seen.

Von Dadelszen et al. (38) reported three cases of endometrial carcinoma, one case of atypical hyperplasia, and two of simple hyperplasia on patients taking tibolone for an average of 12 months (range 7–18). These were the only six cases known to have occurred in an estimated population of 1732 women taking tibolone at the time.

SELECTIVE ESTROGEN RECEPTOR MODULATORS (SERMs)

Antiestrogens act as partial estrogen antagonists. They bind to and compete with endogenous estrogen for estrogen receptors in the nuclei of estrogen-responsive tissues. In clinical practice, antiestrogens are used for ovulation induction (clomiphene), for the treatment or prevention of breast cancer (tamoxifen and toremifene), and can be used as an alternative to HRT for the prevention of osteoporosis (e.g., raloxifene).

It is well established that tamoxifen is associated with an increased risk of endometrial cancer in women (39,40) with reports demonstrating a 2–5 fold increase (40–44). In contrast, the available reports on raloxifene suggest that it has no proliferating or carcinogenic action on human endometrium (45–47). A recent report combined two identically designed, prospective, double-blinded five-year trials including postmenopausal women (mean age, 55 years) randomly assigned to either placebo ($n = 143$) or raloxifene (60 mg/day; $n = 185$). The endometrium was assessed by transvaginal ultrasonography or biopsy and clinical diagnoses of endometrial hyperplasia or endometrial cancer were confirmed by blinded review of histopathology reports. The incidence of mean endometrial thickness of more than 5 mm did not differ between the two groups. No diagnoses of endometrial hyperplasia or endometrial cancer were made in either treatment group (47).

ERT USE IN WOMEN WITH PREVIOUS ENDOMETRIAL CARCINOMA

Clinicians are understandably reluctant to administer ERP therapy in patients treated for endometrial cancer. A chief concern is that an occult or quiescent focus of metastatic disease could be activated by estrogen therapy. However, nonrandomized, uncontrolled studies involving more than 250 women treated with estrogens have shown no increased risk of recurrence in selected low-risk endometrial cancer survivors treated with HRT (48–52).

Creasman et al. (48) reported follow-up of 47 selected women (of a total of 220 treated women) who had received estrogen after their cancer therapy. Risk factors for recurrence were reported to be similar between the two groups. After controlling for these known risk factors, the estimated distributions of time to recurrence for the two groups showed a longer disease-free survival within the estrogen group.

Lee et al. (49) undertook a retrospective analysis of 144 patients with clinical stage I endometrial adenocarcinoma who were treated over an 11-year period. After surgical staging, 44 selected patients were placed on oral ERT for a median duration of 64 months. Patients treated with ERT had low-risk factors for recurrence, e.g., low tumor grade (grades 1 and 2), less than 1/2 myometrial invasion, and no metastases to lymph nodes or other organs. In these women, there were no recurrent endometrial cancers and no intercurrent deaths. Chapman et al. (50) performed a retrospective review of 123 women with surgical stage I and II endometrial adenocarcinoma treated between 1984 and 1994; 62 received ERP after treatment. The ERT group had earlier stage disease ($p = 0.04$) and less severe depth of invasion ($p = 0.003$) than those not given treatment. The total number of deaths in each group was not different. The overall recurrence rate was 6.5%, with an overall death rate of 1.6%. The disease-free survival did not differ between the groups.

More recently, Surriano et al. (51) reported results from 249 women with surgical stage I, II, and III endometrial cancer who were treated between 1984 and 1998; 130 received estrogen replacement after their primary cancer treatments. Forty-nine percent received progesterone in addition to estrogen. Among the cohort, 75 matched treatment-control pairs were identified. The two groups were matched by using decade of age at diagnosis and stage of disease. Both groups were comparable in terms of parity, grade of tumor, depth of invasion, histology, surgical treatment, lymph node status, postoperative radiation, and concurrent diseases. The HRT users were followed for a mean interval of 83 months and the non-HRT users for a mean of 69 months. For the 75 women who received estrogen replacement, 57% initiated hormonal supplementation within six months of primary surgery (mean interval, 2.2 months). Within one year of follow-up, an additional 16% of the subjects were taking HRT; the remaining 27% were started on HRT later (range, 1.1–5.0 years). Most patients used a daily dose of 0.625 mg oral conjugated equine estrogens. Medroxyprogesterone 2.5 mg/day acetate was routinely offered to women taking HRT, and 49% of the subjects elected to include this medication in their daily regimen. There were two recurrences (1%) among the 75 estrogen users compared with 11 (14%) recurrences in the 75 non-HRT users. Hormone users had a statistically significant longer disease-free interval than non-HRT users ($p = 0.006$). Because the number of recurrences among the current hormone users was small ($n = 2$), the data were insufficient to examine any effects of progestogen on disease-free interval or disease-free survival.

A criticism common to all the available studies of the effects of estrogen on endometrial cancer recurrence is that selection bias may have profoundly affected the results. It is possible and likely that women who were deemed low risk for recurrence were more likely to have been offered estrogens. However, it appears that for women who have had early stage low-grade endometrial cancer treatment, HRT could be considered for patients suffering from menopausal symptoms. Such women should be made aware of the current deficiencies in our knowledge of its effects.

SUMMARY POINTS

Unopposed exposure to exogenous estrogens, whether interrupted or continuous, increases the risk of endometrial cancer.

The risk of developing endometrial cancer is proportional to the dose and duration of estrogen therapy.

Adding a progestogen to ERT will reduce the risk of endometrial hyperstimulation in women with an intact uterus, and addition of an appropriate dose of a progestin for an adequate time significantly reduces the incidence of endometrial cancer associated with ERT.

For sequential progestogen administration, the duration of progestogen use is at least as important as the dose and needs to be administered for 12–14 days or more per month.

Tibolone and raloxifene do not appear to increase the risk of endometrial carcinoma in postmenopausal women.

For women who have completed appropriate treatment for early stage low-grade endometrial cancer, HRT could be considered for patients suffering from menopausal symptoms after alternative treatments and the unknown risks of HRT have been discussed.

There is a wide variety of estrogens and progestins used in different doses and via different routes of administration. Different estrogens do not show the same bioavailability and tissue effects. Data available at the moment do not take into account all these variations, and it may be inappropriate to extrapolate from known effects of one HRT type to another. Women should be made aware of this diversity of effect when HRT and cancer of the endometrium are discussed.

REFERENCES

1. Beral V, Banks E, Reeves G. Evidence from randomised trials on the long-term effects of hormone replacement therapy. Lancet 2002; 360:942–944.
2. Beral V, Banks E, Reeves G, Appleby P. Use of HRT and the subsequent risk of cancer. J Epidemiol Biostat 1999; 4:191–210.
3. Lethaby A, Farquhar C, Sarkis A, et al. Hormone replacement therapy in postmenopausal women: endometrial hyperplasia and irregular bleeding. Cochrane Database Syst Rev 2000; 2:CD000402.

4.   Jick SS, Walker AM, Jick H. Estrogens, progesterone, and endometrial cancer. Epidemiology 1993; 4:20–24.
5.   Antunes CM, Strolley PD, Rosenshein NB, et al. Endometrial cancer and estrogen use: report of a large case–control study. N Engl J Med 1979; 300:9–13.
6.   Brinton LA, Hoover RN. Estrogen replacement therapy and endomctrial cancer risk: unresolved issues. The Endometrial Cancer Collaborative Group. Obstet Gynecol 1993; 81:265–271.
7.   Grady D, Gebretsadik T, Kerlikowske K, Ernster V, Petitti D. Hormone replacement therapy and endometrial cancer risk: a meta-analysis. Obstet Gynecol 1995; 85(2):304–313.
8.   Ferenczy A, Gelfand M. The biologic significance of cytological atypia in progestogen-treated endometrial hyperplasia. Am J Obstet Gynecol 1989; 160:126–131.
9.   Hill DA, Weiss NS, Beresford SA, et al. Continuous combined hormone replacement therapy and risk of endometrial cancer. Am J Obstet Gynecol 2000; 183:1456–1461.
10. Shapiro S, Kelly JP, Rosenberg L, et al. Risk of localized and widespread endometrial cancer in relation to recent and discontinued use of conjugated estrogens. N Engl J Med 1985; 313:969–972.
11. Kurman RJ, Kaminski PF, Norris HJ. The behaviour of endometrial hyperplasia. A long-term review of untreated hyperplasia in 170 patients. Cancer 1985; 56:403–412.
12. Cushing KL, Weiss NS, Voigt LF, et al. Risk of endometrial cancer in relation to use of low-dose, unopposed estrogens. Obstet Gynecol 1998; 91:35–39.
13. Weiderpass E, Baron JA, Adami HO, et al. Low-potency oestrogen and risk of endometrial cancer: a case–control study. Lancet 1999; 353:1824–1828.
14. Persson I, Yuen J, Bergkvist L, Schairer C. Cancer incidence and mortality in women receiving estrogen and estrogen-progestin replacement therapy—long-term follow-up of a Swedish cohort. Int J Cancer 1996; 67:327–332.
15. Shiff I, Sela HK, Cramer D, et al. Endometrial hyperplasia in women on cyclic or continuous estrogen regimens. Fertil Steril 1982; 37, 79–82.
16. Hulka BS, Fowler WC Jr, Kaufman DG, et al. Estrogen and endometrial cancer: cases and two control groups from North Carolina. Am J Obset Gynecol 1980; 137:92–101.
17. Mack TM, Pike MC, Hjenderson BE, et al. Estrogens and endometrial cancer in a retirement community. N Engl J Med 1976; 294:1262–1267.
18. Rubin GL, Peterson HB, Lee NC, et al. Estrogen replacement therapy and the risk of endometrial cancer: remaining controversies. Am J Obstet Gynecol 1990; 162:148–154.
19. Stavraky KM, Collins JA, Donner A, Wells GA. A comparison of estrogen use by women with endometrial cancer, gynecologic disorders, and other illnesses. Am J Obstet Gynecol 1981; 141:547–555.
20. Kelsey JL. LiVolsi VA. Holford TR, et al. A case–control study of cancer of the endometrium. Am J Epidemiol 1982; 116:333–342.
21. Dyer GI, Young O, Townsend PT, Collins WP, Whitehead MI, Jelowitz J. Dose-related changes in vaginal cytology after topical conjugated equine oestrogens. Br Med J 1982; 284:789.

22. Vooijs GP, Geurts TBP. Review of the endometrial safety during intravaginal treatment with estriol. Eur J Obstet Gynecol. 1995; 62:101–106.
23. Pike MC, Peters RK, Cozen W, et al. Estrogen-progestin replacement therapy and endometrial cancer. J Natl Cancer Inst 1997; 89:1110–1116.
24. Grady D, Ernster VL. Hormone replacement therapy and endometrial cancer: are current regimens safe? J Natl Cancer Inst 1997; 89:1088–1089
25. The Scandinavian Long Cycle Study Group, Bjarnason K, Cerin A, Lindgren R, Weber T. Adverse endometrial effects during long cycle hormone replacement therapy. Maturitas 1999; 32:61–170.
26. The Writing Group for the PEPI Trial, Effects of HRT on endometrial histology in postmenopausal women. The PEPI trial. J Am Med Assoc 1996; 275:370–375.
27. Woodruff JD, Pickar JH. Incidence of endometrial hyperplasia in postmenopausal women taking conjugated estrogens (Premarin) with medroxyprogesterone acetate versus conjugated estrogens alone. Am J Obstet Gynecol 1994; 170:1213–1223.
28. Ferenczy A, Gelfand MM. Endometrial histology and bleeding patterns in postmenopausal women taking sequential, combined E2 and dydrogesterone. Maturitas 1997; 26:219–226.
29. Van der Mooren MJ, Hanselaar AGJM, Borm GF, et al. Changes in the withdrawal bleeding pattern and endometrial histology during 17-estradiol-dydrogesterone therapy in postmenopausal women: a 2-year prospective study. Maturitas 1995; 20:175–180.
30. Beresford SA, Weiss NS, Voigt LF, et al. Risk of endometrial cancer in relation to use of oestrogen combined with cyclic progestagen therapy in postmenopausal women. Lancet 1997; 349:458–461.
31. Weiderpass E, Adami HO, Baron JA, et al. Risk of endometrial cancer following estrogen replacement with and without progestins. J Natl Cancer Inst 1999; 91:1131–1137.
32. Hawthorn RJS, Spowart K, Walsh D, et al. The endometrial status of women on long-term continuous combined hormone replacement therapy. Br J Obstet Gynaecol 1991; 98:939–940.
33. Piegsa K, Calder A, Davis JA, et al. Endometrial status in postmenopausal women on long term continuous combined HRT (Kliofem). A comparative study of endometrial biopsy, outpatient hysteroscopy and TVU. Eur J Obstet Gynecol 1997; 72:175–180.
34. Writing Group for the Women's Health Initiative Investigators. Risks and benefits of estrogen plus progestin in healthy post-menopausal women: principal results from the Women's Health Initiative randomized controlled trial. J Am Med Assoc 2002; 288:321–333.
35. Hulley S, Furberg C, Barrett-Connor E, et al. Noncardiovascular disease outcomes during 6.8 years of hormone therapy: Heart and Estrogen/progestin Replacement Study follow-up (HERS II). JAMA 2002; 288:58 66.
36. Collaborative Group on Hormonal Factors in Breast Cancer. Breast cancer and hormone replacement therapy: collaborative reanalysis of data from 51 epidemiological studies of 52,705 women with breast cancer and 108,411 women without breast cancer. Lancet 1997; 350:1047–1059.

37. Volker W. Effects of Tibolone on the endometrium. Climateric 2001; 4(3):203–208.
38. von Dadelszen P, Gillmer MD, Gray MD, et al. Endometrial hyperplasia and adenocarcinoma during tibolone (Livial) therapy. Br J Obstet Gynaecol 1994; 101(2):158–161.
39. White NH. The tamoxifen dilemma. Carcinogenesis 1999; 20:1153–1160.
40. IARC. Tamoxifen. In: Some pharmaceutical drugs. Lyon: IARC. 1996:253–365.
41. Rutqvist LE, Johansson H, Signomklao T, et al. Adjuvant tamoxifen therapy for early stage breast cancer and second primary malignancies: Stockholm Breast Cancer Study Group. J Natl Cancer Inst 1995; 87:645–651.
42. Poirier D, Auger S, Merand Y, Simard J, Labrie F. Synthesis and antiestrogenic activity of diaryl thioether derivatives. J Med Chem 1994; 37:1115–1125.
43. Curtis RE, Boice JD Jr, Shriner DA, Hankey BF, Fraumeni JF Jr. Second cancers after adjuvant tamoxifen therapy for breast cancer. J Natl Cancer Inst 1996; 88:832–834.
44. Fisher B, Constantino JP, Wickerham DL, et al. Tamoxifen for prevention of breast cancer: report of the National Surgical Adjuvant Breast and Bowel Project P-1 study. J Natl Cancer Inst 1998; 90:1371–1388.
45. Cummings SR, Eckert S, Krueger KA. The effects of raloxifene on risk of breast cancer in postmenopausal women. JAMA 1999; 281:2189–2197.
46. Kauffman RF, Bryant HU, Yang N, et al. Preventing postmenopausal osteoporosis: an update on raloxifene. Drug News Perspect 1999; 12:223–233.
47. Jolly EE, Bjarnason NH, Neven P, Plouffe L Jr, Johnston CC Jr, Watts SD, Arnaud CD, Mason TM, Crans G, Akers R, Draper MW. Prevention of osteoporosis and uterine effects in postmenopausal women taking raloxifene for 5 years. Menopause 2003; 10(4):337–344.
48. Creasman WT, Henderson D, Hinshaw W, Clarke-Pearson DL. Estrogen replacement therapy in the patient treated for endometrial cancer. Obstet Gynecol 1986; 67:326–330.
49. Lee RB, Burke TW, Park RC. Estrogen replacement therapy following treatment for stage I endometrial carcinoma. Gynecol Oncol 1990; 36:189–191.
50. Chapman JA, DiSaia PJ, Osann K, et al. Estrogen replacement in surgical stage I and II endometrial cancer survivors. Am J Gynecol 1996; 175: 1195–1200.
51. Surriano KA, McHale M, McLaren CE, et al. Estrogen replacement therapy in endometrial cancer patients: a matched control study. Obster Gynecol 2001; 97:555–560.

15

Future Developments in Radiation Therapy for Endometrial Carcinoma

Carien L. Creutzberg

Department of Clinical Oncology, Leiden University Medical Center, Leiden, The Netherlands

Jan G. Aalders

Department of Gynecological Oncology, University Medical Center Groningen, Groningen, The Netherlands

The role of radiotherapy (RT) for endometrial carcinoma has evolved over the course of many years, from being the mainstay of treatment before the era of modern surgical techniques to an adjunctive to surgery based on the presence of adverse prognostic factors. The need to tailor the indication for RT to prognostic factors became increasingly clear when many authors recognized the disadvantages in terms of morbidity of possible overtreatment for the large majority of low-risk endometrial cancers. In Chapter 9 an overview of the indications for RT and standards of treatment has been given. In this chapter the current developments and major controversies are discussed, which are relevant to future perspectives in the treatment of endometrial cancer.

Current trends and fields of research on radiotherapy in endometrial carcinoma include:

1. Reducing indications for pelvic RT,
2. The role of lymphadenectomy and its combination with RT,
3. The increasing use of brachytherapy alone,

4. Increasing use of both adjuvant RT and chemotherapy in high-risk disease, and

5. Developing new RT techniques to reduce morbidity.

REDUCING INDICATIONS FOR PELVIC RADIOTHERAPY

What has been learned from randomized trials and large non-randomized studies of pelvic RT in stage I endometrial carcinoma?

- Pelvic RT provides a highly significant improvement of local control (1–3).
- Pelvic failure rates in patients with high-risk uterus-confined disease without RT are over 15% (1,2,4,5).
- RT does not increase overall survival rates (1,2).
- The use of pelvic RT should be limited to patients at increased risk of loco-regional relapse based on the presence of major risk factors (grade 3, deep myometrial invasion, age >60) (1,4,6).
- RT does not reduce the risk of distant metastases (1,2).
- RT is a very effective salvage treatment for vaginal relapse in patients not previously irradiated, with 80–90% complete remissions, five-year local control rates of 65–77%, and five-year overall survival rates of 45–65% (7–10).

It is clear that a large proportion of endometrial cancer patients have a very favorable prognosis and no adjuvant therapy is warranted (1,4,6,11). The inclusion of such low-risk cases in clinical studies of the role of RT or of lymphadenectomy reduces the likelihood of observing a potential benefit for the higher risk subsets, and subjects these patients to increased risks of toxicity. Stage IA and stage IB, grade 1 and grade 2 cases should be observed after total abdominal hysterectomy and bilateral salpingo-oophorectomy (TAH-BSO) (1,4,6,12).

It can thus be stated that the role of pelvic RT for stage I endometrial carcinoma is the reduction of the risk of loco-regional relapse, and that RT is not indicated if the a priori risk of loco-regional recurrence at five years is less than 15%, as effective salvage treatment is available. The use of post-operative RT should be limited to the group of patients at sufficiently high risk of loco-regional recurrence (15% or over) to warrant the risk of treatment-associated morbidity in order to maximize initial local control and relapse-free survival. Thus, pelvic RT should be limited to those subgroups of stage I endometrial cancer where at least two of the following three major risk factors are present: grade 3, age 60 and over, or outer 50% myometrial invasion. For these subgroups (two of the three risk factors) combined, the rate of loco-regional relapse in the control arm of the Postoperative Radiation Therapy in Endometrial Carcinoma (PORTEC) trial was 19%. Omitting RT in these subgroups leaves these patients at a significant risk of relapse.

However, recent data suggest that vaginal brachytherapy may be used instead of external beam RT to optimize local control with less side effects and better quality of life (13,14). This is the rationale of the currently ongoing randomized PORTEC-2 trial.

THE ROLE OF LYMPHADENECTOMY AND ITS COMBINATION WITH RADIOTHERAPY

There is sample evidence that the standard management of endometrial carcinoma consists of surgery, followed by RT if adverse prognostic factors are found. There is, however, controversy as to the optimal extent of surgery and the use of external beam RT. Since the landmark Gynecologic Oncology Group (GOG) staging study (15), and the inclusion of surgical and pathologic features in the International Federation of Gynecology and Obstetrics (FIGO) staging, there has been debate as to the indication (which risk factors) and extent (pelvic and/or para-aortic, complete or sampling) of lymphadenectomy. Most authors advocating lymphadenectomy (16–18) presented small, single-institutional, retrospective studies with both patient selection bias and stage migration. Often, the justification for lymphadenectomy has been the assumption that in the absence of pelvic node metastases, RT could be omitted. However, the safety of this approach has never been proven in a randomized or multi-institutional study. First data from the randomized GOG-99 trial (3) show a similarly increased risk of local failure if RT is omitted as in the control arm of the PORTEC trial. In the GOG-99 trial, all patients underwent TAH-BSO with lymphadenectomy. Patients without pelvic node metastases were randomized to pelvic RT or no further treatment. The two-year relapse-free survival rates were 88% in the control group (17 loco-regional, mainly vaginal, recurrences in 200 patients) and 96% in the RT group (3 recurrences in 190 patients). These results are strikingly similar to those obtained in the PORTEC study without lymphadenectomy. However, the rate of severe complications was 8%, compared to 3% in the PORTEC trial, which underlines the increased risk of toxicity when combining extended surgery with pelvic RT.

It should be noted that the potential benefit of lymphadenectomy depends on the risk of microscopic nodal disease, and that the procedure would be most effective in cases with a substantial risk of pelvic lymph node metastases. Most series, however, included mainly low- and intermediate-risk patients, for whom the risk ranges from well below 5% to 10% (15,16). For the present time there is insufficient evidence to support the standard use of lymphadenectomy for low- and intermediate-risk endometrial carcinoma. In the United Kingdom, the randomized MRC-ASTEC study is nearing its completion and will hopefully provide essential information as to the role of lymphadenectomy in stage I endometrial cancer.

The true benefit of lymphadenectomy can only be determined in high-risk and advanced stage disease. As advanced stage endometrial carcinoma is relatively rare, only small series have been reported. In a study by Rose et al. (19), microscopic para-aortic nodal metastases were diagnosed in 26 of 144 patients, 10%, 22%, and 71% of patients with clinical stage I (with risk factors grade 3 and/or deep invasion), stage II and stage III disease, respectively. If macroscopic or microscopic para-aortic lymph node metastases have been diagnosed, the radiation target volume can be extended to include the para-aortic region, which is potentially curative therapy. Hicks et al. (20) reported 27% five-year disease-free survival (DFS) among 11 patients with microscopic para-aortic nodal disease treated with extended field RT, while none of eight patients treated with pelvic RT combined with progestins survived. Complete removal of macroscopic or microscopic para-aortic nodal disease followed by extended field RT resulted in five-year survival rates of 46% and 53% among 50 and 17 patients, respectively, while patients with residual macroscopic nodal disease or omission of para-aortic field radiation had significantly decreased survival rates (13–18%) (19,21). The combination of extended surgery and extended field RT has, however, a substantial complication rate with reported intestinal obstruction rates of 12–27% (19,20). Extended field RT should, therefore, be reserved for patients with suspected or proven para-aortic lymph node involvement.

THE INCREASING USE OF VAGINAL BRACHYTHERAPY ALONE

Several authors have reported that for patients with intermediate-risk disease, vaginal brachytherapy can be used instead of pelvic RT to obtain equally high local control rates with less side effects and, consequently, to obtain optimal disease-free and overall survival rates as well as best quality of life (11,13,14,22). Data from (mostly retrospective) studies which used vaginal brachytherapy alone in stage I endometrial cancer have shown the five-year risk of vaginal relapse to be 0–7% (2,5,14,16,22–28). In most series vaginal control rates of over 95% were reported, even with modest doses of vaginal brachytherapy. Pelvic and distant failure rates and overall survival, however, remain similar to those of patients treated with surgery alone, which is the reason that most studies included only or mainly low-risk patients (grades 1 and 2 with no or superficial invasion).

High-risk stage I and stage II patients were included in some studies. Elliott et al. (5) compared 435 stage I and stage II endometrial patients treated with 60 Gy low-dose rate (LDR) brachytherapy to 492 patients treated with surgery alone. The 10-year vaginal recurrence rates were 2.8% in low-risk patients, 9.3% in high-risk stage I patients and 11.2% in stage II patients. Only 8 of the 435 patients treated with brachytherapy had a vaginal recurrence, four of whom were stage II patients. In the randomized trial by Aalders et al. (2), 261 of the 518 stage I patients had high-risk features (grade 3 and/or outer 50% invasion). In the control group treated with 60 Gy LDR vaginal brachytherapy, the vaginal and pelvic recurrence rate was 7%, as compared to 2% in the patients treated with pelvic RT after brachytherapy.

The advantages of high-dose rate (HDR) brachytherapy (increased patient convenience, no hospitalization with bed rest, decreased risk of acute thrombo embolic events, improved stability of the applicators during treatment, possibility of optimization of dose distributions) prompted its use in many centers. Despite the theoretical biological disadvantages of HDR brachytherapy, reported vaginal control and complications rates for vaginal HDR brachytherapy are comparable to those of LDR (27,29). Petercit and Pearcey (30) reviewed the results of HDR-brachytherapy in stage I endometrial cancer patients and concluded that local control rates of 98% and over were obtained with modest doses (e.g., 35 Gy HDR to the surface or 21 Gy to 5 mm depth in three fractions). The use of higher doses did not further increase local control, while complication rates were higher. The studies by Weiss et al. (22), Chadha et al. (14), and Anderson et al. (28), using HDR brachytherapy, all included some 30% of patients with high-risk stage I or stage II disease, and reported vaginal control rates of 98.4%, 100%, and 98%. However, pelvic and distant relapses were higher in the high-risk stage I and stage II patients, yielding five-year DFS rates of 93–94% and 74%, respectively.

In summary, moderate, convenient dose fractionation schedules of vaginal brachytherapy provide vaginal control rates of over 95% with very low morbidity rates. In patients with higher risk disease, however, overall and DFS rates are decreased by pelvic and distant relapse. The challenge is to effectively select the high-risk patients who would benefit from more extensive treatment.

THE USE OF BOTH ADJUVANT RADIOTHERAPY AND CHEMOTHERAPY IN HIGH-RISK DISEASE

Increasing evidence has accumulated that among stage I endometrial carcinoma patients, the IC grade 3 category should be regarded separately, as this subgroup is at increased risk of pelvic and distant metastases and has a lower survival rate (2,31,32).

During the inclusion period of the PORTEC trial, patients who had stage I endometrial carcinoma, grade 3 with deep myometrial invasion, were not eligible for randomization, but were registered in a separate database and received postoperative RT. Of the 104 IC grade 3 patients registered, 99 were evaluable. The five-year actuarial vaginal and pelvic relapse rate of the IC grade 3 patients was 13%, clearly higher than the other stage I patients, who had excellent pelvic control rates after pelvic RT (97–99%).

The five-year rates of distant metastases were increased in both subgroups with grade 3 tumors: 20% for grade 3 with superficial invasion and 31% for grade 3 with deep myometrial invasion, compared to 3–8% for grade 1 and stage II disease. Overall survival at five years was 58% for the IC grade 3 patients, compared to 74% for those with IB grade 3, and 83–86% for IB grade 2 and IC grade 1 and stage II disease ($p < 0.001$). In multivariate analyses grade 3 was the most important adverse prognostic factor with hazard ratios for any relapse and for endometrial carcinoma related death of 5.4 ($p = 0.0001$) and 5.5 ($p = 0.0004$), respectively (33).

Stage IC grade 3 patients have a significantly increased recurrence rate compared to other stage I patients, and are especially at risk of distant metastases and of endometrial cancer death. The predominant type of relapse for stage IC grade 3 patients following adjuvant radiation is distant metastases. In the randomized Norwegian trial (2), only the IC grade 3 patients seemed to have potential survival benefit from additional pelvic RT. However, the numbers were too small to draw conclusions.

Whether or not surgical staging has been performed, pelvic RT is generally recommended for grade 3 tumors with deep myometrial invasion (32,34–37). Straughn et al. (38) analyzed the outcome of 220 stage IC endometrial cancer patients who had surgical staging including pelvic and para-aortic lymphadenectomy, comparing 99 patients (45%) treated with RT (20% pelvic RT and 25% brachytherapy alone) with 121 (55%) who did not receive RT. The selection criteria for RT were unclear. Five-year DFS rates were significantly lower in the observation group (75% vs. 93%), while overall survival rates were similar (90% and 92%). Among the 47 patients with IC grade 3 diseases, five-year DFS rates were 90% after RT and 59% in the observation group.

The disease-free and overall survival rates of stage IC grade 3 endometrial cancer patients are strongly influenced by the increased distant relapse rates. This raises the question whether adjuvant chemotherapy would lower the risk of distant metastases and thus improve survival. Problems encountered when considering the use of adjuvant chemotherapy, however, are the elderly age and concurrent morbidities of the endometrial cancer population, which might lead to selection bias by including younger, relatively favorable patients in chemotherapy trials. In metastatic disease, multi-agent chemotherapy has been shown to have superior response rates and duration as compared with single-agent therapy (39). Several schemes have been investigated (doxorubicin and cisplatin; paclitaxel and cisplatin or carboplatin) and have response rates of 35–75% and time to progression of 4–6 months.

Two randomized trials have been published which evaluated the efficacy of chemotherapy in the adjuvant setting. The first trial, using single-agent doxorubicin, did not show any benefit of adjuvant chemotherapy (40). The first results of GOG 122, a randomized trial comparing whole abdominal radiotherapy (WAI) with combination doxorubicin-cisplatin chemotherapy (AP) in advanced (stages III and IV) endometrial carcinoma, have recently been presented (41). Combination chemotherapy was shown to improve both progression-free and overall survival rates, with a predicted difference in DFS of 13% at two years (59% in the AP arm and 46% in the WAI arm), and in overall two-year survival of 11% (AP: 70% and WAI: 59%). However, recurrences remained very frequent (55%), predominantly in the pelvis and abdomen in both arms, and adverse effects were substantial, especially in the AP arm. Further results of this and other current trials have to be awaited to assess the impact of chemotherapy on overall survival, and the cost in terms of added morbidity or even mortality in this elderly patient group.

Controversy exists as to whether high-risk patients receiving adjuvant chemotherapy should receive pelvic RT, or vault brachytherapy alone. The omission of pelvic RT might leave the patients at substantial risk of pelvic failure. Mundt et al. (42) reported increased pelvic relapse rates when using adjuvant chemotherapy alone in patients with high-risk and/or advanced stage endometrial carcinoma. Of the 67% who relapsed, 40% had pelvic recurrence and 56% distant relapse. The three-year pelvic failure rate was 47%, and in 31% the pelvis was the first or only site of recurrence.

As these data support the use of pelvic RT in high-risk patients undergoing adjuvant chemotherapy, future trials should explore the optimal sequencing of therapy and the use of concurrent RT and chemotherapy.

THE USE OF NEW RT TECHNIQUES TO REDUCE MORBIDITY

In view of the addition of toxicities when combining surgery, external beam RT, and chemotherapy in high-risk endometrial cancer patients, several groups are investigating the use of intensity-modulated radiotherapy (IMRT) to reduce the dose to critical organs surrounding the target tissues. Pelvic RT results in the irradiation of large volumes of the small bowel and rectum, and leads to gastrointestinal (GI) toxicity in a significant proportion of the patients. Severe complications requiring surgery occur in 3% of patients treated with pelvic RT, but some 20% experience GI side effects which are considered mild (grades 1 and 2), but do influence their quality of life (43–46). Complication rates are dose-dependent and are higher for the combination of pelvic RT with vaginal brachytherapy, with chemotherapy, and after lymphadenectomy (45–49).

IMRT utilizes multiple beams of varying intensity that conform the high-dose region to the shape of the target tissues in three dimensions, thereby minimizing the dose to the surrounding organs. Treatment planning studies (50–52) have shown that a substantial reduction of the doses to the small bowel, rectum, and the pelvic bone marrow can be realized. The volume of small bowel irradiated to the prescription dose is reduced by a factor of two as compared to a computed tomography (CT) based conventional three-dimensional (3D), four-field box technique (50,52). First results of clinical studies have shown a reduction of acute GI toxicity in patients treated with pelvic IMRT (50), and of acute hematologic toxicity in gynecologic cancer patients receiving pelvic IMRT combined with chemotherapy (53). In an analysis of 36 gynecologic cancer patients treated with pelvic RT with or without chemotherapy and/or brachytherapy, IMRT also resulted in a significant reduction of patients experiencing chronic GI toxicity (11% mild symptoms, as compared to 50% in a historical series of pelvic RT patients) and less severe GI complications (0% and 3%) (54). Especially for the increasing number of high-risk endometrial carcinoma patients treated with surgery, RT, and chemotherapy, IMRT will be an essential tool in reducing the chronic toxicities of multi-modality treatment.

CONCLUSIONS

The main recent developments in RT for endometrial carcinomas have been the reduction of indications for pelvic RT, shifting the role of RT in low-risk disease towards treatment reserved for patients with vaginal or pelvic relapse, the increasing use of brachytherapy alone for intermediate-risk disease, and the use of both adjuvant chemotherapy and RT in high-risk and advanced disease. Research efforts should be directed towards defining the optimal treatment for high-risk and advanced disease, especially the combined use of (concurrent) RT and chemotherapy and the role of lymphadenectomy, and to quality of life and cost-effectiveness analyses. New RT techniques are being developed which reduce the risk of complications, especially for patients receiving multi-modality treatment. The ultimate goal of treatment for endometrial cancer patients remains the maximization of both event-free and complication-free survival.

REFERENCES

1. Creutzberg CL, van Putten WL, Koper PC, Lybeert ML, Jobsen JJ, Warlam-Rodenhuis CC, De Winter KA, Lutgens LC, van den Bergh AC, Steen-Banasik E, Beerman H, van Lent M. Surgery and postoperative radiotherapy versus surgery alone for patients with stage-1 endometrial carcinoma: multicentre randomised trial. PORTEC Study Group. Post Operative Radiation Therapy in Endometrial Carcinoma. Lancet 2000; 355:1404–1411.
2. Aalders J, Abeler V, Kolstad P, Onsrud M. Postoperative external irradiation and prognostic parameters in stage I endometrial carcinoma: clinical and histopathologic study of 540 patients. Obstet Gynecol 1980; 56:419–427.
3. Keys HM, Roberts JA, Brunetto VL, Zaino RJ, Spirtos NM, Bloss JD, Pearlman A, Maiman MA, Bell JG. A phase III trial of surgery with or without adjunctive external pelvic radiation therapy in intermediate risk endometrial

adenocarcinoma: a Gynecologic Oncology Group study. Gynecol Oncol 2004; 92:744–751.

4. Carey MS, O'Connell GJ, Johanson CR, Goodyear MD, Murphy KJ, Daya DM, Schepansky A, Peloquin A, Lumsden BJ. Good outcome associated with a standardized treatment protocol using selective postoperative radiation in patients with clinical stage I adenocarcinoma of the endometrium. Gynecol Oncol 1995; 57:138–144.

5. Elliott P, Green D, Coates A, Krieger M, Russell P, Coppleson M, Solomon J, Tattersall M. The efficacy of postoperative vaginal irradiation in preventing vaginal recurrence in endometrial cancer. Int J Gynecol Cancer 1994; 4:84–93.

6. Poulsen HK, Jacobsen M, Bertelsen K, Andersen JE, Ahrons S, Bock J, Bostofte E, Engelholm SA, Holund B, Jakobsen A, Kiaer H, Nyland M, Pedersen PH, Stroyer I. Adjuvant radiation therapy is not necessary in the management of endometrial carcinoma stage I, low-risk cases. Int J Gynecol Cancer 1996; 6:38–43.

7. Creutzberg CL, van Putten WLJ, Koper PC, Lybeert MLM, Jobsen JJ, Warlam-Rodenhuis CC, De Winter KAJ, Lutgens LCHW, van den Bergh ACM, Steen-Banasik E, Beerman H, van Lent M. Survival after relapse in patients with endometrial cancer: results from a randomized trial. Gynecologic Oncology 2003; 89:201–209.

8. Pai HH, Souhami L, Clark BG, Roman T. Isolated vaginal recurrences in endometrial carcinoma: treatment results using high-dose-rate intracavitary brachytherapy and external beam radiotherapy. Gynecol Oncol 1997; 66:300–307.

9. Wylie J, Irwin C, Pintilie M, Levin W, Manchul L, Milosevic M, Fyles A. Results of radical radiotherapy for recurrent endometrial cancer. Gynecol Oncol 2000; 77:66–72.

10. Curran WJ, Jr., Whittington R, Peters AJ, Fanning J. Vaginal recurrences of endometrial carcinoma: the prognostic value of staging by a primary vaginal carcinoma system. Int J Radiat Oncol Biol Phys 1988; 15:803–808.

11. Alektiar KM, McKee A, Venkatraman E, McKee B, Zelefsky MJ, Mychalczak BR, Hoskins WJ, Barakat RR. Intravaginal high-dose-rate brachytherapy for Stage IB (FIGO Grade 1, 2) endometrial cancer. Int J Radiat Oncol Biol Phys 2002; 53:707–713.

12. Mariani A, Webb MJ, Keeney GL, Haddock MG, Calori G, Podratz KC. Low-risk corpus cancer: Is lymphadenectomy or radiotherapy necessary? Am J Obstet Gynecol 2000; 182:1506–1516.

13. Rittenberg PV, Lotocki RJ, Heywood MS, Jones KD, Krepart GV. High-risk surgical stage 1 endometrial cancer: outcomes with vault brachytherapy alone. Gynecol Oncol 2003; 89:288–294.

14. Chadha M, Nanavati PJ, Liu P, Fanning J, Jacobs A. Patterns of failure in endometrial carcinoma stage IB grade 3 and IC patients treated with postoperative vaginal vault brachytherapy. Gynecol Oncol 1999; 75:103–107.

15. Creasman WT, Morrow CP, Bundy BN, Homesley HD, Graham JE, Heller PB. Surgical pathologic spread patterns of endometrial cancer. A Gynecologic Oncology Group Study. Cancer 1987; 60:2035–2041.

16. COSA-NZ-UK endometrial cancer study group. Pelvic lymphadenectomy in high risk endometrial cancer. Int J Gynecol Cancer 1996; 6:102–107.

17. Mohan DS, Samuels MA, Selim MA, Shalodi AD, Ellis RJ, Samuels JR, Yun HJ. Long-term outcomes of therapeutic pelvic lymphadenectomy for stage I endometrial adenocarcinoma [see comments]. Gynecol Oncol 1998; 70:165–171.

18. Fanning J, Nanavati PJ, Hilgers RD. Surgical staging and high dose rate brachytherapy for endometrial cancer: limiting external radiotherapy to node-positive tumors. Obstet Gynecol 1996; 87:1041–1044.

19. Rose PG, Cha SD, Tak WK, Fitzgerald T, Reale F, Hunter RE. Radiation-Therapy for Surgically Proven Paraaortic Node Metastasis in Endometrial Carcinoma. Int J Radiat Oncol Biol Phys 1992; 24:229–233.

20. Hicks ML, Piver MS, Puretz JL, Hempling RE, Baker TR, Mcauley M, Walsh DL. Survival in Patients with Paraaortic Lymph-Node Metastases from Endometrial Adenocarcinoma Clinically Limited to the Uterus. Int J Radiat Oncol Biol Phys 1993; 26:607–611.

21. Corn BW, Lanciano RM, Greven KM, Schultz DJ, Reisinger SA, Stafford PM, Hanks GE. Endometrial Cancer with Paraaortic Adenopathy-Patterns of Failure and Opportunities for Cure. Int J Radiat Oncol Biol Phys 1992; 24:223–227.

22. Weiss E, Hirnle P, Arnold-Bofinger H, Hess CF, Bamberg M. Adjuvant vaginal high-dose-rate afterloading alone in endometrial carcinoma: patterns of relapse and side effects following low-dose therapy. Gynecol Oncol 1998; 71:72–76.

23. Bond WH. Early uterine body carcinoma: has post-operative vaginal irradiation any value?. Clin Radiol 1985; 36:619–623.

24. Eltabbakh GH, Piver MS, Hempling RE, Shin KH. Excellent long-term survival and absence of vaginal recurrences in 332 patients with low-risk stage I endometrial adenocarcinoma treated with hysterectomy and vaginal brachytherapy without formal staging lymph node sampling: report of a prospective trial. Int J Radiat Oncol Biol Phys 1997; 38:373–380.

25. Rose PG, Tak WK, Fitzgerald TJ, Reale FR, Hunter RE, Nelson BE. Brachytherapy for early endometrial carcinoma: a comparative study with long-term follow-up. Int J Gynecol Cancer 1999; 9:105–109.

26. Petereit DG, Tannehill SP, Grosen EA, Hartenbach EM, Schink JC. Outpatient vaginal cuff brachytherapy for endometrial cancer. Int J Gynecol Cancer 1999; 9:456–462.

27. Pearcey RG, Petereit DG. Post-operative high dose rate brachytherapy in patients with low to intermediate risk endometrial cancer. Radiother Oncol 2000; 56:17–22.

28. Anderson JM, Stea B, Hallum AV, Rogoff E, Childers J. High-dose-rate post-operative vaginal cuff irradiation alone for stage IB and IC endometrial cancer. Int J Radiat Oncol Biol Phys 2000; 46:417–425.

29. Petereit DG, Sarkaria JN, Potter DM, Schink JC. High-dose-rate versus low-dose-rate brachytherapy in the treatment of cervical cancer: analysis of tumor recurrence–the University of Wisconsin experience. Int J Radiat Oncol Biol Phys 1999; 45:1267–1274.

30. Petereit DG, Pearcey R. Literature analysis of high dose rate brachytherapy fractionation schedules in the treatment of cervical cancer: is there an optimal fractionation schedule? Int J Radiat Oncol Biol Phys 1999; 43:359–366.

31. Meerwaldt JH, Hoekstra CJ, van Putten WL, Tjokrowardojo AJ, Koper PC. Endometrial adenocarcinoma, adjuvant radiotherapy tailored to prognostic factors. Int J Radiat Oncol Biol Phys 1990; 18:299–304.
32. Koh WJ, Tran AB, Douglas JG, Stelzer KJ. Radiation therapy in endometrial cancer. Best Pract Res Clin Obstet Gynaecol 2001; 15:417–432.
33. Creutzberg CL, van Putten WL, Warlam-Rodenhuis CC, van den Bergh AC, De Winter KA, Koper PC, Lybeert ML, Slot A, Lutgens LC, Stenfert Kroese MC, Beerman H, van Lent M. Outcome of high-risk stage IC, grade 3, compared with stage I endometrial carcinoma patients: the Postoperative Radiation Therapy in Endometrial Carcinoma Trial. J Clin Oncol 2004; 22:1234–1241.
34. Naumann RW, Higgins RV, Hall JB. The use of adjuvant radiation therapy by members of the Society of Gynecologic Oncologists. Gynecol Oncol 1999; 75:4–9.
35. Greven KM, Corn BW. Endometrial cancer. Curr Probl Cancer 1997; 21:65–127.
36. Jereczek-Fossa BA. Postoperative irradiation in endometrial cancer: still a matter of controversy. Cancer Treat Rev 2001; 27:19–33.
37. Greven KM, Randall M, Fanning J, Bahktar M, Duray P, Peters A, Curran WJ, Jr. Patterns of failure in patients with stage I, grade 3 carcinoma of the endometrium. Int J Radiat Oncol Biol Phys 1990; 19:529–534.
38. Straughn JM, Huh WK, Orr JW, Kelly FJ, Roland PY, Gold MA, Powell M, Mutch DG, Partridge EE, Kilgore LC, Barnes MN, Austin JM, Alvarez RD. Stage IC adenocarcinoma of the endometrium: survival comparisons of surgically staged patients with and without adjuvant radiation therapy small star, filled. Gynecol Oncol 2003; 89:295–300.
39. Aapro MS, Van Wijk FH, Bolis G, Chevallier B, Van Der Burg ME, Poveda A, De Oliveira CF, Tumolo S, Scotto DP, Piccart VM, Franchi M, Zanaboni F, Lacave AJ, Fontanelli R, Favalli G, Zola P, Guastalla JP, Rosso R, Marth C, Nooij M, Presti M, Scarabelli C, Splinter TA, Ploch E, Beex LV, Ten Bokkel HW, Forni M, Melpignano M, Blake P, Kerbrat P, Mendiola C, Cervantes A, Goupil A, Harper PG, Madronal C, Namer M, Scarfone G, Stoot JE, Teodorovic I, Coens C, Vergote I, Vermorken JB. Doxorubicin versus doxorubicin and cisplatin in endometrial carcinoma: definitive results of a randomised study (55872) by the EORTC Gynaecological Cancer Group. Ann Oncol 2003; 14:441–448.
40. Morrow CP, Bundy BN, Homesley HD, Creasman WT, Hornback NB, Kurman R, Thigpen JT. Doxorubicin as an adjuvant following surgery and radiation therapy in patients with high-risk endometrial carcinoma, stage I and occult stage II: a Gynecologic Oncology Group Study. Gynecol Oncol 1990; 36:166–171.
41. Randall ME, Brunetto VL, Muss H. Whole abdominal radiotherapy versus combination doxorubicin-cisplatin chemotherapy in advanced endometrial carcinoma: A randomized phase III trial of the Gynecologic Oncology Group. Proc Am Soc Clin Oncol 22, 2 (Abstract 3). 2003.
42. Mundt AJ, McBride R, Rotmensch J, Waggoner SE, Yamada SD, Connell PP. Significant pelvic recurrence in high-risk pathologic stage I–IV endometrial carcinoma patients after adjuvant chemotherapy alone: implications for adjuvant radiation therapy. Int J Radiat Oncol Biol Phys 2001; 50:1145–1153.

43. Creutzberg CL, van Putten WL, Koper PC, Lybeert ML, Jobsen JJ, Warlam-Rodenhuis CC, De Winter KA, Lutgens LC, van den Bergh AC, Steen-Banasik E, Beerman H, van Lent M. The morbidity of treatment for patients with Stage I endometrial cancer: results from a randomized trial. Int J Radiat Oncol Biol Phys 2001; 51:1246–1255.

44. Weiss E, Hirnle P, Arnold-Bofinger H, Hess CF, Bamberg M. Therapeutic outcome and relation of acute and late side effects in the adjuvant radiotherapy of endometrial carcinoma stage I and II. Radiother Oncol 1999; 53:37–44.

45. Jereczek-Fossa B, Jassem J, Nowak R, Badzio A. Late complications after post-operative radiotherapy in endometrial cancer: analysis of 317 consecutive cases with application of linear-quadratic model. Int J Radiat Oncol Biol Phys 1998; 41:329–338.

46. Corn BW, Lanciano RM, Greven KM, Noumoff J, Schultz D, Hanks GE, Fowble BL. Impact of improved irradiation technique, age, and lymph node sampling on the severe complication rate of surgically staged endometrial cancer patients: a multivariate analysis. J Clin Oncol 1994; 12:510–515.

47. Greven KM, Lanciano RM, Herbert SH, Hogan PE. Analysis of complications in patients with endometrial carcinoma receiving adjuvant irradiation. Int J Radiat Oncol Biol Phys 1991; 21:919–923.

48. Lewandowski G, Torrisi J, Potkul RK, Holloway RW, Popescu G, Whitfield G, Delgado G. Hysterectomy with extended surgical staging and radiotherapy versus hysterectomy alone and radiotherapy in stage I endometrial cancer: a comparison of complication rates. Gynecol Oncol 1990; 36:401–404.

49. Potish RA, Dusenbery KE. Enteric morbidity of postoperative pelvic external beam and brachytherapy for uterine cancer. Int J Radiat Oncol Biol Phys 1990; 18:1005–1010.

50. Mundt AJ, Lujan AE, Rotmensch J, Waggoner SE, Yamada SD, Fleming G, Roeske JC. Intensity-modulated whole pelvic radiotherapy in women with gynecologic malignancies. Int J Radiat Oncol Biol Phys 2002; 52:1330–1337.

51. Lujan AE, Mundt AJ, Yamada SD, Rotmensch J, Roeske JC. Intensity-modulated radiotherapy as a means of reducing dose to bone marrow in gynecologic patients receiving whole pelvic radiotherapy. Int J Radiat Oncol Biol Phys 2003; 57:516–521.

52. Heron DE, Gerszten K, Selvaraj RN, King GC, Sonnik D, Gallion H, Comerci J, Edwards RP, Wu A, Andrade RS, Kalnicki S. Conventional 3D conformal versus intensity-modulated radiotherapy for the adjuvant treatment of gynecologic malignancies: a comparative dosimetric study of dose-volume histograms. Gynecologic Oncology 2003; 91:39–45.

53. Brixey CJ, Roeske JC, Lujan AE, Yamada SD, Rotmensch J, Mundt AJ. Impact of intensity-modulated radiotherapy on acute hematologic toxicity in women with gynecologic malignancies. Int J Radiat Oncol Biol Phys 2002; 54:1388–1396.

54. Mundt AJ, Mell LK, Roeske JC. Preliminary analysis of chronic gastrointestinal toxicity in gynecology patients treated with intensity-modulated whole pelvic radiation therapy. Int J Radiat Oncol Biol Phys 2003; 56:1354–1360.

Future Directions: Chemotherapy and Novel Agents for Uterine Cancer

Stacy D. D'Andre

Department of Hematology–Oncology, University of California, Davis, California, U.S.A.

Karl C. Podratz

Division of Gynecologic Surgery, Mayo Clinic, Rochester, Minnesota, U.S.A

INTRODUCTION

The role of chemotherapy in the treatment of endometrial cancer is evolving rapidly. For many years, the mainstay of treatment for uterine cancer was surgery with or without radiotherapy depending on the stage of disease. Chemotherapy was mainly used in the palliative setting, with little benefit. Newer combination chemotherapy regimens developed over the past few years have shown high response rates which will hopefully translate into longer survival with acceptable toxicity for patients with advanced disease. Novel agents are also being extensively tested in clinical trials. Chemotherapy is now moving into first-line treatment for patients with stage III and IV disease, and often for those with high-risk features such as serous papillary and clear cell histology. The major questions that need answers include:

1. What is the role of radiation therapy when chemotherapy is given in the adjuvant setting?
2. What is the best sequence of chemotherapy and radiotherapy in the adjuvant setting?
3. What is the tolerability and benefit of radiosensitizing chemotherapy?

4. What is the most effective and tolerable chemotherapy regimen for patients with advanced disease?
5. How will new targeted therapies be incorporated into treatment regimens, with or without chemotherapy?

ADJUVANT CHEMOTHERAPY

Gynecologic Oncology Group (GOG) 122 was recently reported at the American Society of Clinical Oncology (ASCO), in which patients with stage III/IV resected uterine cancer were randomized to WART (whole abdominal radiotherapy) versus seven cycles of doxorubicin/cisplatin (1). At a median follow-up of 52 months, there was an improvement in both progression-free and overall survival in those receiving chemotherapy. This study was important in finally showing a benefit of chemotherapy in the adjuvant setting. However, patients receiving chemotherapy had more long-term toxicity with peripheral neuropathy. Ongoing and planned studies will determine what is the most effective and well-tolerated chemotherapy in the adjuvant setting, and also explore the role of consolidative radiation given after chemotherapy. Another important issue that needs more study is defining the optimal sequence of chemotherapy and radiation. Table 1 lists examples of possible sequences and potential advantages/disadvantages to each approach (2–6). Ongoing studies will address the tolerability of delivering chemotherapy up front, followed by radiation.

COMBINED MODALITY THERAPY: RADIOSENSITIZING CHEMOTHERAPY

Combined modality therapy with chemotherapy and radiation is used in treating a wide variety of gynecologic malignancies, either as primary therapy, or as adjuvant treatment. For example, combined chemo-radiation has been shown to improve survival and is now the standard of care for many patients with cervical cancer (7,8). Radiation is commonly employed as adjuvant therapy for many women with endometrial cancer; however, concomitant chemotherapy radiation has not been well studied in this setting. Agents that are commonly employed as radiosensitizers in the treatment of other cancers include cisplatin, paclitaxel, carboplatin, 5-fluorouracil, and gemcitabine. Pilot studies using either paclitaxel or cisplatin in patients with endometrial cancer have shown good tolerability (5,6).

CHEMOTHERAPY FOR ADVANCED DISEASE

The number of active agents in the treatment of advanced or recurrent uterine cancer is ever-expanding. Many of these drugs have been combined, producing higher response rates, but often with more toxicity. Table 2 lists

Table 1 Different Sequences of Chemotherapy and Radiation (RT) in the Adjuvant Treatment of Endometrial Cancer

Treatment sequence	Advantages	Disadvantages	Example
RT→Chemo	Able to deliver RT early, without possibility of increased toxicity from chemo	Not treating micrometastasis early enough; not able to deliver full doses of chemotherapy	GOG 184: RT followed by either doxorubicin-cisplatin or doxorubicin-cisplatin-paclitaxel
Chemo→RT	Able to get in full doses of chemotherapy early, treat micrometastasis	May add to toxicity of radiation and prevent full delivery of local therapy	GOG 1198: phase-I study of three cycles of doxorubicin-cisplatin followed by WART; Katz et al. (2): paclitaxel-carboplatin × 6 followed by RT
Chemo→RT→Chemo	Allows early delivery of some chemotherapy to treat micrometastasis before radiation	Chemo may add to toxicity of radiation; post-RT chemotherapy may need dose-reduction	Khabele et al. (3): paclitaxel-carboplatin/cisplatin × 3, followed by 45–50 Gy, followed by three more cycles of chemotherapy Duska et al. (4): Paclitaxel-doxorubicin-carboplatin × 3 followed by 4500 Gy to pelvis
Concurrent Chemo-RT	Chemo may enhance effects of radiation, and potentially treat micrometastasis	Enhanced radiation toxicity	Frigerio et al. (5): paclitaxel 60 mg/m^2 weekly during radiation (50 Gy), followed by paclitaxel 80 mg/m^2 wk × 3 Reisinger et al. (6): cisplatin 15 mg/m^2/wk with radiation (30 Gy)

Table 2 New Cytotoxic Agents and Combinations in the Treatment of Advanced Endometrial Cancer

New agents/combinations	Reference	RR
Paclitaxel	9–11	27–37%
Weekly paclitaxel	16	67%
Topotecan	21,22	9–20%
Doxil	25,26	9.5–21%
Docetaxel	27	Case reports of activity
Carboplatin	58,59	13–30%
Oral etoposide	60	14%
Paclitaxel/cisplatin	15	67%
Paclitaxel/carboplatin	12–14	35–78%
Paclitaxel/adriamycin/cisplatin	19	57%
Paclitaxel/epirubicin/carboplatin	61	77%
Paclitaxel/epirubicin/cisplatin	62	73%
Cisplatin/vinorelbine	63	57%
Docetaxel/carboplatin	28	Case report

some of the newer agents and combination regimens which are discussed below.

PACLITAXEL

Paclitaxel has been shown to have activity in multiple phase-II trials, both as a single agent and in combination with either cisplatin or carboplatin (9–15). Weekly paclitaxel is also active in endometrial cancer, and may be better tolerated with less neuropathy and myalgias (16). A number of trials have been performed recently to determine if other combinations are better. Doxorubicin-cisplatin (AC) was compared to doxorubicin +24 hour paclitaxel (GOG 163) and no difference in response rates or survival was shown (17). A small randomized phase-II trial of paclitaxel-carboplatin versus

Table 3 Novel Therapies for the Treatment of Advanced Endometrial Cancer

Investigations agent	Mechanism of action
Thalidomide	Antiangiogenesis
Suramin	Antiangiogenesis
Herceptin	Monoclonal antibody against HER-2/neu
Iressa	EGFR inhibitor
Erlotinib	small molecule that inhibits HER/EGFR tyrosine kinase
CCI-779	mTOR inhibitor

doxorubicin-cisplatin showed higher response rates (35.3% vs. 27.6%), disease-free survival (DFS) (15 months 34.7% vs. 23.5%), and overall survival (OS) (40.5% vs. 27.1%) (18). Finally, the addition of paclitaxel to doxorubicin and cisplatin (TAP) as reported from GOG 177 improved response rates (57% vs. 33%) and improved progression-free survival (PFS) (five months PFS of 67% for TAP vs. 50% for AP) (19).

However, TAP required growth factor support, and produced more peripheral neuropathy and heart failure. An ongoing GOG study is randomizing patients with stage III/IV measurable disease to TAP with granulocyte colony-stimulating factor (G-CSF) versus carboplatin-paclitaxel (20). This study will provide important information about the most effective combination and the associated toxicities.

TOPOTECAN

Topotecan is a topoisomerase I inhibitor that is active against ovarian, lung, and other cancers. It can be given daily for five days every three weeks, or as a weekly infusion. A phase-II GOG study of patients with advanced, pretreated disease in which topotecan was given daily for five days, every three weeks, showed a response rate of 9% (21). Eastern Cooperative Oncology Group (ECOG) recently reported better results in untreated patients with advanced disease, again given 1.2–1.5 mg/m^2 daily for five days, every three weeks, which eventually was dose reduced due to toxicity (22). Overall response rate was 20%, with a reported median survival of 6.5 months. Weekly regimens are being studied as well, and may be better tolerated (23). A new oral formulation of topotecan has been developed and may provide patients with an alternative that is more convenient. Ongoing studies are combining topotecan with other agents such as cisplatin (24).

DOXIL®

Pegylated liposomal doxorubicin (Doxil®) has been tested in patients with advanced endometrial cancer. In pretreated patients, doxil at 50 mg/m^2 q four weeks produced a response rate of only 9.5% (25). Escobar et al. reported a higher response rate of 21% in a smaller trial of pretreated patients (26). The dose in this trial was 40 mg/m^2 every four weeks, and toxicities were very mild. Older patients may tolerate this drug better than doxorubicin, and it may be worth studying in combination with other agents.

DOCETAXEL

Docetaxel has been studied extensively in ovarian cancer, and has similar efficacy but a different toxicity profile than paclitaxel (less neurotoxicity). It has not been studied in clinical trials in endometrial cancer, but does appear to have activity (27,28). Future studies could take advantage of the different spectrum of toxicities, especially when combining cytotoxic agents.

OXALIPLATIN

Oxaliplatin is a platinum derivative with fairly broad spectrum activity that differs from cisplatin, and has been approved for the treatment of metastatic colorectal cancer in combination with 5FU (29). Oxaliplatin has some activity in breast cancer and ovarian cancer both as a single agent and in combination with other agents (30–32). The primary toxicities are hematologic and neuropathic. In contrast to cisplatin, there are no major nephrotoxic effects. Oxaliplatin is currently being studied in patients with advanced refractory endometrial cancer, given at $130 \, mg/m^2$ q three weeks. The non-cross-resistance and differing toxicity pattern compared to cisplatin makes this drug interesting, especially in combination with other agents.

NOVEL AGENTS

There are a number of novel agents that have been studied or are in clinical trials for patients with advanced endometrial cancer (Table 3). Many of these agents target growth factors or their receptors but we do not know how, if at all, to use these agents in combination with cytotoxic chemotherapy. Should we, for instance, combine targeted agents with each other, since the pathways involved are very complex, and may require blocking at multiple levels? Combining biologic agents that have different targets may also prove useful with or without chemotherapy, and this approach is already being tested in clinical trials.

Targeting Growth Factors and Their Receptors

Trastuzumab (Herceptin®)

Trastuzumab is a monoclonal antibody that binds to the human epidermal growth factor receptor (EGFR) 2 protein, HER-2. Trastuzumab has been extensively studied in breast cancer, both as a single agent and in combination with cytotoxic chemotherapy (33). In endometrial cancer, HER-2/neu (an EGFR family member) is overexpressed in some patients; the rates of overexpression vary widely in the literature due to different assay and reporting methods (34–36). The overexpression of this gene has been associated with poor prognostic indicators (higher stage, deep myometrial invasion), and inferior outcomes, similar to observations with breast cancer. A phase-II study of trastuzumab in patients with advanced/recurrent endometrial cancer was recently reported at ASCO (37). Trastuzumab has little activity as a single agent in this population, but for patients with overexpression of HER-2/FISH+, future studies will need to determine if trastuzumab in combination with chemotherapy provides any additional benefit. In breast cancer, combining chemotherapy with trastuzumab can produce higher response rates than are seen with either agent alone (38). Serous papillary cancers have higher reported rates of HER-2 overexpression and may represent a population that could benefit more from trastuzumab therapy (39).

Gefitinib (Iressa®)

Gefitinib is an inhibitor of EGFR tyrosine kinase activity which has been extensively studied in lung cancer (40–42). This oral drug is generally well tolerated with side effects including skin changes, nausea/vomiting, and diarrhea. EGFR is overexpressed in endometrial cancer, which may confer a worse prognosis (43–45). However, the pathways that are involved with growth factors and their receptors are complex, and more work needs to be done to clarify what markers can be studied to determine response to therapy. This agent is currently being tested in patients with advanced refractory endometrial cancer in an ongoing phase-II trial (GOG 229C). Translational studies will help to determine if overexpression of EGFR or increased levels of circulating EGFR correlate with clinical response to gefitinib.

Erlotinib

Erlotinib (Tarceva®) is a small molecule that inhibits HER/EGFR-tyrosine kinase. This drug has shown activity in lung cancer, and ongoing studies are combining erlotinib with paclitaxel/carboplatin, and gemcitabine/cisplatin (46). In gynecologic cancer, the National Cancer Institute of Canada is conducting a phase-II trial using erlotinib for untreated patients with locally advanced/metastatic disease that is measurable. If active in this setting, this drug could then be combined with cytotoxic agents as in the lung cancer trials.

Rapamycin

CCI-779 (rapamycin) is a novel agent which targets a serine/threonine kinase (mTOR) that plays a role in many cellular functions (47). Tumor cells with p53 or PTEN mutations, as are often seen in endometrial cancer, may be more sensitive to mTOR inhibitors (48,49). This agent will be studied in an NCI-Canada trial for previously untreated patients with measurable locally advanced or metastatic disease.

Targeting Angiogenesis

Targeting angiogenesis has been an active area of research in the last few years. Angiogenesis is a complex pathway involving vascular endothelial growth factors and their receptors, fibroblast growth factors, platelet-derived growth factor (PDGF), matrix metalloproteinases, and interleukins and others (50). Studies have shown that the degree of angiogenesis (as determined by microvessel density) correlates with survival (51). The vascular endothelial growth factor (VEGF)/receptor system is a very complex one; there are multiple types of VEGF/receptors that are involved in angiogenesis, some of which are elevated/expressed in endometrial cancer (52,53).

VEGF can be targeted by antibodies, such as bevacizumab (Avastin®). This drug has mainly been studied in colorectal cancer, with promising results (54). Studies are currently being conducted in patients with ovarian cancer and cervical cancer using antiangiogenesis agents both as single agents and in combination with chemotherapy. In uterine cancer, phase-II trials using suramin (an antiparasitic drug with antigrowth factor properties) and thalidomide have recently been completed. Thalidomide is an immuno-modulatory agent that has anti-angiogenic properties. In some studies, reduction in growth factors such as vascular endothelial growth factor (VEGF) and basic fibroblast growth factor is seen after treatment with thalidomide, which may be a marker for the anti-angiogenic effect (55,56). A recently completed GOG trial (229B) using thalidomide for advanced disease has unfortunately shown minimal activity (PR 12%) (57). However, given the mechanism of action of this drug, it may work better in combination with chemotherapy, or perhaps even in the adjuvant setting when only microscopic disease may be present. Other anti-angiogenesis inhibitors are currently still in clinical trials and may eventually become an important part of our treatment for many solid tumors.

CONCLUSIONS

Cytotoxic chemotherapy is playing a more prominent role in the treatment of endometrial cancers. Ongoing trials will determine the most effective agents and will define the sequence of chemotherapy and radiation in the adjuvant setting. Combined chemotherapy–radiotherapy is tolerable and deserving of further study. Certainly, the most exciting new therapies are the targeted drugs, especially given the potential for use in combination with chemotherapy. Many agents that target growth factors and their receptors and agents targeting angiogenesis are currently being studied in clinical trials. Defining the molecular basis of this disease, determining what markers correlate with response to these agents, and combining these new agents with cytotoxic chemotherapy represent the goals and challenges ahead. Once these goals are accomplished in the metastatic setting, it will be important to test these new therapies in women with earlier stage but high-risk disease in the adjuvant setting.

REFERENCES

1. Randall ME, Brunetto G, Muss H, Mannel N, Spirtos F, Jeffrey J, Thigpen T, Benda J. Whole abdominal radiotherapy versus combination doxonibicin-cis-platin chemotherapy in advanced endometrial carcinoma: a randomized phase III trial of the Gynecologic Oncology Group. Proc Am Soc Clin Oncol 2003; 22:[abstr. #3].
2. Katz LA, Andrews SJ, Fanning J. Survival after multimodality treatment for stage IIIC endometrial cancer. Am J Obstet Gynecol 2001; 184(6):1071–1073.

3. Khabele D, Goldman N, Danish A, Anderson S, Goldberg GL, Fields AL. RT sandwiched between chemotherapy in uterine papillary serous carcinoma. Proc ASCO 2003; 22:492 [abstr. #1975].
4. Duska LR, Berkowitz R, Matulonis U, Muto M, Goodman A, McIntyre JF, Klein A, Atkinson T, Seiden MV, Campos S. A pilot trial of TAC (paclitaxel, doxorubicin, and carboplatin) chemotherapy with filgastrim r(metHuG-CSF) support followed by radiotherapy in patients with "high-risk" endometrial cancer. Gynecol Oncol 2005; 96(1):198–203.
5. Frigerio L, Mangili G, Aletti G, Carnelli M, Garavaglia E, Beatrice S, Ferrari A. Concomitant radiotherapy and paclitaxel for high risk endometrial cancer: first feasibility study. Gynecol Oncol 2001; 81:53–57.
6. Reisinger SA, Asbury R, Liao SY, Homesley HD. A phase I study of weekly cisplatin and whole abdominal radiation for the treatment of stage III and IV endometrial carcinoma: a Gynecologic Oncology Group pilot study. Gynecol Oncol 1996; 63(3):299–303.
7. Rose PG, Bundy BN, Watkins EB, Thigpen JT, Deppe G, Maiman MA, Clarke-Pearson DL, Insalaco S. Concurrent cisplatin-based radiotherapy and chemotherapy for locally advanced cervical cancer. N Engl J Med 1999; 340(15):1144–1153.
8. Green JA, Kirwan JM, Tiemey JF, Symonds P, Fresco L, Collingwood M, Williams CJ. Survival and recurrence after concomitant chemotherapy and radiotherapy for cancer of the uterine cervix: a systematic review and meta-analysis. Lancet 2001; 358(9284):781–786.
9. Lincoln S, Blessing JA, Lee RB, Rocereto TF. Activity of paclitaxel as second-line chemotherapy in endometrial carcinoma: A GOG study. Gyne Oncol 2003; 88:277–281.
10. Zanetta G, Lissoni A, Gabriele A, Landoni F, Colombo A, Perego P, Mangioni C. Phase II study of paclitaxel as salvage treatment in advanced endometrial cancer. Ann Oncol 1996; 7(8):861–863.
11. Ball HG, Blessing JA, Lentz SS, Mutch DG. A Phase II trial of paclitaxel in patients with advanced or recurrent adenocarcinoma of the endometrium: a GOG study. Gyne Onc 1996; 62:278–281.
12. Hoskins PJ, Swenerton KD, Pike JA, Wong F, Lim P, Acquino-Parsons C, Lee N. Paclitaxel and carboplatin, alone, or with radiation, in advanced or recurrent endometrial cancer: a phase II study. J Clin Onc 2001; 19(20): 48–53.
13. Price FV, Edwards RP, Kelley JL, Kunschner AJ, Hart LA. A trial of outpatient paclitaxel and carboplatin for advanced, recurrent, and histologic high-risk endometrial carcinoma: preliminary report. Semin Oncol 1997; 24(5 suppl 15):S1578–S1582.
14. Onishi Y, Nakamura T, Yamamoto F, Hatae M. Evaluation of paclitaxel and carboplatin in patients with endometrial cancer. Proc ASCO 2003; 22:487 #1958.
15. Dimopoulos MA, Papadimitriou CA, Sarris K, Aravantinos G, Kalofonos C, Gika D, Gourgoulis GM, Efstathiou E, Skarlos D, Bafaloukos P. Paclitaxel and cisplatin in advanced or recurrent carcinoma of the endometrium: long term results of a phase II multicenter study. Gyne Onc 2000; 78(1):52–57.

16. Nishio S, Ota S, Sugiyama T, Matsuo G, Kawagoe H, Kurnagai S, Ushijima K, Nishida T, Kamura T. Weekly 1-h paclitaxel infusion in patients with recurrent endometrial cancer: a preliminary study. Int Jo Clin One 2003; 8(1): 45–48.
17. Fleming GF, Filiaci VL, Bentley RC, Herzog T, Sorosky J, Vaccarello L, Gallion H. Phase III randomized trial of doxorubicin + cisplatin versus doxorubicin + 24-h paclitaxel + filgrastim in endometrial carcinoma: a Gynecologic Oncology Group study. Ann Oncol 2004; 15(8):1173–1178.
18. Weber B, Mayer F, Bougnoux P, Lesimple T, Joly F, Fabbro M, Troufleau P, Luporsi E, Mefti F, Ferrero JM. What is the best chemotherapy regimen in recurrent or advanced endometrial carcinoma? Preliminary results. Proc ASCO 2003; 22:453#1819.
19. Fleming GF, Brunetto VL, Cella D, Look KY, Reid GC, Munkarah AR, Kline R, Burger RA, Goodman A, Burks RT. Phase III trial of doxorubicin plus cisplatin with or without paclitaxel plus filgrastim in advanced endometrial carcinoma: a Gynecologic Oncology Group Study. J Clin Oncol 2004; 22(11): 2159–2166.
20. http://www.cancer.gov/clinicaltrials/.
21. Miller DS, Blessing JA, Lentz SS, Waggoner SE. A Phase II trial of topotecan in patients with advanced, persistent, or recurrent endometrial cancer: A GOG Study. Gyne Onc 2002; 87:247–251.
22. Wadler S, Levy DE, Lincoln ST, Soori GS, Schink JC, Goldberg G. Topotecan is active agent in the first-line treatment of metastatic or recurrent endometrial carcinoma: ECOG E3E93. Jo Clin Onc 2003; 21(11):2110–2114.
23. Morris RT. Weekly topotecan in the management of ovarian cancer. Gyne Onc 2003; 90(3):S34–S38.
24. Gelderblom H, Sparreboom A, de Jonge MJ, Loos WJ, Wilms E, Mantel MA, Hennis B, Camlett I, Verweij J, van der Burg ME. Dose and schedule-finding study of oral topotecan and weekly cisplatin in patients with recurrent ovarian cancer. Br J Cancer 2001; 85(8):1124–1129.
25. Muggia FM, Blessing JA, Sorosky J, Reid GC. Phase II trial of the pegylated liposomal doxorubicin in previously treated metastatic endometrial cancer: a Gynecologic Oncology Group study. J Clin Oncol 2002; 20(9):2360–2364.
26. Escobar PF, Markman M, Zanotti K, Webster K, Belinson J. Phase 2 trial of pegylated liposomal doxorubicin in advanced endometrial cancer. J Cancer Res Clin Oncol 2003; 129(11):651–654.
27. Gunthert AR, Pilz S, Kuhn W, Emons G, Meden H. Docetaxel is effective in the treatment of metastatic endometrial cancer. Anticancer Res 1999; 19(4C): 3459–3461.
28. Obata H, Aoki Y, Watanabe M, Matsushita H, Yahata T, Fujita K, Kurata H, Tanaka K. Docetaxel and carboplatin combination chemotherapy for recurrent endometrial cancer. Int J Clin Oncol 2003; 8(1):53–55.
29. Goldberg RM, Sargenu DJ, Morton RF, Fuchs CS, Ramanathan RK, Williamson SK, Findlay BP, Pilot HC, Albens SR. A randomized controlled trial of fluorouracil plus leucovorin, irinotecan, and oxaliplatin combinations in patients with previously untreated metastatic colorectal cancer. J Clin Oncol 2004; 22(1):23–30.

30. Dieras V, Bougnoux P, Petit T, Chollet P, Beuzeboc P, Borel C, Husseini F, Goupil A, Kerbrat P, Missei JL, Bensmaine MA, Tabah-Fiseh I, Pouillart P. Multicentre phase II study of Oxaliplatin as a single-agent in cisplatin/ carboplatin +/- taxane-pretreated ovarian cancer patients. Ann Oncol 2002; 13(2):258–266.

31. Piccart MJ, Green JA, Lacave AJ, Reed N, Vergote I, Benedetti-Panici P, Bonetti A, Kristeller-Tome V, Fernandez CM, Curran D, Van Glabbeke M, Lacombe D, Pinel MC, Pecorelli S. Oxaliplatin or paclitaxel in patients with platinum-pretreated advanced ovarian cancer: a randomized phase II study of the European Organization for Research and Treatment of Cancer Gynecology Group. J Clin Oncol 2000; 18(6):1193–1202.

32. Garufi C, Nistico C, Brienza S, Vaccaro A, D'Ottavino A, Zappala AR, Aschelter AM, Terzoli E. Single-agent oxaliplatin in pretreated advanced breast cancer patients: a phase II study. Ann Oncol 2001; 12(2):179–182.

33. Slamon DJ, Leyland-Jones B, Shak S, Fuchs H, Paton V, Bajamonde A, Fleming T, Eiermann W, Wolter J, Pegram M, Baselga J, Norton L. Use of chemotherapy plus a monoclonal antibody against HER2 for metastatic breast cancer that overexpresses HER2. N Engl J Mcd 2001; 344(11):783–792.

34. Hetzel DJ, Wilson TO, Keeney GL, Roche PC, Cha SS, Podratz KC. HER-2/ neu expression: a major prognostic factor in endometrial cancer. Gynecol Oncol 1992; 47:179–185.

35. Berchuck A, Boyd J. Molecular basis of endometrial cancer. Cancer 1995; 76(10 suppl):2034–2040; Saffari B, Jones LA, el-Naggar A, et al. Amplification and overexpression of HER-2/neu in endometrial cancers: correlation with overall survival. Cancer Res 1995; 23:5693–5698.

36. Cianciulli AM, Guadagni F, Marzano R, Benevolo M, Merola R, Giannarelli D, Marandino F, Vocaturo G, Mariani L, Mottolese M. HER-2/neu oncogene amplification and chromosome 17 aneusomy in endometrial carcinoma: correlation with oncoprotein expression and conventional pathologic parameters. J Exp Clin Ca Res 2003; 22(2):265–271.

37. Fleming GF, Sill MA, Thigpen JT, et al. Phase II evaluation of trastuzumab in patients with advanced or recurrent endometrial carcinoma: a report on GOG. 181B. Proc ASCO 2003#1821;453.

38. Leyland-Jones B, Gelmon K, Ayoub JP, Arnold A, Verma S, Dias R, Ghahramani P. Pharmacokinetics, safety, and efficacy of trastuzumab administered every three weeks in combination with paclitaxel. J Clin Oncol 2003; 21(21): 3965–3971.

39. Slomovitz BM, Broaddus RR, Schmandt R, Wu W, Oh JC, Ramondetta LM, Burke TW, Gershenson DM, Lu KH. Her-2/neu expression and amplification in uterine papillary serous carcinoma (UPSC). Gynecol Oncolo 2004; 92:435 [abstr#93].

40. Wakeling AE, Guy SP, Woodburn JR, Ashton SE, Curry BJ, Barker AJ, Gibson KH. ZD1839 (Iressa): an orally active inhibitor of epidermal growth factor signaling with potential for cancer therapy. Cancer Res 2002; 62:5749–5754.

41. Kris MG, Natale RB, Herbst RS, Lynch TJ Jr, Prager D, Belani CP, Schiller JH, Kelly K, Spiridonidis H, Sandler A, Albain KS, Cella D, Wolf MK, Averbuch SD, Ochs JJ, Kay AC. Efficacy of gefitinib, an inhibitor of the epider-

mal growth factor receptor tyrosine kinase, in symptomatic patients with non-small cell lung cancer: a randomized trial. JAMA 2003; 290(16):2149–2158.

42. Hainsworth JD, Mainwaring MG, Thomas M, Porter LL 3rd, Gian VG, Jones SF, Greco FA. Gefitinib in the treatment of advanced, refractory non-small-cell lung cancer: results in 124 patients. Clin Lung Cancer 2003; 4(6):347–355.

43. Niikura H, Sasano H, Kaga K, Sato S, Yajima A. Expression of epidermal growth factor family proteins and epidermal growth factor receptor in human endometrium. Hum Pathol 1996; 27(3):282–289.

44. Scambia G, Benedetti Panici P, Ferrandina G, Battaglia F, Distefano M, D'Andrea G, De Vincenzo R, Maneschi R, Ranellerri FO, Mancuso S. Significance of epidermal growth factor receptor expression in primary human endometrial cancer. In Jo Cancer 1994; 56(1):26–30.

45. Khalifa MA, Mannel RS, Haraway SD, Walker J, Min KW. Expression of EGFR, HER-2new, P53, and PCNA in endometrioid, seous papillary, and clear cell endometrial adenocarcinoma. Gynecol Oncol 1994; 53(l):84–94.

46. Ciardiello F, De Vita F, Orditura M, De Placido S, Tortora G. Epidermal growth factor receptor tyrosine kinase inhibitors in late stage clinical trials. Expert Opin Emerg Drugs 2003; 8(2):501–514.

47. Huang S, Houghton PJ. Targeting mTOR signaling for cancer therapy. Curr Opin Pharm 2003; 3:371–377.

48. Neshat MS, Mellinghoff IK, Tran C Stiles B, Thomas G, Petersen R, Frost P, Gibbons JJ, Wu H, Sawyers CL. Enhanced sensitivity of PTEN-deficient tumors to inhibition of FRAP/mTOR. Proc Natl Acad Sci 2001; 98:10314–10319.

49. Slomovitz BM, Wu W, Broaddus RR. Preclinical assessment of mTOR inhibition: a novel therapeutic target for the treatment of endometrial cancer. Rapamyciycin inhibits mTOR. Gynecol Oncol 2004; 92:477 (abstr #188).

50. Stadler W, Wilding G. Angiogenesis inhibitors in genitourinary cancers. Crit Rev in Onc/Hem 2003; 46(suppl l):41–47.

51. Kirschner CV, Alanis-Amezcua JM, Martin VG, Luna N, Morgan E, Yang JJ, Yordan EL. Angiogenesis factor in endometrial carcinoma: a new prognostic indicator? Am J Obstet Gynecol 1996; 174(6):1879–1882.

52. Holland CM, Day K, Evans A, Smith SK. Expression of the VEGF and angiopoeitin genes in endometrial atypical endometrial cancer. Br Jo Can 2003; 89:891–898.

53. Fujimoto J, Ichigo S, Hirose R, Sakaguchi H, Tamaya T. Expressions of vascular endothelial growth (VEGF) and its mRNA in uterine endometrial cancers. Cancer Lett 1998; 134:15–22.

54. Giantonio BJ, Levy D, O'Dwyer PJ, Meropol NJ, Catalano PJ, Benson AB. Bevacizumab (anti-VEGF) plus IFL as from line therapy for advanced colorectal cancer: results from the ECOG study E2200. Proc ASCO 2003; 22:255 [abstr #1024].

55. Abramson N, Stokes P. Ovarian and peritoneal papillary-serous carcinoma: pilot study using thalidomide. Proc Am Soc Clin Oncol 2001; 20:179b [abstr 2466].

56. Eisen T, Boshoff C, Mak I, Sapunar F, Vaughan MM, Pyle L, Johnston SR, Ahern R, Smith LE, Gore ME. Continuous low dose thalidomide: a phase II study in advanced melanoma, renal cell, ovarian and breast cancer. Br J Cancer 2000; 82:812–817.

57. McMeekiu SD, Sill M, Benbrook D, et al. A Phase II study of thalidomaide in patients with recurrent or persistent endometrial carcinoma: a GOG study. Gynecol Oncol 2004; 92:438 [abstr #99].
58. van Wijk FH, Lhomme C, Bolis G, Scotto di Palumbo V, Tumolo S, Nooij M, de Oliveira CF, Vermorken JB; Europaan Organization for Research. Treatment of Cancer, Gynaecological Cancer Group. Phase II study of carboplatin in patients with advanced or recurrent endometrial cancer: a trial of the EORTC Gynaecological Cancer Group. Eur Jo Cancer 2003; 39:78–85.
59. Long HJ, Pfeifle DM, Wieand HS, Krook JE, Edmonson JH, Buckner JC. Phase II evaluation of carboplatin in advanced endometrial carcinoma. J Natl Cancer Inst 1998; 80(4):276–278.
60. Poplin EA, Liu PY, Delmore JB, Wilczynski S, Moore DF Jr, Potkul RK, Fine BA, Hannigan EV, Alberts DS. Phase II trial of oral etoposide in recurrent or refractory endometrial adenocarcinoma: a Southwest Oncology Group study. Gyne Oncol 1999; 74:432–435.
61. Nakashima R, Enomoto T, Matsuzaki N, Kameda T, Ogawa H, Miyatake F, Saji Y, Murata Y. Paclitaxel, epirubicin and carboplatin in advanced and recurrent endometrial carcinoma: a preliminary report of phase I/II trial. Proc Am Soc Clin Oncol 2003; 22:#1963.
62. Lissoni A, Gabriele A, Gorga G, Tumolo S, Landoni F, Mangioni C, Sessa C. Cisplatin, epirubicin- and paclitaxel-containing chemotherapy in uterine adenocardnoima. Ann Oncol 1997; (10):969–972.
63. Gebbia V, Testa A, Borsellino N, Ferrara P, Tirrito M, Palmeri S. Cisplatin and vinorelbine in advanced and/or metastatic adenocarcinoma of the endometrium: a new highly active chemotherapeutic regimen. Ann Oncol 2001; 12(6): 767–772.

17

Combined Therapy in Uterine Cancer: Future Directions

Howard D. Homesley

Clinical Professor, Brody School of Medicine, East Carolina University, Greenville, North Carolina, U.S.A.

Women with advanced or recurrent endometrial cancer live less than one year largely unimpacted by current management. Combining chemotherapy and radiation therapy to improve outcome in patients with advanced endometrial cancer has been a consideration of the Gynecologic Oncology Group (GOG) for some years. Radiation targeted to prevent pelvic recurrence coupled with chemotherapy directed against intra-abdominal and systemic metastases is the current strategy. Yet, if one gave any substantial number of cycles of chemotherapy first, radiation could be delayed for weeks and greatly compromised. On the other hand, radiation given upfront could markedly reduce the ability to later give effective doses of chemotherapy. Concurrent radiation and chemotherapy does not allow for full dose chemotherapy. Radiation has to be limited to small volume residual disease (<2 cm residual tumor sites), microscopic disease, or high-risk-of-recurrence patients, while chemotherapy has no such limitations. Future directions will be guided by the culmination of findings from recent studies.

WHOLE ABDOMINAL RADIATION VERSUS CHEMOTHERAPY

The GOG has just reported on a prospective, randomized comparison of whole abdominal irradiation (WAI) versus chemotherapy with doxorubicin and cisplatin (DC) in endometrial cancer patients with stages III and IV disease confined to the abdomen with no residual disease greater than 2 cm at any one site (1). Four hundred twenty-two patients were entered from 1992 to 2000. Of the 388 evaluable patients, 198 were to receive WAI and 190, DC. The WAI employed 30 Gray (Gy) in 20 fractions and a pelvic boost of 15 Gy. Patients with pathologically positive para-aortic lymph nodes (PALN) or positive pelvic lymph nodes (PLN) without PALN surgical assessment received this same dose to the PALNs. The DC arm consisted of doxorubicin (60 mg/m^2) and cisplatin (50 mg/m^2) every three weeks for seven courses, with an additional course of cisplatin. The treatment arms were balanced in terms of patient and tumor characteristics, although the DC arm had more patients with positive PLN and PALN. In the WAI arm, 43 (21.3%) and 7 (3.5%) of tumors were serous and clear cell, respectively. In the DC arm, 40 (20.6%) and 10 (5.2%) were serous and clear cell, respectively. Median follow-up was 52 months (range: 2–116). There are significant differences in progression-free survival (PFS) and overall survival between the two regimens. The PFS hazard relative to WAI adjusted for stage is 0.68 [95% confidence interval (CI) is 0.52–0.89; $p < 0.01$]. Using the adjusted hazard ratio, there is a 13% predicted difference in the proportion disease-free at 24 months (WAI: 46%, DC: 59%). Similarly, the hazard of death relative to WAI adjusted for stage is 0.67 (95% CI is 0.51–0.89; $p < 0.01$) with an 11% predicted difference in the percent alive at 24 months (WAI: 59%, AP: 70%). Recurrences were frequent, predominantly in the pelvis and abdomen in both arms. Adverse effects were much more common in the DC arm. As delivered in this study, DC chemotherapy improves PFS and survival when compared with WAI. Still, approximately 55% of patients with advanced endometrial carcinoma recurred.

It is unlikely that whole abdominal radiation alone will be employed again for advanced endometrial cancer in the future. If nearly one half of the patients were effectively treated with chemotherapy alone, then what should the future strategy be? Should radiation be abandoned? Should there be a concentration only on improving chemotherapy? Does radiation still have a role in controlling pelvic disease but not upper abdominal disease? Are there other treatment options that should be considered?

HIGH-RISK STAGE I ENDOMETRIAL CARCINOMA

Over the past decade, in spite of aggressive therapy with new chemotherapy combinations or use of various radiation techniques such as whole abdominal or extended pelvic field, survival rates have remained low for high-risk stage I endometrial carcinoma. Endometrial cancer patients with early stage disease and poor prognostic factors such as high grade, lymphoinvasion, or deep myometrial invasion have survivals of less than 50%.

There was an intergroup randomized trial of the GOG (0194) and the Radiation Therapy Oncology Group (99–105) in post-hysterectomy high-risk stage I patients defined as grade 2 or 3 with greater than 50% myoinvasion or stromal invasion of the cervix. In one arm, patients received radiotherapy of 50.4 Gy in 5.5 weeks (1.8 Gy once a day, five times a week in 28 fractions) with optional vaginal brachytherapy boost. In the other arm, patients received the same radiation plus cisplatin 50 mg/m^2 intravenously on days 1 and 28 followed by cisplatin 50 mg/m^2 and paclitaxel 160 mg/m^2 on days 56, 84, 112, and 140 from the start of radiation.

The trial was closed early, as accrual was slow largely because the criteria restricted this to a small group of high-risk patients. Conclusive progress in the future may never be made in small high-risk subsets.

HORMONAL THERAPY

What role in the future might hormonal therapy have in combined therapy? In advanced disease, progestin therapy alone offers a 15–25% response rate and survival of less than one year while there is no role for adjuvant progestin-only therapy in early stage disease (2). The GOG has conducted a number of hormonal trials in treatment of advanced endometrial cancer (Table 1) (3–10). In the GOG comparison of low-dose (200 mg) medroxy-progesterone to high-dose (1000 mg), the median durations of PFSs were 3.2 and 2.5 months for the low-dose and high-dose regimens, respectively (4). Median survival durations were 11.1 and 7.0 months, respectively. The adjusted relative odds of response to the high-dose regimen compared with the low-dose regimen were 0.61. Prognostic factors having a significant impact on the probability of response included initial performance status, age, histologic grade, and progesterone receptor concentration. Response to progestin therapy was more frequent among patients with a well-differentiated histology and/or progesterone receptor-positive (>50 fmol/mg cytosol protein). Patients with poorly differentiated and/or progesterone receptor levels <50 fmol/mg cytosol protein had only an 8–9% response rate.

Continuous tamoxifen and alternate week medroxyprogesterone acetate [overall response rate of 34% (GOG 0119)] did not offer an advantage over progestin alone (6). Unfortunately, to date, no data have been published pertaining to the prospective value of knowing hormone receptor status and predicted response rate to progestin in a clinical trial setting. Megestrol acetate (80 mg orally twice daily for three weeks) alternating with tamoxifen (20 mg orally twice a day for three weeks) in a subsequent GOG trial did have a high complete response rate and a high sustained no evidence of disease rate of 14% (8).

The reason for reviewing progestin response is that there have been two pilot studies that would indicate there has been increased benefit using the combination of hormonal therapy and chemotherapy. Using one of the most active hormonal regimens of alternating megestrol and tamoxifen combined with carboplatin 300 mg/m^2, a response rate of 77% was noted

Table 1 Gynecologic Oncology Group Endometrial Hormonal Trials

Protocol no. (years)	Regimen	Response		Response rate	Median progression-free (months)	Median survival (months)	NED
		PR	CR				
048 Ref. (3) (1979–1985)	Provera 150 mg/day	25	34		4.0	10.4	
081 Ref. (4) (1985–1989)	Medroxy-progesterone 200 mg/day	13	23	36/138, 26%			
	Medroxy-progesterone 1000 mg/day	14	11	25/140, 18%			
081F Ref. (5) (1985–1992)	Tamoxifen 40 mg/day; progestin responders	4	3	7/63, 10%	1.9	8.8	
119 Ref. (6) (1991–1996)	Continuous tamoxifen provera 200 mg every other week	13	6	19/57, 34%			2%
0121 Ref. (7) (1991–1992)	Megestrol 800 mg/day	7	6	13/49, 26%	2.4	7.6	
0153 Ref. (8) (1994–1995)	Megestrol 160 mg/day × 3 weeks; tamoxifen 40 mg/day × 3 weeks	3	12	15/56, 27%			14%
0168 Ref. (9) (1997–1998)	Anastrozole 1 mg/day	2	0	2/23, 9%	1.0	6.0	
0180 Ref. (10) (1999–2000)	Danazol 100 mg four times a day	0	0	0/21			

Abbreviations: PR, partial response; CR, complete response.

with a 31% complete response rate in 18 evaluable patients (11). In a supporting study, 23 patients were treated with daily medroxyprogesterone acetate 300 mg daily orally and carboplatin 300 mg/m^2, methotrexate 30 mg/m^2, and 5-fluoruracil 500 mg/m^2 given every three weeks, and 74% had an objective response (12). The median progression free interval (PFI) was 10 months and the median survival 17 months.

If a large randomized trial in the future substantiated increased effectiveness of chemotherapy when combined with progestins, then perhaps the optimal combination would be radiation, chemotherapy, and hormonal therapy. Although not confirmed in clinical trials, patients receiving progestin therapy with quality of life instruments may possibly be proven to have an improved quality of life with increased appetite and more vigor.

THE GOG CHEMOTHERAPY TRIALS IN ENDOMETRIAL CANCER

Only recently has it become more evident what the most effective chemotherapy combinations might be and what might be optimal and tolerable radiation combined with chemotherapy. Before combining these two approaches, randomized chemotherapy trials in the next few years will be necessary to better define the most effective regimens.

The four first-line GOG chemotherapy trials for advanced endometrial carcinoma have confirmed a higher response rate and longer survival for combination chemotherapy (Table 2) (4,13–15). Unfortunately, the median progression-free interval remains in the range of six months with a median survival of about 9–12 months. The most active chemotherapeutic agents are ifosfamide, cisplatin, carboplatin, doxorubicin, and paclitaxel. The combination of cisplatin, doxorubicin, and paclitaxel at this time appears to be the superior combination, but randomized trials comparing this combination to the combination of carboplatin and paclitaxel are in progress by the GOG.

ALTERNATIVE CHEMOTHERAPY COMBINATIONS

Carboplatin and paclitaxel have been found in 63 patients to be an efficacious, low-toxicity regimen for managing primarily advanced or recurrent endometrial cancers (16). In another study, using granulocyte colony-stimulating factor (G-CSF) support with a regimen of paclitaxel 175 mg/m^2 and cisplatin 75 mg/m^2 a response rate of 67% was noted in 16 patients (17). Likewise another regimen, cisplatin 80 mg/m^2 on day 1 plus vinorelbine on days 1 and 8 were noted to have high activity (57% overall response rate with 11% complete response (CR) in 35 patients) against recurrent and/or metastatic endometrial adenocarcinoma (18). However, duration of objective response and median overall survival are in the disappointing range reported for other regimens.

Where cisplatin and doxorubicin chemotherapy alone was given adjunctively to 43 high-risk stages I–IV endometrial cancer patients as

Table 2 Gynecologic Oncology Group Endometrial Chemotherapy First Line Trials

Protocol no. (years trial active)	Arm	Regimen	Response		Response rate (responders/ entries per arm)	Median progression-free interval (months)	Median survival (months)	NED
			PR	CR				
049 Ref. (4) (1981–1985)	1	Doxorubicin			22%			
	2	Doxorubicin + Cyclophosphamide			30%			
0107 Ref. (13) (1988–1992)	1	Doxorubicin	26	12	25% (38/150)	3.8	9.2	
	2	Doxorubicin + Cisplatin	30	25	42% (55/131)	5.7	9	
0163 Ref. (14) (1996–1998)	1	Doxorubicin + Cisplatin	40	23	41% (63/157)			9%
	2	Doxorubicin + Paclitaxel	42	27	46% (69/160)			11%
0177 Ref. (15) (1998–2000)	1	Doxorubicin + Cisplatin	35	9	34% (44/131)			
	2	Doxorubicin + Cisplatin + Paclitaxel	48	29	56% (77/134)	Higher PFI	Higher survival	

Abbreviations: PR, partial response; CR, complete response.

adjuvant chemotherapy alone, there was a 40% pelvic recurrence rate indicating a need for loco-regional control with radiation (19).

CURRENT GOG COMBINED RADIATION AND CHEMOTHERAPY TRIAL

In designing the current GOG trial of combined radiation and chemotherapy, many alternative trial options were considered without the final conclusions available from the GOG whole pelvic irradiation versus chemotherapy trial. Many would now argue that if whole abdomen radiation with pelvic boost was inferior to chemotherapy alone, what need is there for pelvic radiation? The current combination of radiation and chemotherapy trial is not a comparison of these two modalities, but an effort to assess the effectiveness of attacking the pelvic disease primarily with full dose tumor volume directed radiation and all tumor sites, especially the upper abdomen, with full dose chemotherapy.

The radiation regimen is tumor volume directed where the radiation therapist guidelines are flexible and extended field radiation is used when para-aortic nodal involvement is suspected. Upon completion of 5040 cGy to the pelvis and 4350 cGy to the para-aortic area, the patient is randomized to doxorubicin 45 mg/m^2 and cisplatin 50 mg/m^2, with or without paclitaxel 160 mg/m^2 every three weeks for six courses, with all patients now receiving pegfilgrastim. This regimen has been well tolerated by the vast majority of patients. The study has been closed with entry of 659 patients and analysis will be completed soon.

It is likely that this study (GOG 0184) may well show no difference between the two chemotherapy arms. If there is no improvement over the prior GOG study (0122) comparing whole abdominal radiation to chemotherapy alone, then by inference one might conclude that combined therapy is not superior.

In the future, the ultimate trial that may be necessary to judge the value of combined therapy would be a trial comparing the most active chemotherapy available to some combination of chemotherapy plus radiation. A major problem in the present trial is that chemotherapy was not given prior to the radiation where better vascularity may accelerate chemotherapy responsiveness. A prospective randomized trial comparing pre- and post-radiation chemotherapy to chemotherapy only is needed. It is likely that a molecular targeting agent will also be added to the next clinical trial.

COMBINED HORMONAL, CHEMOTHERAPY, AND RADIATION THERAPY

There have been reports of higher response rates by combining hormonal therapy with chemotherapy, but no large randomized trials have addressed the benefits of adding progesterone to chemotherapy. One could envision that the most aggressive approach may be combining best hormonal therapy, best chemotherapy, and best radiation.

REFERENCES

1. Randall ME, Brunetto G, Muss H, Manner RS, Spirtos N, Jeffrey F, Thigpen JT, Benda J. Whole Abdominal Radiotherapy versus Combination Doxorubicin-Cisplatin Chemotherapy in Advanced Endometrial Carcinoma: A Randomized Phase III Trial of the Gynecologic Oncology Group. ASCO Proceedings, 2003.
2. von Minckwitz G, Loibl S, Brunnert K, Kreienberg R, Melchert F, Mosch R, Neises M, Schermann J, Seufert R, Stiglmayer R, Stosiek U, Kaufmann M. Adjuvant endocrine treatment with medroxyprogesterone acetate or tamoxifen in stages I and II endometrial cancer–a multicentre, open, controlled, prospectively randomized trial. Eur J Cancer 2002; 38(17):2265–2271.
3. Thigpen JT, Blessing JA, DiSaia PJ, Yordan E, Carson LF, Evers C. A randomized comparison of doxorubicin alone versus doxorubicin plus cyclophosphamide in the management of advanced or recurrent endometrial carcinoma: a Gynecologic Oncology Group study. J Clin Oncol 1994; 12(7): 1408–1414.
4. Thigpen JT, Brady MF, Alvarez RD, Adelson MD, Homesley HD, Manetta A, Soper JT, Given FT. Oral medroxyprogesterone acetate in the treatment of advanced or recurrent endometrial carcinoma: a dose-response study by the Gynecologic Oncology Group. J Clin Oncol 1999; 17(6):1736–1744.
5. Thigpen T, Brady MF, Homesley HD, Soper JT, Bell J. Tamoxifen in the treatment of advanced or recurrent endometrial carcinoma: a Gynecologic Oncology Group study. J Clin Oncol 2001; 19(2):364–367.
6. Whitney CW, Brunetto VL, Zaino RJ, Lentz SS, Sorosky J, Armstrong DK, Lee RB. Gynecologic Oncology Group study. Phase II study of medroxyprogesterone acetate plus tamoxifen in advanced endometrial carcinoma: a Gynecologic Oncology Group study. [see comment]. Gynecol Oncol 2004; 92(1):4–9.
7. Lentz SS, Brady MF, Major FJ, Reid GC, Soper JT. High-dose megestrol acetate in advanced or recurrent endometrial carcinoma: a Gynecologic Oncology Group Study. J Clin Oncol 1996; 14(2):357–361.
8. Fiorica JV, Brunetto VL, Hanjani P, Lentz SS, Mannel R, Andersen W. Gynecologic Oncology Group study. Phase II trial of alternating courses of megestrol acetate and tamoxifen in advanced endometrial carcinoma: a Gynecologic Oncology Group study. Gynecol Oncol 2004; 92(1):10–14.
9. Rose PG, Brunetto VL, VanLe L, Bell J, Walker JL, Lee RB. A phase II trial of anastrozole in advanced recurrent or persistent endometrial carcinoma: a Gynecologic Oncology Group study. Gynecol Oncol 2000; 78(2):212–216.
10. Covens A, Brunetto VL, Markman M, Orr JW, Lentz SS, Benda J. Gynecologic Oncology Group. Phase II trial of danazol in advanced, recurrent, or persistent endometrial cancer: a Gynecologic Oncology Group study. Gynecol Oncol 2003; 89(3):470–474.

11. Pinelli DM, Fiorica JV, Roberts WS, Hoffman MS, Nicosia SV, Cavanagh D. Chemotherapy plus sequential hormonal therapy for advanced and recurrent endometrial carcinoma: a phase II study. Gynecol Oncol 1996; 60(3):462–467.

12. Bafaloukos D, Aravantinos G, Samonis G, Katsifis G, Bakoyiannis C, Skarlos D, Kosmidis P. Carboplatin, methotrexate and 5-fluorouracil in combination with medroxyprogesterone acetate (JMF-M) in the treatment of advanced or recurrent endometrial carcinoma: a Hellenic cooperative oncology group study. Oncology 1999; 56(3):198–201.

13. Thigpen JT. A randomized study of doxorubicin vs doxorubicin plus cisplatin in patients with primary stage III and IV and recurrent endometrial adenocarcinoma, phase III. J Clin Oncol 1993; 12:261 ASCO Abstract #830.

14. Fleming GF, Filiaci VL, Bentley RC, Herzog T, Sorosky J, Vaccarello L, Gallion H. Phase III randomized trial of doxorubicin + cisplatin versus doxorubicin + 24-h paclitaxel + filgrastim in endometrial carcinoma: a Gynecologic Oncology Group study. Annal Oncol 2004; 15(8):1173–1178.

15. Fleming J. A randomized study of doxorubicin plus cisplatin versus doxorubicin plus cisplatin plus 3-hour paclitaxel with G-CSF support in patients with primary stage III & IV or recurrent endometrial carcinoma. J Clin Oncol 2002; ASCO Abstract #807.

16. Hoskins PJ, Swenerton KD, Pike JA, Wong F, Lim P, Acquino-Parsons C, Lee N. Paclitaxel and carboplatin, alone or with irradiation, in advanced or recurrent endometrial cancer: a phase II study. J Clin Oncol 2001; 19(20): 4048–4053.

17. Dimopoulos MA, Papadimitriou CA, Georgoulias V, Moulopoulos LA, Aravantinos G, Gika D, Karpathios S, Stamatelopoulos S. Paclitaxel and cisplatin in advanced or recurrent carcinoma of the endometrium: long-term results of a phase II multicenter study. Gyn Oncol 2000; 78(1):52–57.

18. Gebbia V, Testa A, Borsellino N, Ferrera P, Tirrito M, Palmeri S. Cisplatin and vinorelbine in advanced and/or metastatic adenocarcinoma of the endometrium: a new highly active chemotherapeutic regimen. Ann Oncol 2001; 12(6):767–772.

19. Mundt AJ, McBride R, Rotmensch J, Waggoner SE, Yamada SD, Connell PP. Significant pelvic recurrence in high-risk pathologic stage I–IV endometrial carcinoma patients after adjuvant chemotherapy alone: implications for adjuvant radiation therapy. Int J Radiat Oncol Biol Phys 2001; 50(5):1145–1153.

Index

Abdominal radiation, 281–282
Adjuvant chemotherapy, 182
  endometrioid adenocarcinoma,
    181–182
  serous carcinoma, 182–184
  stage I disease, 152–153
  uterine cancer, 268
Adjuvant radiotherapy, endometrial
  carcinoma, 259–261
Alcohol, risk factors, 5–6
Angiogenesis research, endometrial
  cancer, 273
Architectural grading, endometrial
  carcinomas, 44
Atypia hyperplasia, distinctions, 46–47

β-catenin, 72
Blind endometrial biopsy, as
  endometrial sampling, 92–93
Body mass, risk factors related to, 4
Brachytherapy, vaginal, 258
Breast cancer, 43

Carcinoma, 41
  mixed, 42
  mucinous, 38–39
  undifferentiated, 43
Carcinosarcoma, chemotherapy,
  185–188
Cervical involvement, for pathologic
  prognostic factors, 46

Chemotherapy, 181–182
  adjuvant, 182
  advanced disease, uterine cancer,
    268–270
  combined therapy, 179–181
    future direction, 281–282
  endometrial carcinoma, 259–261
  endometrioid adenocarcinoma,
    178–182
  novel agents, future uses, uterine
    cancer, 267–274
  radiation therapy, combined therapy,
    hormonal therapy, 287–288
  radiotherapy, uterine cancer, adjuvant
    treatment, 269
  serous carcinoma, 182–184
    adjuvant therapy, 183–184
  single agent therapy, 178–179
  uterine cancer, 177–188, 268
  uterine sarcomas, 184–188
    carcinosarcoma, 185–186
    leiomyosarcoma, 187–188
  whole abdominal radiation, 281–282
Chemotherapy combinations, future
  direction, 285, 287
Classification, of endometrial
  carcinoma, 32–34
Clear cell carcinoma, 41–42
Clinical phenotype molecular profiles,
  endometrial cancer, 81–83
Combination regimens, chemotherapy,
  179–181

Combined modality therapy, uterine
cancer, 268
Combined therapy, 283
chemotherapy combinations, 285, 287
endometrial carcinoma
stage I, 282–283
future directions, 285–287
GOG chemotherapy trials, 285
whole abdominal radiation,
281–282
hormonal therapy, 287–288
Complex hyperplasia, atypical, 46
Cytoreductive results, advanced
disease, 238
Cytotoxic agents, 270–272
docetaxel, 271–272
doxil, 271
paclitaxel, 270–271
topotecan, 271

Detection, uterine cancer, recurrence,
223–228
Diabetes, risk factors, 4–5
Diagnosis, of endometrial cancer,
136–137
Diet, risk factors, 5–6
Docetaxel, endometrial cancer,
271–272
Doxil, endometrial cancer, 271

Endometrial biopsies, interpretation of,
47
Endometrial cancer
clinical phenotype, 70
molecular profiles, 82
cytotoxic agents, 270–272
diagnosis, 136–137
epidemiology, 1–6
epignetics, 76–77
estrogen replacement therapy,
249–251
FIGO staging, 133–134, 150–151
genetics, 69–83
hormone replacement therapy, 109
imaging, 107–126

[Endometrial cancer]
laparoscopic surgery, 205–208
methylation epigenetic silencing, 78
minimal access surgery, 199–208
mucinous carcinoma, 38–39
novel agents, 272
pelvic exenteration, 239
premalignant conditions, 19, 22
preoperative work-up, 137
radiotherapy, 149–168
rare types, 43
risk factors, 2–6
screening studies, 13–26
surgery for, 133–142, 233–240
Endometrial cancer, advanced disease,
cytoreductive results, 238
primary cytoreductive surgery,
235–237
relapse, radical hysterectomy,
233–235
surgery for, 233–234
Endometrial hyperplasia, 46
complex hyperplasia, 46
pathology, 31–48
simple hyperplasia, 46
Endometrial intraepithelial
carcinoma, 47
Endometrial neoplasia, 46–48
Endometrial sampling
blind endometrial biopsy, 92–93
hysteroscopy, 91–100
rapid access clinic, 97–100
vaginal ultrasound, 91–100
Endometrial stromal sarcoma
diagnosis, from curettage material, 58
gross pathology, 56
classification controversies,
55–56
microscopic pathology, 56–58
uterine sarcoma, 54–58
Endometrioid adenocarcinoma,
178–182
adjuvant chemotherapy, 182
chemotherapy, 178–182
combination regimens, 179–181
single agent therapy, 178–179
whole abdominal radiotherapy, 181

Endometrioid carcinoma, 38
  endometrial carcinoma, 38–40
  variants, 39–40
Endometrium, metastatic tumors of, 43
Epidemiology, of endometrial cancer, 1–6
Epigenetics, of endometrial cancer, 76
  APC methylation, 77–78
  hormones, 79–80
  MLH1 methylation, 77
Epithelial tumors, World Health Organization classifications, 33
Epithelioid leiomyoscarcoma, 62
ERBB2. *See* Eryhthroblastic leukemia viral oncogene homolog.
Erlotinib, for endometrial cancer, 273
  Tarceva, 273
ERP. *See* Estrogen receptor protein.
ERT. *See* Estrogen replacement therapy.
Erythroblastic leukemia viral oncogene homolog (ERBB2), 71–72
Estrogen receptor protein (ERP), 248
Estrogen replacement therapy (ERT), 249–251
  endometrial carcinoma, 249–251
  hormone replacement therapy, 243
Estrogen/progestogen continuous combinations, 248
Estrogen/progestogen sequential combinations, 246
Exercise, risk factors, 5–6

FIGO clinical staging, 133, 150
  recurrence rate, 213
FIGO surgical staging
  endometrial cancer, 134, 151
FIGO. *See* International Federation of Gynecology Obstetrics, 44–45

Gefitinib, endometrial cancer, 273
  Iressa, 273
Genetics, 69
  endometrial cancer, 69–83
  epigenetics, 76–80
  hereditary endometrial cancer, 76

[Genetics]
  microarray, 80–82
  risk factors, 6
  somatic genetic alterations, 70–76
GOG chemotherapy trials, combined therapy, 285
GOG first line trials, combined therapy, 285
GOG radiation and chemotherapy trial, 287
GOG. *See* Gynecologic Oncology Group.
Grading, FIGO, 44
Gynecologic Oncology Group (GOG), 281

Herceptin, 272
Hereditary endometrial cancer, genetics of, 76
Histologic type, surgical prognostic factors, 134–135
Hormonal aspects, leiomyosarcoma, 59–60
Hormone replacement therapy, 243
  endometrial carcinoma, 243–251
  estrogen replacement therapy, 243
  estrogen/progestogen continuous combinations, 248
  estrogen/progestogen sequential combinations, 246
  progestogen addition, 245–248
  risk factors of, 3
  selective estrogen receptor modulators, 249
  tibolene, endometrial cancer, 248–249
  unopposed estrogen use, 243–244
  vaginal estrogen treatment, 244–245
Hormones, epigenetics, 79–80
Hyperplasia, 46
Hypertension, risk factors of, 4–5
Hysteroscopy, 91
  endometrial sampling, 91–100
  outpatient, 95–97
  rapid access clinic, 97–100

[Hysteroscopy]
  saline infusion sonohysterography,
    94–95
  vaginal ultrasound, 91–100

Imaging, endometrial cancer, 107–126
Immunohistochemistry, of uterine
    sarcoma, 58–59
In-randomized trials, 15
International Federation of Gynecology
    Obstetrics (FIGO), grading, 44
Iressa, 273
Irradiation, dose and technique, 166–167
Isolated pelvic recurrences, radiotherapy
    for, 158–159

Laparoscopic lymphadenectromy,
    201
Laparoscopic surgery, procedure,
    205–208
Laparoscopic-assisted vaginal
    hysterectomy, 200–202
Laparoscopy
  clinical outcome, 203
  complications, 202
  contraindications, 204
  cost benefit, 203–204
  pre-surgical procedures, 204–205
Leiomyosarcoma
  appearance, 60
  chemotherapy, 186–188
  histological features, 61
  hormonal aspects, 59–60
Lymph node metastase, pathologic
    prognostic factors, 46
Lymphadenoectomy, endometrial
    carcinoma, 257–258

Magnetic resonance imaging, 112–126
Menstrual factors, in cancer risk, 2
Methylation epigenetic silencing, 78
Microarray, endometrial cancer genetics
    studies, 80–81

Minimal access surgery, 199–208
  clinical outcome, 203
  complications, 202
  cost benefit, 203–204
  laparoscopic lymphadenectomy,
    201–202
  laparoscopic-assisted vaginal
    hysterectomy, 200–202
  vaginal hysterectomy, 200
Mixed carcinomas, endometrial, 42
MLH1 methylation, 77
Mucinous carcinoma, 38–39
Myometrial invasion, pathologic
    prognostic factors, 45
Myxoid leiomyosarcoma, 61–62

Neoplasia, pathology of, 31–48
Non-randomized trials, 14–15
Novel agents, in treatment, 272
  Erlotinib, 273
  Gefitinib, 273
  Rapamycin, 273
  Trastuzumab, 272–273

Oncogenes
  β-catenin, 72
  erythroblastic leukemia viral
    homolog, 71–72
  retrovirus associated sequence
    genes, 71
  somatic genetic alterations, 70
Oral contraceptives, risk factors, 4

p53 protein, tumor suppressor genes, 73
Paclitaxel, 270–271
Palliative, radiotherapy, 165
Pathologic prognostic factors
  cervical involvement, 46
  endometrial carcinomas, 43
  grading, 44
  lymph node metastases, 46
  myometrial invasion, 45
  peritoneal cytology, 46
  stage, 44

Pelvic exenteration, for endometrial
  cancer, relapse, 239
Pelvic radiotherapy, indications of
  reduction, 256–257
Peritoneal cytology
  pathologic prognostic factors, 44
  surgical prognostic factors, 133
Phenotype, molecular profiles for
  cancer, 82
Phosphatase and tensin homolog
  (PTEN), 74–75
Primary cytoreductive surgery,
  advanced disease, 235–237
Progestogen addition, endometrial
  cancer, prognostic factors,
  245–248
Prognostic factors, 44–46
  cervical involvement, 46
  grading, 44–45
  lymph node metastases, 46
  myometrial invasion, 45
  peritoneal cytology, 46
  stage, 44
PTEN. *See* Phosphatase and tensin
  homolog.

Radiation therapy
  adjuvant, 259–261
  combined therapy, 287
  future developments, 255–262
Radical hysterectomy, for advanced
  disease and relapse, 234–235
Radical radiation, stage I disease, 157,
  160
Radiotherapy, 149–168
  dose and technique, 166–167
  history, 149–150
  lymphadenoectomy, 257–258
  new techniques, 261–262
  palliative, 165
  pelvic recurrences, 157
  prognostic factors, 150–153
  stage I disease, 153–160
    adjuvant brachytherapy, 154–156
    radical radiation, 157, 160
    recurrence treatment, 156–157

[Radiotherapy]
  vaginal brachytherapy, 154
  stage II disease, 160
  staging factors, 150–153
  toxicity, 167–168
  uterine cancer, 268
  uterine papillary serous carcinoma,
    165–166
  vaginal brachytherapy, 258
Rapamycin, 273
Rapid access clinic, 97–100
RAS genes. *See* Retrovirus associated
  sequence genes.
Recurrence, 213–228
  detection, 223–228
  of uterine cancer, 223–228
  prognosis, 218–220
  rate, 213
  surveillance programs, 220–222
  time, 213–214
  tumor risk factors, 217
Reproductive risk factors, 2–3
Retrovirus associated sequence genes,
  oncogenes, 71–72
Risk factors
  body mass, 4
  diabetes, 4–5
  diet/alcohol/exercise, 5–6
  genetics, 6
  hormone replacement therapy and, 3
  hypertension, 4–5
  menstrual factors, 2
  of endometrial cancer, 2–6
  oral contraceptives, 4
  reproductive factors, 2–3
  smoking, 5

Saline infusion sonohysterography
  (SIS), 94–95
Screening studies, 13–26
  advantages, 18–19
  basic principles, 15–16
  preliminary trials, 22–25
  risk groups, 22
  traps, 14–15
  trials, 14–15

Selective estrogen receptor modulators (SERMs), 249
SERMs. *See* Selective estrogen receptor modulators.
Serous carcinoma (UPSC), 39–41
  adjuvant therapy, 183–184
  chemotherapy, 182–184
  endometrial carcinoma, 43
Simple hyperplasia
  atypia, 46
  complex hyperplasia, 46
Single agent therapy, chemotherapy, 178–179
SIS. *See* Saline infusion sonohysterography, 94
Smoking, risk factors, 5
Somatic genetic alterations, 70–76
  oncogenes, 70–72
  tumor suppressor genes, 72–73
Stage I disease, 153–160
  combined therapy, future direction, 282–283
Stage II disease, 160–161
Stage III disease, 161–165
Stage IV disease, 161–165
Surgery, 131–144
  post-hysterectomy, 142
  procedures, 137–142
  recurrent, 141–142
  stage II disease, 140
  stage III disease, 140–141
  stage IV disease, 141
Surgical prognostic factors
  age, 133–134
  histologic type, 134–135
  peritoneal cytology, 136
  tumor grade/depth/size, 135–136
Surveillance programs
  follow-up protocol, 222
  recurrence, 220–222

Tamoxifen, 63
Tarceva, 273
Tibolene , 248
  hormone replacement therapy, 246, 248

Topotecan, 271
Toxicity, to radiotherapy, 167–168
Transvaginal ultrasound, 93–94
Trasuzumab, 272–273
  herceptin, 272
Tumor risk factors, recurrence rates, 216
Tumor suppressor genes
  p53 protein, 73
  phosphatase and tensin homolog, 74–75
  somatic genetic alterations, 70

Undifferentiated carcinoma, 43
Unopposed estrogen use, endometrial cancer, 243–244
UPSC. *See* Uterine papillary serous carcinoma.
Uterine cancer
  adjuvant chemotherapy, 268
  chemotherapy, 177–188
    advanced disease, 268, 271
  combined modality therapy, 281–288
  endometrial cancer, 131–133
  novel agents, 267–274
  radiosensitizing chemotherapy, 268
  radiotherapy, 267–268
  relapse, 211–231
    detection, 223–228
    FIGO stage, 213
    prognosis, 218–220
    risk groups, 216–218
    site, 214–216
    surveillance programs, 220–222
    time characteristics, 213–214
  surgery, 131–144
  surveillance programs, 220
Uterine corpus lesions, World Health Organization classifications, 32
  epithelial tumors, 32
Uterine papillary serous carcinoma, radiotherapy for, 165–166
Uterine sarcoma
  chemotherapy, 184–186
  endometrial stromal sarcoma, 54–57
  epithelioid leiomyoscarcoma, 62
  hormonal aspects, 59–60

[Uterine sarcoma]
  immunohistochemistry, 58–59
  leiomyosarcoma, 187–188
  myxoid leiomyosarcoma, 61–62
  pathology, 53–62
  radiotherapy, 166
  stages of, 54
  tamoxifen, 63

Vaginal brachytherapy, 258
  stage I disease, 153
Vaginal estrogen treatment, 244–245
Vaginal hysterectomy, 200

Vaginal ultrasound
  endometrial sampling, 91–100
  hysteroscopy, 91–100
  rapid access clinic, 97–100
  transvaginal ultrasound, 93–94

Whole abdominal radiation
  combined therapy, future direction,
    281–282
  for endometrioid adencarcinoma, 181
World Health Organization
  classifications, 32